Pharmacological Activities of Flavonoids and Its Analogues

Pharmacological Activities of Flavonoids and Its Analogues

Guest Editors

Fernando Calzada
Miguel Valdes

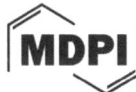

Basel • Beijing • Wuhan • Barcelona • Belgrade • Novi Sad • Cluj • Manchester

Guest Editors

Fernando Calzada
Medical Research Unit
in Pharmacology
Mexican Institute of
Social Security
Mexico City
Mexico

Miguel Valdes
Medical Research Unit
in Pharmacology
Mexican Institute of
Social Security
Mexico City
Mexico

Editorial Office
MDPI AG
Grosspeteranlage 5
4052 Basel, Switzerland

This is a reprint of the Special Issue, published open access by the journal *Pharmaceuticals* (ISSN 1424-8247), freely accessible at: www.mdpi.com/journal/pharmaceuticals/special_issues/pharmacological_flavonoids.

For citation purposes, cite each article independently as indicated on the article page online and using the guide below:

Lastname, A.A.; Lastname, B.B. Article Title. *Journal Name* **Year**, *Volume Number*, Page Range.

ISBN 978-3-7258-2824-1 (Hbk)
ISBN 978-3-7258-2823-4 (PDF)
https://doi.org/10.3390/books978-3-7258-2823-4

© 2024 by the authors. Articles in this book are Open Access and distributed under the Creative Commons Attribution (CC BY) license. The book as a whole is distributed by MDPI under the terms and conditions of the Creative Commons Attribution-NonCommercial-NoDerivs (CC BY-NC-ND) license (https://creativecommons.org/licenses/by-nc-nd/4.0/).

Contents

About the Editors vii

Preface ix

Francisco Canindé Ferreira de Luna, Wallax Augusto Silva Ferreira, Samir Mansour Moraes Casseb and Edivaldo Herculano Correa de Oliveira
Anticancer Potential of Flavonoids: An Overview with an Emphasis on Tangeretin
Reprinted from: *Pharmaceuticals* **2023**, *16*, 1229, https://doi.org/10.3390/ph16091229 1

Hao Li and Qi Zhang
Research Progress of Flavonoids Regulating Endothelial Function
Reprinted from: *Pharmaceuticals* **2023**, *16*, 1201, https://doi.org/10.3390/ph16091201 22

Fahad F. Albaqami, Hassan N. Althurwi, Khalid M. Alharthy, Abubaker M. Hamad and Fatin A. Awartani
Rutin Gel with Bone Graft Accelerates Bone Formation in a Rabbit Model by Inhibiting MMPs and Enhancing Collagen Activities
Reprinted from: *Pharmaceuticals* **2023**, *16*, 774, https://doi.org/10.3390/ph16050774 45

Fernando Calzada, Miguel Valdes, Jesús Martínez-Solís, Claudia Velázquez and Elizabeth Barbosa
Annona cherimola Miller and Its Flavonoids, an Important Source of Products for the Treatment of Diabetes Mellitus: In Vivo and In Silico Evaluations
Reprinted from: *Pharmaceuticals* **2023**, *16*, 724, https://doi.org/10.3390/ph16050724 58

Tarek Khamis, Abdelmonem Awad Hegazy, Samaa Salah Abd El-Fatah, Eman Ramadan Abdelfattah, Marwa Mohamed Mahmoud Abdelfattah and Liana Mihaela Fericean et al.
Hesperidin Mitigates Cyclophosphamide-Induced Testicular Dysfunction via Altering the Hypothalamic Pituitary Gonadal Axis and Testicular Steroidogenesis, Inflammation, and Apoptosis in Male Rats
Reprinted from: *Pharmaceuticals* **2023**, *16*, 301, https://doi.org/10.3390/ph16020301 75

Batoul Alallam, Abd Almonem Doolaanea, Mulham Alfatama and Vuanghao Lim
Phytofabrication and Characterisation of Zinc Oxide Nanoparticles Using Pure Curcumin
Reprinted from: *Pharmaceuticals* **2023**, *16*, 269, https://doi.org/10.3390/ph16020269 95

Miguel Valdes, Fernando Calzada, Jesús Martínez-Solís and Julita Martínez-Rodríguez
Antihyperglycemic Effects of *Annona cherimola* Miller and the Flavonoid Rutin in Combination with Oral Antidiabetic Drugs on Streptozocin-Induced Diabetic Mice
Reprinted from: *Pharmaceuticals* **2023**, *16*, 112, https://doi.org/10.3390/ph16010112 118

Tong Zhang, Yun-Hong Xiu, Hui Xue, Yan-Nan Li, Jing-Long Cao and Wen-Shuang Hou et al.
A Mechanism of Isoorientin-Induced Apoptosis and Migration Inhibition in Gastric Cancer AGS Cells
Reprinted from: *Pharmaceuticals* **2022**, *15*, 1541, https://doi.org/10.3390/ph15121541 135

Ganjun Yuan, Xuexue Xia, Yingying Guan, Houqin Yi, Shan Lai and Yifei Sun et al.
Antimicrobial Quantitative Relationship and Mechanism of Plant Flavonoids to Gram-Positive Bacteria
Reprinted from: *Pharmaceuticals* **2022**, *15*, 1190, https://doi.org/10.3390/ph15101190 149

Amin Gasmi, Pavan Kumar Mujawdiya, Roman Lysiuk, Mariia Shanaida, Massimiliano Peana and Asma Gasmi Benahmed et al.
Quercetin in the Prevention and Treatment of Coronavirus Infections: A Focus on SARS-CoV-2
Reprinted from: *Pharmaceuticals* **2022**, *15*, 1049, https://doi.org/10.3390/ph15091049 . . . . **163**

Jirapak Ruttanapattanakul, Nitwara Wikan, Saranyapin Potikanond and Wutigri Nimlamool
Molecular Targets of Pinocembrin Underlying Its Regenerative Activities in Human Keratinocytes
Reprinted from: *Pharmaceuticals* **2022**, *15*, 954, https://doi.org/10.3390/ph15080954 . . . . **178**

Violeta Popovici, Laura Bucur, Cerasela Elena Gîrd, Antoanela Popescu, Elena Matei and Georgeta Camelia Cozaru et al.
Phenolic Secondary Metabolites and Antiradical and Antibacterial Activities of Different Extracts of *Usnea barbata* (L.) Weber ex F.H.Wigg from Climani Mountains, Romania
Reprinted from: *Pharmaceuticals* **2022**, *15*, 829, https://doi.org/10.3390/ph15070829 . . . . **193**

About the Editors

Fernando Calzada

Dr. Fernando Calzada is a researcher studying the pharmacological evaluation of selected medicinal plants from Mexican folk medicine, focusing on antidiabetic, anticancer, ancidiarrheal, and antiobesity properties. He belongs to the National System of Researchers (SNII) Level 3 from Mexico.

Miguel Valdes

Dr. Miguel Valdes is a researcher focused on the pharmacological evaluation of natural products as antidiabetic agents, with a special interest in the isolation of pure compounds and their evaluation in vivo, ex vivo, in vitro, and in silico in order to elucidate their action mechanism. He belong to the National System of Researchers (SNII) Level 1 from Mexico.

Preface

Dear Colleagues,

The development of new drugs continues to be an important point for global society. In recent years, there has been increased interest in the study of polyphenols due to the multiple pharmacological activities that they have demonstrated. Flavonoids are a class of polyphenols that have been widely studied; they are characterized as having a 15-carbon skeleton with a 2-phenylbenzopyranone core structure. They are classified as flavones, isoflavones, flavonols, anthocyanidins, flavanones, flavanols, chalcones, and aurones. Within the various classes, further differentiation is possible based on the number and nature of substituent groups attached to the rings; moreover, flavonoids can exist as free aglycones or conjugated glycosidic bonds. Flavonoids are present in almost all types of nourishment, and recent studies have focused on their biological, nutritional, pharmacological, and medicinal relevance. These kind of molecules, as well as their analogues, are of utmost relevance due to their multiple applications. Considering the above, we invite researchers to publish their findings on the pharmacological applications of flavonoids, as well as their analogs, while highlighting the importance of using these molecules as a basis for the development of new drugs.

Fernando Calzada and Miguel Valdes
Guest Editors

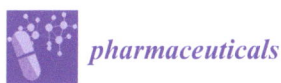

Review

Anticancer Potential of Flavonoids: An Overview with an Emphasis on Tangeretin

Francisco Canindé Ferreira de Luna [1,*], Wallax Augusto Silva Ferreira [1], Samir Mansour Moraes Casseb [2] and Edivaldo Herculano Correa de Oliveira [1,3]

[1] Laboratory of Cytogenomics and Environmental Mutagenesis, Environment Section (SEAMB), Evandro Chagas Institute (IEC), BR 316, KM 7, s/n, Levilândia, Ananindeua 67030-000, Brazil; wallaxaugusto@gmail.com (W.A.S.F.); ehco@ufpa.br (E.H.C.d.O.)
[2] Oncology Research Center, Federal University of Pará, Belém 66073-000, Brazil; samircasseb@ufpa.br
[3] Faculty of Natural Sciences, Institute of Exact and Natural Sciences, Federal University of Pará (UFPA), Rua Augusto Correa, 01, Belém 66075-990, Brazil
* Correspondence: lunafcf@gmail.com

Abstract: Natural compounds with pharmacological activity, flavonoids have been the subject of an exponential increase in studies in the field of scientific research focused on therapeutic purposes due to their bioactive properties, such as antioxidant, anti-inflammatory, anti-aging, antibacterial, antiviral, neuroprotective, radioprotective, and antitumor activities. The biological potential of flavonoids, added to their bioavailability, cost-effectiveness, and minimal side effects, direct them as promising cytotoxic anticancer compounds in the optimization of therapies and the search for new drugs in the treatment of cancer, since some extensively antineoplastic therapeutic approaches have become less effective due to tumor resistance to drugs commonly used in chemotherapy. In this review, we emphasize the antitumor properties of tangeretin, a flavonoid found in citrus fruits that has shown activity against some hallmarks of cancer in several types of cancerous cell lines, such as antiproliferative, apoptotic, anti-inflammatory, anti-metastatic, anti-angiogenic, antioxidant, regulatory expression of tumor-suppressor genes, and epigenetic modulation.

Keywords: flavonoids; tangeretin; cancer; anti-cancer; anti-proliferative; anti-metastatic

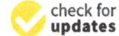

Citation: de Luna, F.C.F.; Ferreira, W.A.S.; Casseb, S.M.M.; de Oliveira, E.H.C. Anticancer Potential of Flavonoids: An Overview with an Emphasis on Tangeretin. *Pharmaceuticals* **2023**, *16*, 1229. https://doi.org/10.3390/ph16091229

Academic Editors: Fernando Calzada and Miguel Valdes

Received: 26 July 2023
Revised: 18 August 2023
Accepted: 25 August 2023
Published: 30 August 2023

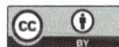

Copyright: © 2023 by the authors. Licensee MDPI, Basel, Switzerland. This article is an open access article distributed under the terms and conditions of the Creative Commons Attribution (CC BY) license (https:// creativecommons.org/licenses/by/ 4.0/).

1. Introduction

Cancer cells possess biological properties that confer the ability to develop and become malignant. The spread of these cells occurs through a variety of tumor physiological strategies, including the maintenance of proliferative signaling, evasion of growth suppressor genes, evasion of immune destruction, induction of replicative immortality, activation of invasion and metastasis, promotion of angiogenesis, resistance to cell death, deregulation of cellular energy and metabolism, unlocking of phenotypic plasticity, and cellular senescence. These properties are acquired at different stages of neoplasia in diverse types of cancer. This ability is triggered by strong genomic instability caused by successive mutations of regulatory genes, the infiltration of tumor-promoting immune cells, non-mutational epigenetic reprogramming, and polymorphic microbiomes [1–3]. Elucidating these "hallmarks" of cancer is the subject of intense experimentation to explore cancer therapies, as the effective intervention of any of these tumor characteristics can potentially improve and refine anticancer therapeutic treatments against cancer.

Within the therapeutic approaches to various types of cancers, the resistance to multiple drugs (MDRs) exhibited by tumor cells is considered the main cause of chemotherapy effectiveness failure. This occurs due to cellular physiological responses triggered by the tumor, including the evasion of drug-induced apoptosis, activation of detoxification pathways, reduction in drug uptake, and activation of DNA repair mechanisms [4]. From this perspective, the use of natural products in clinical trials has been instrumental in suppressing resistance mechanisms, and hence of utmost importance in the search for new genotoxic therapeutic approaches against tumors. These products have enabled the development of more effective strategic combinations with fewer side effects for the treatment of various types of cancer, in addition to improving our understanding of cancer cell defense and resistance mechanisms [5]. The alteration of gene expression patterns in tumor cells is linked to genetic and epigenetic events. Aberrant epigenetic modifications through DNA methylation, nucleosome remodeling, histone modifications, and non-coding microRNAs play a crucial role in tumor initiation and uncontrolled cellular progression. The understanding and discovery of drugs capable of restoring or inhibiting these abnormal epigenetic mechanisms represent a significant advance in the means of cancer control [6–9]. In this context, natural phenolic compounds have gained prominence in anticancer pharmaceutical studies. These compounds, found in plants and fruits, are described as potent epigenetic agents that regulate DNA methylation, histone modification, and microRNAs in cancer therapy. They have shown effectiveness when combined with chemotherapy drugs or even when used in combination with other natural compounds. These promising findings have driven research and the development of new therapeutic strategies for cancer treatment [10,11]. This review article aims to provide an overview of the main anticancer properties of flavonoids demonstrated in various scientific studies, considering the prominent characteristics of cancer, with an emphasis on tangeretin.

2. Polyphenols

Polyphenols constitute a diverse group of phytochemicals associated with secondary metabolism in plants. They have antidiabetic, antiosteoporotic, cardioprotective, neuroprotective, antioxidant, anti-inflammatory, antimicrobial, immunomodulatory, and anticancer properties [12,13]. They protect plants from ultraviolet radiation and microbial infections, serve as signaling molecules during the pollination process, and modulate plant growth hormones [14–16]. Based on their structure, polyphenols are classified into non-flavonoids (curcuminoids, lignans, stilbenes, and tannins) and flavonoids [17] (Figure 1).

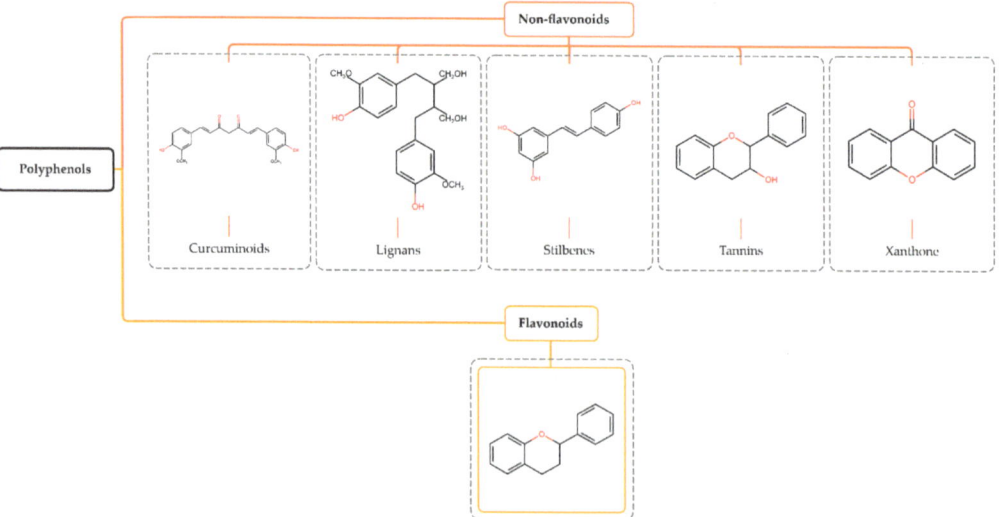

Figure 1. Structure and classification of polyphenols. Polyphenols are phytochemical compounds found in plants, fruits, and natural compounds, divided into non-flavonoids and flavonoids.

Flavonoids (or bioflavonoids) represent an extensive class with over 10,000 described subtypes of compounds [18–20]. They are the most abundant phenolic compounds in the human diet, ubiquitously found in fruits, seeds, roots, cereals, teas, and wines [21–24].

Although some are colorless, their etymology is derived from the Latin word *"flavus,"* which means yellow [25]. In addition, flavonoids exist in various derived forms, including glycosylated, acetylated, methylated, and sulfated aglycones [20,26,27].

3. Structure and Classification of Flavonoids

Structurally, flavonoids have fifteen carbons in their chemical structure (C6-C3-C6), consisting of two benzene rings (A and B) connected by a heterocyclic pyran ring (C) (2-phenyl-1,4-benzopyran) [28,29] (Figure 2).

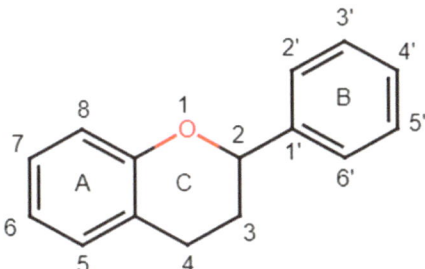

Figure 2. Main molecular structure of flavonoids.

The classification of flavonoids is based on the arrangement of the hydroxyl groups, the degree of unsaturation, and the oxidation of the heterocyclic C-ring. The main subclasses include flavones, flavonols, flavanones, flavanonols, flavanols, isoflavones, anthocyanidins, and chalcones [30–34] (Figure 3). Flavanones and flavanonols show a saturated benzopyran ring, the difference between them being the presence of a hydroxyl group on carbon number three of the benzopyran ring in flavanols. Similarly, flavanols also have a saturated benzopyran ring and hydroxyl groups on carbon number three; however, they differ in the absence of a carbonyl group on carbon number four of the benzopyran ring. Anthocyanins are hydroxylated at carbon number three and have two double bonds. Isoflavones have a double bond between carbon numbers two and three of the benzopyran ring, with the phenyl group attached to carbon number three. Flavonoids that do not have the benzopyran ring are called minor flavonoids. This is true for chalcones, characterized by the absence of the heterocyclic benzopyran ring with oxygen [35–37].

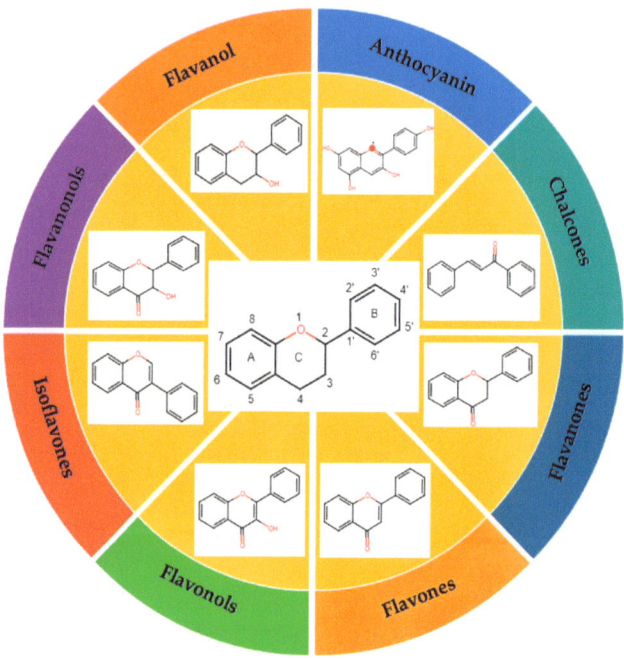

Figure 3. Subclassification of flavonoids.

4. Antitumor Activity of Flavonoids

These bioactive compounds exhibit many biological properties, including antioxidant, antiviral, antifungal, antibacterial, anti-inflammatory, antidiabetic, anti-obesity, antimutagenic, cardioprotective, and anticancer activities [38–42]. Concerning their anticancer activities, the recognized importance of flavonoids has led to efforts and challenges to elucidate the molecular and cellular mechanisms of antitumor effects [43]. This awareness has been accompanied by an increasing number of scientific publications comparing the human health benefits of flavonoids in the field of oncology with those of other medical specialties, such as endocrinology, cardiology, and neurology [44]. Epidemiological studies support the chemopreventive benefits of flavonoids when included in the human diet, with their intake correlated with a lower risk of developing some tumors, such as gastric, breast, prostate, and colorectal cancers [45,46]. Flavonoids mediate anti-neoplastic mechanisms by modulating reactive oxygen species (ROS) levels in tumor cells, inhibiting carcinogens, pro-inflammatory pathways, angiogenesis, autophagy, inducing apoptosis, and inhibiting tumor proliferation and invasion [47–55] (Figure 4).

Even though the anticancer efficacy of flavonoids is described in the literature, the pharmacological activity of these compounds may be limited due to their water insolubility. The low solubility of flavonoids presents a double-edged sword in the therapeutic field. On one hand, their reduced absorption due to low solubility does not confer toxicity to the organism. On the other hand, it also becomes a problem as it may reduce their chemosensitizing effectiveness due to inefficient absorption [55,56].

In order to overcome this disadvantage, nanoparticle-based delivery systems have been developed aiming to improve the bioavailability and absorption of drugs in cancer therapy. These drug-carrying nanocarriers, such as polymeric micelles, liposomes, dendrimers, and carbon nanotubes, have been extensively investigated to ensure the chemotherapeutic and chemosensitizing effectiveness of drugs targeted to cancer cells [57,58]. In this context, the production of flavonoid-loaded phytoparticles has added advantages to the treatment, prevention, and clinical perspectives of cancer. These phytoparticles increase the bioavailability of compounds with low solubility, prolong the half-life of drugs, improve blood absorption, and reduce gastrointestinal degradation. Moreover, this delivery system allows for lower quantities of flavonoids to be used, thereby decreasing the risk of toxicity in non-tumor cells [59–62].

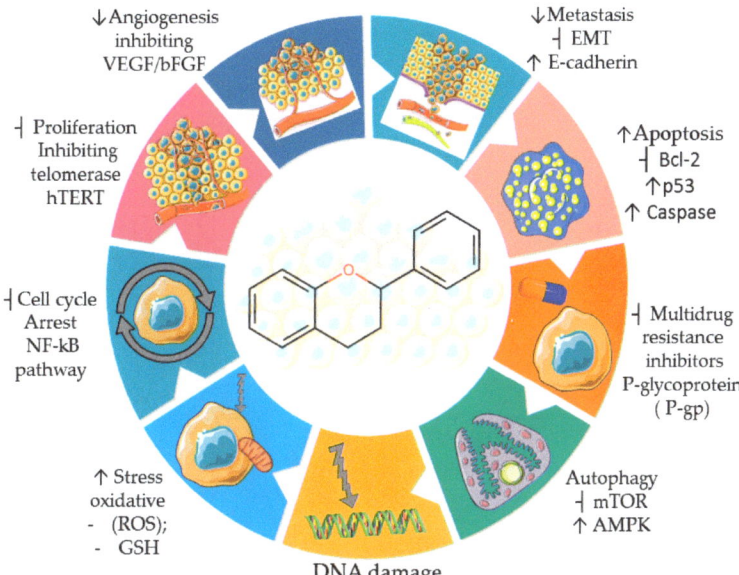

Figure 4. Properties and some anticancer action mechanisms of flavonoids. Parts of the figure are drawn by using pictures from Servier Medical Art. Servier Medical Art by Servier is licensed under a Creative Commons Attribution 3.0 Unported License (https://creativecommons.org/licenses/by/3.0/ accessed on 12 August 2023).

As an example, the effect of an oral nanoparticle delivery system of chitosan containing an encapsulated epigallocatechin-3-O-gallate (EGCG) flavonoid has been described as excellent in vitro in human melanoma cells and in vivo in melanoma tumor xenografts. It promotes cell growth inhibition and the induction of apoptosis in vivo, showing enhanced effectiveness in vitro when compared to native EGCG treatment [63]. These results stem from efforts to improve the bioavailability of EGCG based on previous research focusing on melanoma cancer, aiming to optimize the anticancer effects of antiproliferation and pro-apoptosis physiologically [64]. These findings reaffirm that the encapsulation (nanochemoprevention) of substances with chemopreventive activity in EGCG nanoparticles can be an efficient alternative in cancer treatment [65].

In the same way, treatment with EGCG nano-emulsion (nano-EGCG) in lung cancer cells showed the anti-tumor effects between EGCG and nano-EGCG groups. Both treatment groups blocked tumor cell growth. Importantly, the nano-EGCG treatment inhibited cell migration and invasion in a dose-dependent manner, achieved through the stimulation of the adenosine monophosphate-activated protein kinase (AMPK) signaling pathway [66]. This pathway is altered in the metabolic reprogramming of cancer cells and is responsible for conferring resistance to cancer-fighting drugs, preventing the autophagy of cancer cells [67,68].

Moderate levels of reactive oxygen species (ROS) resulting from mitochondrial activity act as redox signaling molecules in growth, differentiation, and cell proliferation pathways. However, excessive levels of ROS induce DNA mutations, protein and lipid damage, and stimulate pro-oncogenic signaling pathways, thus contributing to carcinogenesis [69,70].

Tumor cells have significantly higher ROS levels in the tumor microenvironment compared to the homeostatic conditions of non-tumor cells. However, excess ROS can be harmful to cancer cells, leading to cell death. Consequently, tumor cells develop adaptive detoxification mechanisms in response to excessive ROS [71,72]. As the elevation of ROS can trigger apoptosis in cancer cells, therapeutic strategies aimed at modulating ROS levels in cancer treatment have shown the efficacy of anticancer drugs [73–75]. In this sense, flavonoids are described to exhibit antioxidant biological activity in non-tumor cells and pro-oxidant activity by inducing increased oxidative stress in cancer cells, thereby inhibiting cell proliferation signaling, suppressing pro-inflammatory cytokines, promoting apoptosis, necrosis, and autophagy activation [28]. The ability to scavenge oxygen reactive species is related to the presence of a large number of phenolic hydroxyl groups in the molecular structure of flavonoids, where intense electron exchange facilitates substitution reactions with free radicals, forming a more stable compound. Therefore, the higher the number of hydroxyl groups, the greater the oxidant and pro-oxidant capacities of the flavonoid [76,77]. Ovarian cancer cells treated with flavonoids apigenin, luteolin, and myricetin showed an intracellular increase in ROS levels in a dose-dependent manner compared to untreated control cells, resulting in the activation of the intrinsic apoptotic pathway, cell cycle arrest, and anti-invasion [78]. Similarly, it was described that the flavonoid quercetin triggered cell death in cancer cells by positively regulating ROS levels [79]. The expression of the transglutaminase 2 (TGM2) gene is generally associated with poor prognosis in pancreatic cancer and is involved in its initiation, inflammation, and progression, making it a target marker in studies analyzing drugs with chemosensitizing activity [80–82]. Treatment with kaempferol suppressed pancreatic cancer growth in vivo and in vitro. It was observed that treated cells had decreased TGM2 expression, and the increase in ROS induced apoptosis through the Akt/mTOR signaling pathway [83]. The therapeutic potential of flavonoids in modulating ROS demonstrates that their pro-oxidant activity can positively contribute to anticancer research.

In order for excessive cell growth to be achieved, cancer cells reprogram their energy metabolism. This reprogramming is directly related to the maintenance and aggressiveness of neoplastic cells [84]. In this sense, glutathione is a ubiquitous endogenous antioxidant tripeptide (γ-Glu-Cys-Gly; GSH) found in eukaryotic cells, being responsible for maintaining cellular redox homeostasis by eliminating reactive oxygen species (ROS), a cellular metabolic byproduct [85–87]. Glutathione (GSH) metabolism has been investigated in tumor progression and explored as a targeted therapeutic strategy for cancer [87,88]. The positive modulation of GSH levels is directly related to the response to cellular detoxification mechanisms. This provides advantages to various types of cancers, as it is crucial for the elimination and detoxification of certain chemotherapeutic agents, thus conferring therapeutic resistance. Moreover, high GSH levels contribute to tumor development and increase metastasis events [89]. On the other hand, the reduction (depletion) in GSH levels leads to certain types of cell death, such as apoptosis, necroptosis, ferroptosis, and autophagy, providing a foundation for studies exploring the suppression of GSH levels in chemosensitization approaches in cancer therapies, making tumor cells prone to the cytotoxic and cytoprotective effects of antineoplastic substances [90]. In this direction, it has been observed that tangeretin is able to reduce oxidative stress in human hepatocellular carcinoma induced by *tert*-Butyl Hydroperoxide (t-BHP) by inhibiting GSH depletion in the cell [91]. Similarly, in cisplatin-induced liver lesions in rats treated with tangeretin, protective activity against cellular oxidative stress was observed, and an increase in antioxidant defense was also observed, as evidenced by elevated GSH levels [92]. Hence, this flavonoid is capable of reducing cellular stress and restoring the antioxidant defense system.

Epigenetic mechanisms are commonly associated with cancer development. In breast cancer, the expression pattern of certain tumor suppressor genes is related to methylation patterns. DNA methylation plays a critical role in controlling gene activity and nuclear architecture, being the most extensively studied epigenetic modification in humans. It is involved in the regulation of various biological processes, such as cell differentiation, embryogenesis, X-chromosome inactivation, microRNA expression, suppression of transposable elements, and genomic imprinting [93–95]. Hence, DNA methylation is an epigenetic mark associated with gene silencing, as it affects chromatin structure and blocks the access of binding factors, preventing the expression of the genes. This pattern can be stably maintained throughout life or undergo changes during aging [96]. Hypermethylation of CpG islands in the promoter region of tumor suppressor genes is an early event in various types of cancer. Consequently, CpG island hypermethylation in the promoter region can affect genes involved in cell control, DNA repair, apoptosis, and angiogenesis. In breast and ovarian cancers, hypermethylation is found in the promoter region of the BRCA1 gene, which acts as a tumor suppressor and is responsible for preventing the uncontrolled proliferation of cells [97,98]. Hypomethylation of DNA also triggers neoplastic transformations when it causes chromosomal instability, thus reactivating or activating oncogenes [99]. The literature highlights flavonoids as epigenetic modifiers in breast cancer. Epigallocatechin-3-gallate (EGCG), genistein, daidzein, resveratrol, and quercetin are capable of restoring the expression pattern of silenced tumor suppressor genes, such as BRCA1 and BRCA2, by inhibiting the enzymes called DNA methyltransferases (DNMTs). These enzymes are responsible for catalyzing the gene silencing process in the promoter region of the genes [99–101]. The restauration of the original expression patterns of these suppressor genes by the flavonoids was observed in different breast cancer cells, resulting in decreased proliferation and cancer cell migration [100]. The knowledge of the antitumor properties and ability of flavonoid subclasses (anthocyanidin—delphinidin, flavones—apigenin, luteolin, tangeretin, isoflavones—genistein, flavanones—hesperetin, silibinin, flavanol—EGCG, flavonols—quercetin, kaempferol, and fisetin) to modulate epigenetic enzymes, such as DNA methyltransferases (DNMTs), acetyltransferases (HATs), histone methyltransferases (HMTs), and histone deacetylases (HDACs), reinforce the incentive for research on therapeutic combination approaches involving these natural compounds that alter the epigenetic marks related to cancer development and progression along with drugs already used for cancer treatment [102].

The study of the mechanisms of action of apoptotic caspases in cancer has been explored through the use of antineoplastic drugs as a therapeutic strategy to overcome resistance and control the proliferation of cancer cells. The modulation of apoptosis under the action of natural products has demonstrated efficacy in inducing neoplastic cell death, representing an additional alternative to common chemotherapeutic agents employed in cancer treatment. It opens up a path for the development of new antineoplastic drugs, focusing on the apoptotic events executed by caspases [103–107]. The deregulation of the caspase cascade is implicated in the disruption of programmed cell death and directly related to the pathophysiology of cancer (evasion of apoptotic programming). The apoptotic imbalance resulting from negative caspase regulation is considered one of the causes of the resistance to tumor death found in cancer treatment [108–110]. The apoptotic proteolytic activation of caspases is executed through intrinsic (mitochondrial) and extrinsic (cytoplasmic) pathways. The intrinsic pathway is activated as feedback in response to cellular stress caused by cytotoxic substances, DNA mutations, hypoxia, cytoskeletal disruption, etc. [111–113]. In lung cancer cells treated with the flavonoid hesperetin, cell death by apoptosis was induced through the extrinsic pathway by increasing the expression levels of death domains genes, such as FADD, caspase-8, and FAS. The same study also mentioned that increased cell death occurred independently of the suppressor protein p53 and the pro-apoptotic protein Bax [114]. Treatment with malvidin and an analysis through flow cytometry showed that apoptotic activity was triggered by increased effector caspase-3 in myeloid and lymphoid leukemia cells in a dose-dependent manner, resulting in cell death [115]. Another study, also using flow cytometry, as well as Western blot and real-time PCR, showed the result of cell death by apoptosis in gastric cancer cells, where silibinin increased the level of caspases-3 and -9, followed by the inhibition of the transducer of signaling and activator of transcription 3 (STAT3) pathway, which is related to tumor growth and metastasis [116].

The molecular protective effect of flavonoids on DNA reduces the damage caused by carcinogens and promotes cellular genomic stability, allowing the development of strategies to treat neoplasms [19]. Table 1 presents the developed studies that describe the antitumor properties of flavonoids in various types of cancers.

Table 1. Subclasses of flavonoids and their compounds with antitumor activity described in cancer cell lines.

Subclasses	Compounds	Antitumor Activity	Cancer/Cell
Anthocyanin	Cyanidin	Anti-proliferative Anti-metastatic Apoptosis ↓ (NF-κB) Anti-metastatic Apoptosis ↓ (NF-κB)	Kidney/ 786-O; ACHN; [117] Colorectal/ HCT116; HT29; SW620; [118]
	Delphinidin	Apoptosis ⊣ (ERK; NF-κB)	Breast/ MDA; MB-453; BT-474; [119]
	Malvidin	Anti-proliferative Apoptosis	Leukemia/ SUP-B15; KG-1; [115]
Chalcones	Phloretin	Anti-proliferative ⊣ Migration ↑ ROS	Prostate/ PC3; DU145; [120]

Table 1. *Cont.*

Subclasses	Compounds	Antitumor Activity	Cancer/Cell
Flavanones	Naringin	Apoptosis ↓ (PI3K/AKT) Anti-proliferative Anti-metastatic ⊣ (Zeb1) Autophagy ↓ (PI3K/AKT/mTOR)	Thyroid/ TPC-1; SW1736; [121] Osteosarcoma/ MG63, U2OS; [122] Gastric/ AGS; [123]
	Hesperidin	Apoptosis ↑ (FADD/caspase-8)	Lung/ H522; [114]
	Eriodictyol	Anti-proliferative Apoptosis ⊣ mTOR/PI3K/Akt Anti-proliferative Apoptosis -Anti-metastatic ⊣ PI3K/Akt/NF-κB	Lung/ A549; [124] Glioma/ U87MG; CHG-5; [125]
Flavones	Baicalein	Induction apoptosis Autophagy ⊣ (PI3K/AKT)	Breast/ MCF-7; MDA-MB-231; [126]
	Tangeretin	Anti-proliferative ⊣ (Cdk2/Cdk4) Anti-proliferative Apoptosis ↓ (MMP) ↑ Caspases-3, -8, -9	Colorectal/ COLO 205; [127] Leukemia/ HL-60 [128] Gastric/ AGS; [129]
	Luteolin	↑ p53 Apoptosis ⊣ DNA metiltransferas	Colo/ HT-29 [130]
	Apegenin	Apoptosis ↑ BAX, CYT c ,SMAC/DIABLO, HTRA2/OMI, CASP-3 and -9	Leukemia/ THP-1; Jukart; [131]

Table 1. Cont.

Subclasses	Compounds	Antitumor Activity	Cancer/Cell
Flavonols	Quercetin	Antioxidant ↓ (ROS)	Ovarian/ C13* cisplatin-resistant (C13*) [132]
	Rutin	Induction apoptosis ↑ (caspases-3, -8, -9)	Colo/ HT-29 [133]
	Kaempferol	Apoptosis ⊣ Akt/mTOR	Pancreas/ PANC-1; Mia PaCa-2; [83]
Isoflavones	Genistein	Anti-proliferative Cell cycle arrest G2/M	Breast/ MCF-7; ERβ1; MDA-MB-231/ERβ1; [134]
	Daidzein	Anti-proliferative ⊣ NF-κB	Lung/ A594 e 95D; [135]
	Formononetin	Anti-proliferative ⊣ EGFR-Akt	Lung/ HCC827; H3255; H1975; A549; H1299; [136]

Table 1. Cont.

Subclasses	Compounds	Antitumor Activity	Cancer/Cell
Flavanonols	Silibinin	Anti-proliferative Induction apoptosis Cell cycle arrest G2/M ⊣ (STAT3)	Gastric/ MGC803; [116]
	Sylimarin	Anti-proliferative Apoptosis ↑ (Caspases-5, -8)	Oral/ HSC-4; YD15; Ca9.22; [137]
	Taxifolin	Anti-proliferative ⊣ (EMT) ↑ E-cadherin Cytotoxicity Cell cycle arrest G2/M	Lung/ A549; H1975; [138] Colorectal/ HCT116; HT29; [139]
Flavanol	Catechin	Anti-metastatic ⊣ (Wnt)	Breast/ MCF-7; HTB-26; Pancreas/ PANC-1; AsPC-1 Colorectal/ HT-29; Caco-2; [140]
	Epicatechin	Apoptosis ↑ (DR4/DR5)	Breast/ MDA-MB-231; MCF-7; [141]
	Epigallocatechin (EGCG)	Anti-proliferative Anti-metastatic ↑ AMPK Anti-proliferative Apoptosis Cell cycle arrest S ⊣ EGFR/RAS/RAF/MEK/ERK	H1299, A549; [66] Thyroid/ TT; TPC-1; ARO; [142]

5. Antineoplastic Activity of Tangeretin

The flavonoid tangeretin (5,6,7,8,4′-pentamethoxyflavone) is found in the peels of citrus fruits, especially oranges and tangerines. Studies have reported the beneficial bioactivities of this flavonoid, including its anti-asthmatic, antioxidant, anti-teratogenic, anti-inflammatory, neuroprotective, and anticancer properties [143–146]. Citrus flavonoids have demonstrated their potential anticarcinogenic activity both in in vivo and in vitro experiments by targeting cancer-related cellular processes, such as carcinogen bioactivation, cell signaling, cell cycle regulation, inflammation, and angiogenesis [147,148]. Tangeretin exhibits pharmacological properties, such as antiproliferative, anti-invasive, and anti-metastatic, and can induce apoptosis in specific cancers [149–153] (Figure 5). Experimental molecular analyses have focused on exploring and elucidating the cellular pathways involved in the metabolic activity of these flavonoids, further supporting their chemotherapeutic potential [147].

Using a proteomic approach, Yumnam et al. [154] investigated the effect of tangeretin on a human gastric cancer cell line. They observed that the treatment inhibited the activity of markers (*PKCs, MAPK4, PI4K, PARP14*) associated with poor prognosis in various cancers related to cell migration, proliferation, chemoresistance, the suppression of apoptosis, and differentiation. Remarkably, this study also sheds light on the importance of the PKC family as a novel biomarker in gastric cancer, as the overexpression of one of its members, PKCε, known for its anti-apoptotic functions, was inhibited by tangeretin treatment, which ultimately induced apoptosis in the gastric cell line. These findings highlight the potential of the PKC family as a promising marker and therapeutic target for treating gastric cancer with tangeretin.

Gliomas are responsible for originating the majority of brain tumors, presenting a high mortality rate, infiltrative growth, and low early detection. Despite intense conventional therapeutic advancements in gliomas, a cure for these tumors is still considered distant [155]. Increasing clinical data and research demonstrate that natural compounds emerge as promising agents in therapies aimed at combating GBM [156]. The potential antineoplastic effect of tangeretin was demonstrated by inducing cell cycle arrest and cell death in GBM. Tangeretin treatment positively modulated the expression of the *PTEN* gene and cell cycle regulating genes, and induced cell cycle arrest in G2/M and apoptosis. This suggests that tangeretin can be used as a chemopreventive agent in treating GBM. This assay reinforces the importance of further studies on the antitumor activity of tangeretin in nervous system tumors [157].

In in vivo experiments conducted on rat mammary carcinogenesis, tangeretin exhibited promising results. After cancer induction by 7,12-dimethylbenz(α)anthracene, oral treatment with this flavonoid affected markers associated with uncontrolled cell growth (PCNA, COX-2, and Ki-67). It effectively arrested the division of tumor cells at the G1/S phase by positively regulating the p53/p21 genes. Additionally, tangeretin demonstrated remarkable antimetastatic and antiangiogenic activities by inhibiting matrix metalloproteinases (MMPs) MMP-2/MMP-9 and the vascular endothelial growth factor (VEGF), respectively [158]. Sangavi and Langeswaran, using in silico approaches [159], investigated the inhibitory effect of natural compounds on liver cancer, targeting cyclooxygenase 2 (COX-2), an enzyme associated with inflammatory and carcinogenic processes (angiogenesis, metastasis, and apoptosis resistance). They found that tangeretin exhibited efficacy, showing a favorable pharmacokinetic profile for absorption, distribution, metabolism, excretion, and toxicity. These properties are essential for synthesizing new antineoplastic drugs and confirming the antitumor activity of this compound on the target cyclooxygenase 2 (COX-2) in hepatocellular carcinoma (HCC). The suppression of cyclooxygenase 2 (COX-2) was also observed in the epidermal cells of mice exposed to ultraviolet-B radiation (UVB). This occurred by blocking mitogen-activated protein kinase (MAPK) signaling and NF-kB activation and inhibiting the increase in ROS levels in cells upon UVB exposure, providing cellular protection against oxidative stress. These results suggest that the anti-inflammatory and modulatory effects of tangeretin may have a chemopreventive effect on skin cancer [160].

In macrophage cells, the process of inflammation induced by lipopolysaccharide (LPS) triggered a substantial increase in pro-inflammatory cytokines (IL-1, IL-6, and TNF-α) that were activated by the messenger molecule nitric oxide (NO). After incubation with tangeretin, the activation of anti-inflammatory cytokines (IL-4, IL-13, TNF-β, and IL-10) was observed, along with significant inhibition of inducible nitric oxide synthase (iNOS) and COX-2 [161]. As LPS is responsible for promoting inflammation and cell migration in certain types of cancer [162–165], the control of cellular inflammation described by the action of tangeretin may contribute to cancer treatment.

Antineoplastic agents administered as part of therapies can induce apoptosis in cancer cells. However, these agents often cause cytotoxicity in noncancerous cells, particularly immature immune system cells (myelocytes) and leukocytes (lymphocytes). In this context, the use of tangeretin in human leukemic cells (HL-60) from promyelocytic leukemia inhibited their growth by inducing apoptosis without promoting cytotoxicity or other side effects in immune system cells [128]. Combining antineoplastic agents (synergistic therapy) has resulted in more effective therapeutic strategies and the mitigation of side effects associated with chemotherapeutic agents commonly used for cancer treatment. When tangeretin was combined with the synthetic 5-fluorouracil (5-FU) and administered in treating certain solid tumors, significant antitumor activity was observed in colon cancer cells. This co-exposure decreased the antioxidant levels in tumor cells, resulting in oxidative stress through the accumulation of reactive oxygen species (ROS), triggering a DNA damage response and directing the cells toward apoptosis via c-Jun N-terminal kinases (JNKs). Significantly, tangeretin synergistically intensified the induction of apoptosis by 5-FU. Similarly, the co-treatment also caused a decrease in mitochondrial activity [166].

Another well-known chemotherapeutic agent commonly used to treat various human cancers is cisplatin, or *cis*-diamindichloroplatin (II). Cisplatin proves its effectiveness by causing DNA damage in tumor cells, leading to apoptosis. However, the side effects, such as kidney problems, weakened immunity, gastrointestinal problems, bleeding, and hearing damage, limit its applicability and effectiveness [167,168]. The use of tangeretin in acute liver injury caused by cisplatin in rats showed a protective effect against these histopathological deformations, underscoring its effect on one of the severe side effects of cisplatin treatment. Moreover, tangeretin reduced inflammatory mechanisms by neutralizing tumor necrosis factor-alpha (TNF-α) and stimulating interleukin-10 (IL-10) [92].

The expression of cell division-retarding tumor suppressor proteins, such as p21, p53, and p27, was increased in colorectal carcinoma cells when treated with tangeretin, thus promoting the inhibition of cell growth by triggering the blocking of enzymes responsible for regulating cell cycle progression and cyclin-dependent kinases (CDK2) and (CDK4) [125]. The elevation of tumor suppressor protein levels, followed by the inhibition of CDK, shows important anticancer effects, preventing neoplastic cells from entering division and ensuring the evasion of the suppression mechanism targeted against carcinogenesis. Considering the anticancer activities exhibited by citrus flavonoids, a study of the effects of a synthetic derivative of tangeretin (5,4′-didemethyltangeretin (PMF2)) in human prostate cancer cells demonstrated the restoration of P21 gene expression through epigenetic mechanisms of demethylation, followed by the blocking of DNMT 3B and HDACs protein expressions, thereby inhibiting cell proliferation [167].

Given the properties demonstrated for the different tumor characteristics in various types of cancer, tangeretin presents itself as a promising agent in the development of anticancer therapeutic strategies.

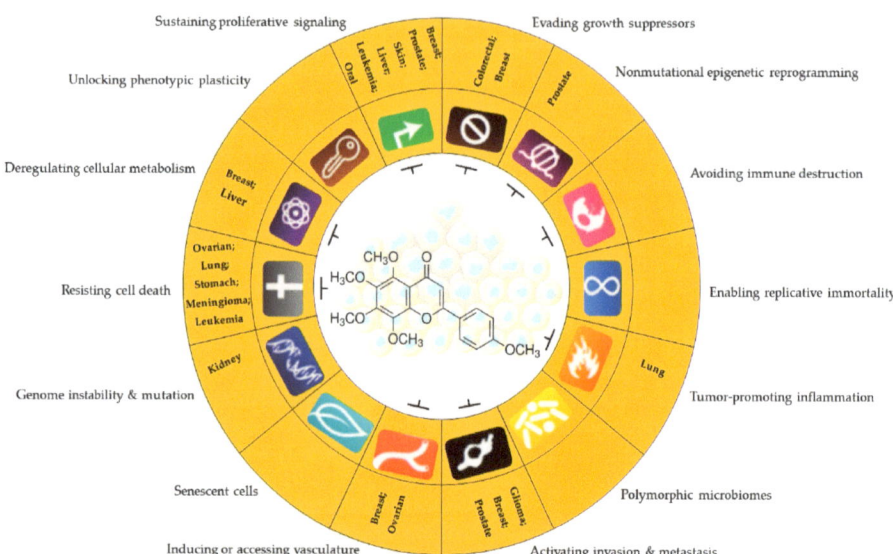

Figure 5. Antitumor potential of tangeretin. Anticancer activity of tangeretin under some cancer characteristics promotes uncontrolled cell progression and resistance to therapies in different types of tumors. Sustaining proliferative signaling: [127,152,160,161,167,168]; evading growth suppressors: [127,167]; nonmutational epigenetic reprogramming: [167]; tumor-promoting inflammation: [161,169]; activating invasion and metastasis: [151,170,171]; inducing or accessing vasculature: [170,172]; genome instability and mutation: [143]; resisting cell death: [128,129,173]; deregulating cellular metabolism: [92,174]. Parts of the figure are drawn by using pictures from Servier Medical Art. Servier Medical Art by Servier is licensed under a Creative Commons Attribution 3.0 Unported License (https://creativecommons.org/licenses/by/3.0/ accessed on 12 August 2023).

6. Conclusions and Future Perspectives

The biological potential, bioavailability, cost-effectiveness, and minimal side effects of flavonoids position them as promising cytotoxic anticancer compounds in the optimization of therapies and in the search for new drugs for the treatment of cancer. However, it is crucial to address the challenges that limit the effectiveness of flavonoids in the field of oncology, including pharmacokinetics (low solubility and stability, interaction with intestinal microflora, and metabolic interaction with receptors), pharmacodynamics, epidemiological studies (long duration, delays in data collection and categorization, absence of participant data, and exposure to heterogeneous factors), and isolation/purification of their natural sources. Among citrus flavonoids, tangeretin exhibited antitumor activities against cell proliferation. In addition, it also synergistically promoted improvements in reducing the side effects and yield when combined with some traditional chemotherapy drugs already implemented in cancer treatments. In order to provide more robust scientific knowledge about the antineoplastic activity of flavonoids, further studies are needed to examine the dosage, bioavailability, efficacy, and safety to establish the clinical use of these promising anticancer therapeutic agents.

Author Contributions: Conceptualization, F.C.F.d.L.; writing—original draft preparation, F.C.F.d.L.; writing—review and editing, F.C.F.d.L., W.A.S.F., S.M.M.C. and E.H.C.d.O.; visualization, supervision, W.A.S.F., S.M.M.C. and E.H.C.d.O. All authors have read and agreed to the published version of the manuscript.

Funding: This research was funded by Evandro Chagas Institute (Brazil)/SVSA/MS.

Institutional Review Board Statement: Not applicable.

Informed Consent Statement: Not applicable.

Data Availability Statement: Data sharing not applicable.

Acknowledgments: Authors would like to thank Pro-reitoria de pesquisa e pós-graduação (PROPESP/UFPA, Brazil) for financial support (publication fees). (Edital 02/2023-PAPQ).

Conflicts of Interest: The authors declare no conflict of interest.

References

1. Hanahan, D. Hallmarks of Cancer: New Dimensions. *Cancer Discov.* **2022**, *12*, 31–46. [CrossRef] [PubMed]
2. Hanahan, D.; Weinberg, R.A. Biological Hallmarks of Cancer. In *Holland-Frei Cancer Medicine*; John Wiley & Sons, Inc.: Hoboken, NJ, USA, 2017. [CrossRef]
3. Hanahan, D.; Weinberg, R.A. Hallmarks of Cancer: The Next Generation. *Cell* **2011**, *144*, 646–674. [CrossRef] [PubMed]
4. Hussain, S.A.; Sulaiman, A.A.; Balch, C.; Chauhan, H.; Alhadidi, Q.M.; Tiwari, A.K. Natural Polyphenols in Cancer Chemoresistance. *Nutr. Cancer* **2016**, *68*, 879–891. [CrossRef] [PubMed]
5. Kumar, A.; Jaitak, V. Natural Products as Multidrug Resistance Modulators in Cancer. *Eur. J. Med. Chem.* **2019**, *176*, 268–291. [CrossRef] [PubMed]
6. Nirmaladevi, R. Epigenetic Alterations in Cancer. *Front. Biosci.* **2020**, *25*, 4847. [CrossRef] [PubMed]
7. Kanwal, R.; Gupta, S. Epigenetic Modifications in Cancer. *Clin. Genet.* **2012**, *81*, 303–311. [CrossRef]
8. Sun, L.; Zhang, H.; Gao, P. Metabolic Reprogramming and Epigenetic Modifications on the Path to Cancer. *Protein Cell* **2022**, *13*, 877–919. [CrossRef]
9. Jones, P.A.; Baylin, S.B. The Epigenomics of Cancer. *Cell* **2007**, *128*, 683–692. [CrossRef]
10. Arora, I.; Sharma, M.; Tollefsbol, T.O. Combinatorial Epigenetics Impact of Polyphenols and Phytochemicals in Cancer Prevention and Therapy. *Int. J. Mol. Sci.* **2019**, *20*, 4567. [CrossRef]
11. Rajendran, P.; Abdelsalam, S.A.; Renu, K.; Veeraraghavan, V.; Ben Ammar, R.; Ahmed, E.A. Polyphenols as Potent Epigenetics Agents for Cancer. *Int. J. Mol. Sci.* **2022**, *23*, 11712. [CrossRef]
12. Tungmunnithum, D.; Thongboonyou, A.; Pholboon, A.; Yangsabai, A. Flavonoids and Other Phenolic Compounds from Medicinal Plants for Pharmaceutical and Medical Aspects: An Overview. *Medicines* **2018**, *5*, 93. [CrossRef] [PubMed]
13. Mutha, R.E.; Tatiya, A.U.; Surana, S.J. Flavonoids as Natural Phenolic Compounds and Their Role in Therapeutics: An Overview. *Future J. Pharm. Sci.* **2021**, *7*, 25. [CrossRef] [PubMed]
14. Kawabata, K.; Yoshioka, Y.; Terao, J. Role of Intestinal Microbiota in the Bioavailability and Physiological Functions of Dietary Polyphenols. *Molecules* **2019**, *24*, 370. [CrossRef] [PubMed]
15. Maleki, S.J.; Crespo, J.F.; Cabanillas, B. Anti-Inflammatory Effects of Flavonoids. *Food Chem.* **2019**, *299*, 125124. [CrossRef] [PubMed]
16. Sandu, M.; Bîrsă, L.M.; Bahrin, L.G. Flavonoids–Small Molecules, High Hopes. *Acta Chem. Iasi* **2017**, *25*, 6–23. [CrossRef]
17. Estrela, J.M.; Mena, S.; Obrador, E.; Benlloch, M.; Castellano, G.; Salvador, R.; Dellinger, R.W. Polyphenolic Phytochemicals in Cancer Prevention and Therapy: Bioavailability versus Bioefficacy. *J. Med. Chem.* **2017**, *60*, 9413–9436. [CrossRef] [PubMed]
18. Afshari, K.; Haddadi, N.; Haj-Mirzaian, A.; Farzaei, M.H.; Rohani, M.M.; Akramian, F.; Naseri, R.; Sureda, A.; Ghanaatian, N.; Abdolghaffari, A.H. Natural Flavonoids for the Prevention of Colon Cancer: A Comprehensive Review of Preclinical and Clinical Studies. *J. Cell. Physiol.* **2019**, *234*, 21519–21546. [CrossRef]
19. George, V.C.; Dellaire, G.; Rupasinghe, H.P.V. Plant Flavonoids in Cancer Chemoprevention: Role in Genome Stability. *J. Nutr. Biochem.* **2017**, *45*, 1–14. [CrossRef]
20. Ross, J.A.; Kasum, C.M. DIETARY FLAVONOIDS: Bioavailability, Metabolic Effects, and Safety. *Annu. Rev. Nutr.* **2002**, *22*, 19–34. [CrossRef]
21. Kasprzak, M.M.; Erxleben, A.; Ochocki, J. Properties and Applications of Flavonoid Metal Complexes. *RSC Adv.* **2015**, *5*, 45853–45877. [CrossRef]
22. Panche, A.N.; Diwan, A.D.; Chandra, S.R. Flavonoids: An Overview. *J. Nutr. Sci.* **2016**, *5*, E47. [CrossRef] [PubMed]
23. Rahnasto-Rilla, M.; Tyni, J.; Huovinen, M.; Jarho, E.; Kulikowicz, T.; Ravichandran, S.; Bohr, V.A.; Ferrucci, L.; Lahtela-Kakkonen, M.; Moaddel, R. Natural Polyphenols as Sirtuin 6 Modulators. *Sci. Rep.* **2018**, *8*, 4163. [CrossRef] [PubMed]
24. Slámová, K.; Kapešová, J.; Valentová, K. "Sweet Flavonoids": Glycosidase-Catalyzed Modifications. *Int. J. Mol. Sci.* **2018**, *19*, 2126. [CrossRef] [PubMed]
25. Jain, V.K.; Vishwavidyalaya, D.A.; Pradesh, M. Flavonoids Impact on Prevention and Treatment of Obesity and Related. *Int. J. Pharm. Sci. Res.* **2019**, *10*, 4420–4429. [CrossRef]
26. Teles, Y.C.F.; Souza, M.S.R.; De Souza, M.d.F.V. Sulphated Flavonoids: Biosynthesis, Structures, and Biological Activities. *Molecules* **2018**, *23*, 480. [CrossRef] [PubMed]
27. Veitch, N.C.; Grayer, R.J. Flavonoids and Their Glycosides, Including Anthocyanins. *Nat. Prod. Rep.* **2011**, *28*, 1626–1695. [CrossRef] [PubMed]

28. Kopustinskiene, D.M.; Jakstas, V.; Savickas, A.; Bernatoniene, J. Flavonoids as Anticancer Agents. *Nutrients* **2020**, *12*, 457. [CrossRef]
29. Wang, T.-y.; Li, Q.; Bi, K.-s. Bioactive Flavonoids in Medicinal Plants: Structure, Activity and Biological Fate. *Asian J. Pharm. Sci.* **2018**, *13*, 12–23. [CrossRef]
30. Brodowska, K.M. European Journal of Biological Research Natural Flavonoids: Classification, Potential Role, and Application of Flavonoid Analogues. *Eur. J. Biol. Res.* **2017**, *7*, 108–123. [CrossRef]
31. Khajuria, R.; Singh, S.; Bahl, A. General Introduction and Sources of Flavonoids. In *Current Aspects of Flavonoids: Their Role in Cancer Treatment*; Springer: Singapore, 2019; pp. 1–7. [CrossRef]
32. Liu, H.; Jiang, W.; Xie, M. Flavonoids: Recent Advances as Anticancer Drugs. *Recent Pat. Anti-Cancer Drug Discov.* **2010**, *5*, 152–164. [CrossRef]
33. Raffa, D.; Maggio, B.; Raimondi, M.V.; Plescia, F.; Daidone, G. Recent Discoveries of Anticancer Flavonoids. *Eur. J. Med. Chem.* **2017**, *142*, 213–228. [CrossRef] [PubMed]
34. Symonowicz, M.; Kolanek, M. Flavonoids and Their Properties to Form Chelate Complexes. *Biotechnol. Food Sci.* **2012**, *76*, 35–41.
35. Ahn-Jarvis, J.H.; Parihar, A.; Doseff, A.I. Dietary Flavonoids for Immunoregulation and Cancer: Food Design for Targeting Disease. *Antioxidants* **2019**, *8*, 202. [CrossRef] [PubMed]
36. Pei, R.; Liu, X.; Bolling, B. Flavonoids and Gut Health. *Curr. Opin. Biotechnol.* **2020**, *61*, 153–159. [CrossRef] [PubMed]
37. Sudhakaran, M.; Sardesai, S.; Doseff, A.I. Flavonoids: New Frontier for Immuno-Regulation and Breast Cancer Control. *Antioxidants* **2019**, *8*, 103. [CrossRef] [PubMed]
38. Al Aboody, M.S.; Mickymaray, S. Anti-Fungal Efficacy and Mechanisms of Flavonoids. *Antibiotics* **2020**, *9*, 45. [CrossRef] [PubMed]
39. Bai, L.; Li, X.; He, L.; Zheng, Y.; Lu, H.; Li, J.; Zhong, L.; Tong, R.; Jiang, Z.; Shi, J.; et al. Antidiabetic Potential of Flavonoids from Traditional Chinese Medicine: A Review. *Am. J. Chin. Med.* **2019**, *47*, 933–957. [CrossRef] [PubMed]
40. Pietta, P.G. Flavonoids as Antioxidants. *J. Nat. Prod.* **2000**, *63*, 1035–1042. [CrossRef]
41. Ren, W.; Qiao, Z.; Wang, H.; Zhu, L.; Zhang, L. Flavonoids: Promising Anticancer Agents. *Med. Res. Rev.* **2003**, *23*, 519–534. [CrossRef]
42. Weston, L.A.; Mathesius, U. Flavonoids: Their Structure, Biosynthesis and Role in the Rhizosphere, Including Allelopathy. *J. Chem. Ecol.* **2013**, *39*, 283–297. [CrossRef]
43. Sharma, N.; Dobhal, M.; Joshi, Y.; Chahar, M. Flavonoids: A Versatile Source of Anticancer Drugs. *Pharmacogn. Rev.* **2011**, *5*, 1–12. [CrossRef] [PubMed]
44. Perez-Vizcaino, F.; Fraga, C.G. Research Trends in Flavonoids and Health. *Arch. Biochem. Biophys.* **2018**, *646*, 107–112. [CrossRef] [PubMed]
45. Rodríguez-García, C.; Sánchez-Quesada, C.; Gaforio, J.J.; Gaforio, J.J. Dietary Flavonoids as Cancer Chemopreventive Agents: An Updated Review of Human Studies. *Antioxidants* **2019**, *8*, 137. [CrossRef] [PubMed]
46. Rudzińska, A.; Juchaniuk, P.; Oberda, J.; Wiśniewska, J.; Wojdan, W.; Szklener, K.; Mańdziuk, S. Phytochemicals in Cancer Treatment and Cancer Prevention—Review on Epidemiological Data and Clinical Trials. *Nutrients* **2023**, *15*, 1896. [CrossRef] [PubMed]
47. Anantharaju, P.G.; Gowda, P.C.; Vimalambike, M.G.; Madhunapantula, S.V. An Overview on the Role of Dietary Phenolics for the Treatment of Cancers. *Nutr. J.* **2016**, *15*, 99. [CrossRef] [PubMed]
48. Mohana, S.; Ganesan, M.; Rajendra Prasad, N.; Ananthakrishnan, D.; Velmurugan, D. Flavonoids Modulate Multidrug Resistance through Wnt Signaling in P-Glycoprotein Overexpressing Cell Lines. *BMC Cancer* **2018**, *18*, 1168. [CrossRef] [PubMed]
49. Hosseinzadeh, A.; Poursoleiman, F.; Biregani, A.N.; Esmailzadeh, A. Flavonoids Target Different Molecules of Autophagic and Metastatic Pathways in Cancer Cells. *Cancer Cell Int.* **2023**, *23*, 114. [CrossRef]
50. De Sousa Silva, G.V.; Lopes, A.L.V.F.G.; Viali, I.C.; Lima, L.Z.M.; Bizuti, M.R.; Haag, F.B.; Tavares de Resende e Silva, D. Therapeutic Properties of Flavonoids in Treatment of Cancer through Autophagic Modulation: A Systematic Review. *Chin. J. Integr. Med.* **2023**, *29*, 268–279. [CrossRef]
51. Parekh, N.; Garg, A.; Choudhary, R.; Gupta, M.; Kaur, G.; Ramniwas, S.; Shahwan, M.; Tuli, H.S.; Sethi, G. The Role of Natural Flavonoids as Telomerase Inhibitors in Suppressing Cancer Growth. *Pharmaceuticals* **2023**, *16*, 605. [CrossRef]
52. Rahman, N.; Khan, H.; Zia, A.; Khan, A.; Fakhri, S.; Aschner, M.; Gul, K.; Saso, L. Bcl-2 Modulation in P53 Signaling Pathway by Flavonoids: A Potential Strategy towards the Treatment of Cancer. *Int. J. Mol. Sci.* **2021**, *22*, 11315. [CrossRef]
53. Kim, M.H. Flavonoids Inhibit VEGF/BFGF-Induced Angiogenesis in Vitro by Inhibiting the Matrix-Degrading Proteases. *J. Cell. Biochem.* **2003**, *89*, 529–538. [CrossRef] [PubMed]
54. Marques, S.M.; Šupolíková, L.; Molčanová, L.; Šmejkal, K.; Bednar, D.; Slaninová, I. Screening of Natural Compounds as P-Glycoprotein Inhibitors against Multidrug Resistance. *Biomedicines* **2021**, *9*, 357. [CrossRef] [PubMed]
55. Li, G.; Ding, K.; Qiao, Y.; Zhang, L.; Zheng, L.; Pan, T.; Zhang, L. Flavonoids Regulate Inflammation and Oxidative Stress in Cancer. *Molecules* **2020**, *25*, 5628. [CrossRef] [PubMed]
56. Zhao, J.; Yang, J.; Xie, Y. Improvement Strategies for the Oral Bioavailability of Poorly Water-Soluble Flavonoids: An Overview. *Int. J. Pharm.* **2019**, *570*, 118642. [CrossRef] [PubMed]

57. Raj, S.; Khurana, S.; Choudhari, R.; Kesari, K.K.; Kamal, M.A.; Garg, N.; Ruokolainen, J.; Das, B.C.; Kumar, D. Specific Targeting Cancer Cells with Nanoparticles and Drug Delivery in Cancer Therapy. *Semin. Cancer Biol.* **2021**, *69*, 166–177. [CrossRef] [PubMed]
58. Pérez-Herrero, E.; Fernández-Medarde, A. Advanced Targeted Therapies in Cancer: Drug Nanocarriers, the Future of Chemotherapy. *Eur. J. Pharm. Biopharm.* **2015**, *93*, 52–79. [CrossRef] [PubMed]
59. Liskova, A.; Samec, M.; Koklesova, L.; Brockmueller, A.; Zhai, K.; Abdellatif, B.; Siddiqui, M.; Biringer, K.; Kudela, E.; Pec, M.; et al. Flavonoids as an Effective Sensitizer for Anti-Cancer Therapy: Insights into Multi-Faceted Mechanisms and Applicability towards Individualized Patient Profiles. *EPMA J.* **2021**, *12*, 155–176. [CrossRef] [PubMed]
60. Ferreira, M.; Costa, D.; Sousa, Â. Flavonoids-Based Delivery Systems towards Cancer Therapies. *Bioengineering* **2022**, *9*, 197. [CrossRef]
61. Khan, H.; Ullah, H.; Martorell, M.; Valdes, S.E.; Belwal, T.; Tejada, S.; Sureda, A.; Kamal, M.A. Flavonoids Nanoparticles in Cancer: Treatment, Prevention and Clinical Prospects. *Semin. Cancer Biol.* **2019**, *69*, 200–211. [CrossRef]
62. Wei, Q.Y.; He, K.M.; Chen, J.L.; Xu, Y.M.; Lau, A.T.Y. Phytofabrication of Nanoparticles as Novel Drugs for Anticancer Applications. *Molecules* **2019**, *24*, 4246. [CrossRef]
63. Siddiqui, I.A.; Bharali, D.J.; Nihal, M.; Adhami, V.M.; Khan, N.; Chamcheu, J.C.; Khan, M.I.; Shabana, S.; Mousa, S.A.; Mukhtar, H. Excellent Anti-Proliferative and pro-Apoptotic Effects of (−)-Epigallocatechin-3-Gallate Encapsulated in Chitosan Nanoparticles on Human Melanoma Cell Growth Both in Vitro and in Vivo. *Nanomed. Nanotechnol. Biol. Med.* **2014**, *10*, 1619–1626. [CrossRef] [PubMed]
64. Nihal, M.; Ahmad, N.; Mukhtar, H.; Wood, G.S. Anti-Proliferative and Proapoptotic Effects of (−)-Epigallocatechin-3-Gallate on Human Melanoma: Possible Implications for the Chemoprevention of Melanoma. *Int. J. Cancer* **2005**, *114*, 513–521. [CrossRef] [PubMed]
65. Siddiqui, I.A.; Adhami, V.M.; Bharali, D.J.; Hafeez, B.B.; Asim, M.; Khwaja, S.I.; Ahmad, N.; Cui, H.; Mousa, S.A.; Mukhtar, H. Introducing Nanochemoprevention as a Novel Approach for Cancer Control: Proof of Principle with Green Tea Polyphenol Epigallocatechin-3-Gallate. *Cancer Res.* **2009**, *69*, 1712–1716. [CrossRef] [PubMed]
66. Chen, B.; Hsieh, C.; Tsai, S.; Wang, C.-Y.; Wang, C. Anticancer Effects of Epigallocatechin-3-Gallate Nanoemulsion on Lung Cancer Cells through the Activation of AMP-Activated Protein Kinase Signaling Pathway. *Sci. Rep.* **2020**, *10*, 5163. [CrossRef] [PubMed]
67. Trefts, E.; Shaw, R.J. AMPK: Restoring Metabolic Homeostasis over Space and Time. *Mol. Cell* **2021**, *81*, 3677–3690. [CrossRef] [PubMed]
68. Thirupathi, A.; Chang, Y.Z. Role of AMPK and Its Molecular Intermediates in Subjugating Cancer Survival Mechanism. *Life Sci.* **2019**, *227*, 30–38. [CrossRef] [PubMed]
69. Gorrini, C.; Harris, I.S.; Mak, T.W. Modulation of Oxidative Stress as an Anticancer Strategy. *Nat. Rev. Drug Discov.* **2013**, *12*, 931–947. [CrossRef]
70. Huang, M.Z.; Li, J.Y. Physiological Regulation of Reactive Oxygen Species in Organisms Based on Their Physicochemical Properties. *Acta Physiol.* **2020**, *228*, e13351. [CrossRef]
71. Marengo, B.; Nitti, M.; Furfaro, A.L.; Colla, R.; De Ciucis, C.; Marinari, U.M.; Pronzato, M.A.; Traverso, N.; Domenicotti, C. Redox Homeostasis and Cellular Antioxidant Systems: Crucial Players in Cancer Growth and Therapy. *Oxid. Med. Cell. Longev.* **2016**, *2016*, 6235641. [CrossRef]
72. Lv, H.; Zhen, C.; Liu, J.; Yang, P.; Hu, L. Unraveling the Potential Role of Glutathione in Multiple Forms of Cell Death in Cancer Therapy. *Oxid. Med. Cell. Longev.* **2019**, *2019*, 3150145. [CrossRef]
73. Zaidieh, T.; Smith, J.R.; Ball, K.E.; An, Q. ROS as a Novel Indicator to Predict Anticancer Drug Efficacy. *BMC Cancer* **2019**, *19*, 1224. [CrossRef] [PubMed]
74. Perillo, B.; Di Donato, M.; Pezone, A.; Di Zazzo, E.; Castoria, G.; Migliaccio, A. ROS in Cancer Therapy: The Bright Side of the Moon. *Exp. Mol. Med.* **2020**, *52*, 192–203. [CrossRef] [PubMed]
75. Liou, G.-Y.; Storz, P. Reactive Oxygen Species in Cancer. *Free Radic. Res.* **2010**, *44*, 479–496. [CrossRef] [PubMed]
76. Cao, G.; Sofic, E.; Prior, R.L. Antioxidant and Prooxidant Behavior of Flavonoids: Structure-Activity Relationships. *Free Radic. Biol. Med.* **1997**, *22*, 749–760. [CrossRef] [PubMed]
77. Havsteen, B.H. The Biochemistry and Medical Significance of the Flavonoids. *Pharmacol. Ther.* **2002**, *96*, 67–202. [CrossRef] [PubMed]
78. Tavsan, Z.; Kayali, H.A. Flavonoids Showed Anticancer Effects on the Ovarian Cancer Cells: Involvement of Reactive Oxygen Species, Apoptosis, Cell Cycle and Invasion. *Biomed. Pharmacother.* **2019**, *116*, 109004. [CrossRef] [PubMed]
79. Biswas, P.; Dey, D.; Biswas, P.K.; Rahaman, T.I.; Saha, S.; Parvez, A.; Khan, D.A.; Lily, N.J.; Saha, K.; Sohel, M.; et al. A Comprehensive Analysis and Anti-Cancer Activities of Quercetin in ROS-Mediated Cancer and Cancer Stem Cells. *Int. J. Mol. Sci.* **2022**, *23*, 11746. [CrossRef] [PubMed]
80. Ai, L.; Kim, W.J.; Demircan, B.; Dyer, L.M.; Bray, K.J.; Skehan, R.R.; Massoll, N.A.; Brown, K.D. The Transglutaminase 2 Gene (TGM2), a Potential Molecular Marker for Chemotherapeutic Drug Sensitivity, Is Epigenetically Silenced in Breast Cancer. *Carcinogenesis* **2008**, *29*, 510–518. [CrossRef]
81. Eckert, R.L. Transglutaminase 2 Takes Center Stage as a Cancer Cell Survival Factor and Therapy Target. *Mol. Carcinog.* **2019**, *58*, 837–853. [CrossRef]

82. Mehta, K.; Han, A. Tissue Transglutaminase (TG2)-Induced Inflammation in Initiation, Progression, and Pathogenesis of Pancreatic Cancer. *Cancers* **2011**, *3*, 897–912. [CrossRef]
83. Wang, F.; Wang, L.; Qu, C.; Chen, L.; Geng, Y.; Cheng, C.; Yu, S.; Wang, D.; Yang, L.; Meng, Z.; et al. Kaempferol Induces ROS-Dependent Apoptosis in Pancreatic Cancer Cells via TGM2-Mediated Akt/MTOR Signaling. *BMC Cancer* **2021**, *21*, 396. [CrossRef]
84. Reyes-Farias, M.; Carrasco-Pozo, C. The Anti-Cancer Effect of Quercetin: Molecular Implications in Cancer Metabolism. *Int. J. Mol. Sci.* **2019**, *20*, 3177. [CrossRef] [PubMed]
85. Ortega, A.L.; Mena, S.; Estrela, J.M. Glutathione in Cancer Cell Death. *Cancers* **2011**, *3*, 1285–1310. [CrossRef] [PubMed]
86. Pakfetrat, A.; Dalirsani, Z.; Hashemy, S.I.; Ghazi, A.; Mostaan, L.V.; Anvari, K.; Pour, A.M. Evaluation of Serum Levels of Oxidized and Reduced Glutathione and Total Antioxidant Capacity in Patients with Head and Neck Squamous Cell Carcinoma. *J. Cancer Res. Ther.* **2018**, *14*, 428–431. [CrossRef] [PubMed]
87. Bansal, A.; Simon, M.C. Glutathione Metabolism in Cancer Progression and Treatment Resistance. *J. Cell Biol.* **2018**, *217*, 2291–2298. [CrossRef] [PubMed]
88. Yoo, D.; Jung, E.; Noh, J.; Hyun, H.; Seon, S.; Hong, S.; Kim, D.; Lee, D. Glutathione-Depleting Pro-Oxidant as a Selective Anticancer Therapeutic Agent. *ACS Omega* **2019**, *4*, 10070–10077. [CrossRef]
89. Traverso, N.; Ricciarelli, R.; Nitti, M.; Marengo, B.; Furfaro, A.L.; Pronzato, M.A.; Marinari, U.M.; Domenicotti, C. Role of Glutathione in Cancer Progression and Chemoresistance. *Oxid. Med. Cell. Longev.* **2013**, *2013*, 972913. [CrossRef]
90. Desideri, E.; Ciccarone, F.; Ciriolo, M.R. Targeting Glutathione Metabolism: Partner in Crime in Anticancer Therapy. *Nutrients* **2019**, *11*, 1926. [CrossRef]
91. Liang, F.; Fang, Y.; Cao, W.; Zhang, Z.; Pan, S.; Xu, X. Attenuation of tert-Butyl Hydroperoxide (t-BHP)-Induced Oxidative Damage in HepG2 Cells by Tangeretin: Relevance of the Nrf2-ARE and MAPK Signaling Pathways. *J. Agric. Food Chem.* **2018**, *66*, 6317–6325. [CrossRef]
92. Omar, H.A.; Mohamed, W.R.; Arab, H.H.; Arafa, E.S.A. Tangeretin Alleviates Cisplatin-Induced Acute Hepatic Injury in Rats: Targeting MAPKs and Apoptosis. *PLoS ONE* **2016**, *11*, e0151649. [CrossRef]
93. Portela, A.; Esteller, M. Epigenetic Modifications and Human Disease. *Nat. Biotechnol.* **2010**, *28*, 1057–1068. [CrossRef]
94. Hernando-Herraez, I.; Garcia-Perez, R.; Sharp, A.J.; Marques-Bonet, T. DNA Methylation: Insights into Human Evolution. *PLoS Genet.* **2015**, *11*, e1005661. [CrossRef] [PubMed]
95. Parry, L.; Clarke, A.R. The Roles of the Methyl-CpG Binding Proteins in Cancer. *Genes Cancer* **2011**, *2*, 618–630. [CrossRef]
96. Bergman, Y.; Cedar, H. DNA Methylation Dynamics in Health and Disease. *Nat. Struct. Mol. Biol.* **2013**, *20*, 274–281. [CrossRef] [PubMed]
97. Ning, B.; Li, W.; Zhao, W.; Wang, R. Targeting Epigenetic Regulations in Cancer. *Acta Biochim. Biophys. Sin.* **2015**, *48*, 97–109. [CrossRef] [PubMed]
98. Stefansson, O.A.; Moran, S.; Gomez, A.; Sayols, S.; Arribas-Jorba, C.; Sandoval, J.; Hilmarsdottir, H.; Olafsdottir, E.; Tryggvadottir, L.; Jonasson, J.G.; et al. A DNA Methylation-Based Definition of Biologically Distinct Breast Cancer Subtypes. *Mol. Oncol.* **2015**, *9*, 555–568. [CrossRef] [PubMed]
99. Zakhari, S. Alcohol Metabolism and Epigenetics Changes. *Alcohol Res.* **2013**, *35*, 6–16. [PubMed]
100. Selvakumar, P.; Badgeley, A.; Murphy, P.; Anwar, H.; Sharma, U.; Lawrence, K.; Lakshmikuttyamma, A. Flavonoids and Other Polyphenols Act as Epigenetic Modifiers in Breast Cancer. *Nutrients* **2020**, *12*, 761. [CrossRef]
101. Cadet, J.; McCoy, M.; Jayanthi, S. Epigenetics and Addiction. *Clin. Pharmacol. Ther.* **2016**, *99*, 502–511. [CrossRef]
102. Fatima, N.; Baqri, S.S.R.; Bhattacharya, A.; Koney, N.K.K.; Husain, K.; Abbas, A.; Ansari, R.A. Role of Flavonoids as Epigenetic Modulators in Cancer Prevention and Therapy. *Front. Genet.* **2021**, *12*, 758733. [CrossRef]
103. Goldar, S.; Khaniani, M.S.; Derakhshan, S.M.; Baradaran, B. Molecular Mechanisms of Apoptosis and Roles in Cancer Development and Treatment. *Asian Pac. J. Cancer Prev.* **2015**, *16*, 2129–2144. [CrossRef] [PubMed]
104. Hassan, M.; Watari, H.; Abualmaaty, A.; Ohba, Y.; Sakuragi, N. Apoptosis and Molecular Targeting Therapy in Cancer. *Biomed Res. Int.* **2014**, *2014*, 150845. [CrossRef] [PubMed]
105. Carneiro, B.A.; El-Deiry, W.S. Targeting Apoptosis in Cancer Therapy. *Nat. Rev. Clin. Oncol.* **2020**, *17*, 395–417. [CrossRef] [PubMed]
106. Tewary, P.; Gunatilaka, A.A.L.; Sayers, T.J. Using Natural Products to Promote Caspase-8-Dependent Cancer Cell Death. *Cancer Immunol. Immunother.* **2017**, *66*, 223–231. [CrossRef] [PubMed]
107. Kong, A.N.T.; Yu, R.; Chen, C.; Mandlekar, S.; Primiano, T. Signal Transduction Events Elicited by Natural Products: Role of MAPK and Caspase Pathways in Homeostatic Response and Induction of Apoptosis. *Arch. Pharm. Res.* **2000**, *23*, 1–16. [CrossRef]
108. McIlwain, D.R.; Berger, T.; Mak, T.W. Caspase Functions in Cell Death and Disease. *Cold Spring Harb. Perspect. Biol.* **2015**, *7*, a026716. [CrossRef] [PubMed]
109. Ghavami, S.; Hashemi, M.; Ande, S.R.; Yeganeh, B.; Xiao, W.; Eshraghi, M.; Bus, C.J.; Kadkhoda, K.; Wiechec, E.; Halayko, A.J.; et al. Apoptosis and Cancer: Mutations within Caspase Genes. *J. Med. Genet.* **2009**, *46*, 497–510. [CrossRef]
110. Xu, D.C.; Arthurton, L.; Baena-Lopez, L.A. Learning on the Fly: The Interplay between Caspases and Cancer. *Biomed Res. Int.* **2018**, *2018*, 5473180. [CrossRef]
111. Pfeffer, C.M.; Singh, A.T.K. Apoptosis: A Target for Anticancer Therapy. *Int. J. Mol. Sci.* **2018**, *19*, 448. [CrossRef]

112. Warren, C.F.A.; Wong-Brown, M.W.; Bowden, N.A. BCL-2 Family Isoforms in Apoptosis and Cancer. *Cell Death Dis.* **2019**, *10*, 177. [CrossRef]
113. Lomonosova, E.; Chinnadurai, G. BH3-Only Proteins in Apoptosis and beyond: An Overview. *Oncogene* **2008**, *27*, S2–S19. [CrossRef] [PubMed]
114. Elango, R.; Athinarayanan, J.; Subbarayan, V.P.; Lei, D.K.Y.; Alshatwi, A.A. Hesperetin Induces an Apoptosis-Triggered Extrinsic Pathway and a P53-Independent Pathway in Human Lung Cancer H522 Cells. *J. Asian Nat. Prod. Res.* **2018**, *20*, 559–569. [CrossRef] [PubMed]
115. Dahlawi, H. Effect of Malvidin on Induction of Apoptosis and Inhibition of Cell Proliferation on Myeloid and Lymphoid Leukemia. *Sch. J. Appl. Med. Sci.* **2022**, *10*, 150–156. [CrossRef]
116. Wang, Y.X.; Cai, H.; Jiang, G.; Zhou, T.B.; Wu, H. Silibinin Inhibits Proliferation, Induces Apoptosis and Causes Cell Cycle Arrest in Human Gastric Cancer MGC803 Cells via STAT3 Pathway Inhibition. *Asian Pac. J. Cancer Prev.* **2014**, *15*, 6791–6798. [CrossRef] [PubMed]
117. Liu, X.; Zhang, D.; Hao, Y.; Liu, Q.; Wu, Y.; Liu, X.; Luo, J.; Zhou, T.; Sun, B.; Luo, X.; et al. Cyanidin Curtails Renal Cell Carcinoma Tumorigenesis. *Cell. Physiol. Biochem.* **2018**, *46*, 2517–2531. [CrossRef] [PubMed]
118. Lee, D.Y.; Yun, S.M.; Song, M.Y.; Jung, K.; Kim, E.H. Cyanidin Chloride Induces Apoptosis by Inhibiting NF-κB Signaling through Activation of Nrf2 in Colorectal Cancer Cells. *Antioxidants* **2020**, *9*, 285. [CrossRef] [PubMed]
119. Wu, A.; Zhu, Y.; Han, B.; Peng, J.; Deng, X.; Chen, W.; Du, J.; Ou, Y.; Peng, X.; Yu, X. Delphinidin Induces Cell Cycle Arrest and Apoptosis in HER-2 Positive Breast Cancer Cell Lines by Regulating the NF-κB and MAPK Signaling Pathways. *Oncol. Lett.* **2021**, *22*, 832. [CrossRef] [PubMed]
120. Kim, U.; Kim, C.-Y.; Lee, J.M.; Oh, H.; Ryu, B.; Kim, J.; Park, J.-H. Phloretin Inhibits the Human Prostate Cancer Cells Through the Generation of Reactive Oxygen Species. *Pathol. Oncol. Res.* **2020**, *26*, 977–984. [CrossRef]
121. Zhou, J.; Xia, L.; Zhang, Y. Naringin Inhibits Thyroid Cancer Cell Proliferation and Induces Cell Apoptosis through Repressing PI3K/AKT Pathway. *Pathol. Res. Pract.* **2019**, *215*, 152707. [CrossRef]
122. He, M.; Qiu, C.; Wang, J.; Li, B.; Wang, G.; Ji, X. Naringin Targets Zeb1 to Suppress Osteosarcoma Cell Proliferation and Metastasis. *Aging* **2018**, *10*, 4141–4151. [CrossRef]
123. Raha, S.; Kim, S.M.; Lee, H.J.; Yumnam, S.; Saralamma, V.V.G.; Ha, S.E.; Lee, W.S.; Kim, G.S. Naringin Induces Lysosomal Permeabilization and Autophagy Cell Death in AGS Gastric Cancer Cells. *Am. J. Chin. Med.* **2020**, *48*, 679–702. [CrossRef] [PubMed]
124. Zhang, Y.; Zhang, R.; Ni, H. Basic Research Eriodictyol Exerts Potent Anticancer Activity against A549 Human Lung Cancer Cell Line by Inducing Mitochondrial-Mediated Apoptosis, G2/M Cell Cycle Arrest and Inhibition of m-TOR/PI3K/Akt Signalling Pathway. *Arch. Med. Sci.* **2020**, *16*, 446–452. [CrossRef]
125. Li, W.; Du, Q.; Li, X.; Zheng, X.; Lv, F.; Xi, X.; Huang, G. Eriodictyol Inhibits Proliferation, Metastasis and Induces Apoptosis of Glioma Cells via PI3K/Akt/NF-κB Signaling Pathway. *Front. Pharmacol.* **2020**, *11*, 114. [CrossRef] [PubMed]
126. Yan, W.; Ma, X.; Zhao, X.; Zhang, S. Baicalein Induces Apoptosis and Autophagy of Breast Cancer Cells via Inhibiting PI3K/AKT Pathway In Vivo and Vitro. *Drug Des. Dev. Ther.* **2018**, *12*, 3961–3972. [CrossRef] [PubMed]
127. Pan, M.H.; Chen, W.J.; Lin-Shiau, S.Y.; Ho, C.T.; Lin, J.K. Tangeretin Induces Cell-Cyle G1 Arrest through Inhibiting Cyclin-Dependent Kinases 2 and 4 Activities as Well as Elevating Cdk Inhibitors P21 and P27 in Human Colorectal Carcinoma Cells. *Carcinogenesis* **2002**, *23*, 1677–1684. [CrossRef] [PubMed]
128. Hirano, T.; Abe, K.; Gotoh, M. Citrus Flavone Tangeretin Inhibits Leukaemic HL-60 Cell Growth Partially through Induction of Apoptosis with Less Cytotoxicity on Normal Lymphocytes. *Br. J. Cancer* **1995**, *72*, 1380–1388. [CrossRef] [PubMed]
129. Dong, Y.; Cao, A.; Shi, J.; Yin, P.; Wang, L.; Ji, G.; Xie, J.; Wu, D. Tangeretin, a Citrus Polymethoxyflavonoid, Induces Apoptosis of Human Gastric Cancer AGS Cells through Extrinsic and Intrinsic Signaling Pathways. *Oncol. Rep.* **2014**, *31*, 1788–1794. [CrossRef] [PubMed]
130. Kang, K.A.; Piao, M.J.; Hyun, Y.J.; Zhen, A.X.; Cho, S.J.; Ahn, M.J.; Yi, J.M.; Hyun, J.W. Luteolin Promotes Apoptotic Cell Death via Upregulation of Nrf2 Expression by DNA Demethylase and the Interaction of Nrf2 with P53 in Human Colon Cancer Cells. *Exp. Mol. Med.* **2019**, *51*, 1–14. [CrossRef]
131. Mahbub, A.A.; Le Maitre, C.L.; Cross, N.A.; Mahy, N.J. The Effect of Apigenin and Chemotherapy Combination Treatments on Apoptosis-Related Genes and Proteins in Acute Leukaemia Cell Lines. *Sci. Rep.* **2022**, *12*, 8858. [CrossRef]
132. Li, N.; Sun, C.; Zhou, B.; Xing, H.; Ma, D.; Chen, G.; Weng, D. Low Concentration of Quercetin Antagonizes the Cytotoxic Effects of Anti-Neoplastic Drugs in Ovarian Cancer. *PLoS ONE* **2014**, *9*, e100314. [CrossRef]
133. Nafees, S.; Mehdi, S.H.; Zafaryab, M.; Zeya, B.; Sarwar, T.; Rizvi, M.A. Synergistic Interaction of Rutin and Silibinin on Human Colon Cancer Cell Line. *Arch. Med. Res.* **2018**, *49*, 226–234. [CrossRef] [PubMed]
134. Jiang, H.; Fan, J.; Cheng, L.; Hu, P.; Liu, R. The Anticancer Activity of Genistein Is Increased in Estrogen Receptor Beta 1-Positive Breast Cancer Cells. *OncoTargets. Ther.* **2018**, *11*, 8153–8163. [CrossRef] [PubMed]
135. Guo, S.; Wang, Y.; Li, Y.; Li, Y.; Feng, C.; Li, Z. Daidzein-Rich Iso Fl Avones Aglycone Inhibits Lung Cancer Growth through Inhibition of NF-κB Signaling Pathway. *Immunol. Lett.* **2020**, *222*, 67–72. [CrossRef] [PubMed]
136. Yu, X.; Gao, F.; Li, W.; Zhou, L.; Liu, W.; Li, M. Formononetin Inhibits Tumor Growth by Suppression of EGFR-Akt-Mcl-1 Axis in Non-Small Cell Lung Cancer. *J. Exp. Clin. Cancer Res.* **2020**, *39*, 62. [CrossRef] [PubMed]

137. Won, D.; Kim, L.; Jang, B.; Yang, I.; Kwon, H.; Jin, B.; Oh, S.H.; Kang, J. In Vitro and in Vivo Anti-Cancer Activity of Silymarin on Oral Cancer. *Tumor Biol.* **2018**, *40*, 1–11. [CrossRef] [PubMed]
138. Wang, R.; Zhu, X.; Wang, Q.; Li, X.; Wang, E.; Zhao, Q.; Wang, Q.; Cao, H. The Anti-Tumor Effect of Taxifolin on Lung Cancer via Suppressing Stemness and Epithelial-Mesenchymal Transition in Vitro and Oncogenesis in Nude Mice. *Ann. Transl. Med.* **2020**, *8*, 590. [CrossRef] [PubMed]
139. Razak, S.; Afsar, T.; Ullah, A.; Almajwal, A.; Alkholief, M.; Alshamsan, A.; Jahan, S. Taxifolin, a Natural Flavonoid Interacts with Cell Cycle Regulators Causes Cell Cycle Arrest and Causes Tumor Regression by Activating Wnt/β-Catenin Signaling Pathway. *BMC Cancer* **2018**, *18*, 1043. [CrossRef]
140. Silva, C.; Correia-Branco, A.; Andrade, N.; Ferreira, A.C.; Soares, M.L.; Sonveaux, P.; Stephenne, J.; Martel, F. Selective Pro-Apoptotic and Antimigratory Effects of Polyphenol Complex Catechin:Lysine 1:2 in Breast, Pancreatic and Colorectal Cancer Cell Lines. *Eur. J. Pharmacol.* **2019**, *859*, 172533. [CrossRef]
141. Pereyra-Vergara, F.; Olivares-Corichi, I.M.; Perez-Ruiz, A.G.; Luna-Arias, J.P.; García-Sánchez, J.R. Apoptosis Induced by (−)-Epicatechin in Human Breast Cancer Cells Is Mediated by Reactive Oxygen Species. *Molecules* **2020**, *25*, 1020. [CrossRef]
142. Wu, D.; Liu, Z.; Li, J.; Zhang, Q.; Zhong, P.; Teng, T.; Chen, M.; Xie, Z.; Ji, A.; Li, Y. Epigallocatechin-3-Gallate Inhibits the Growth and Increases the Apoptosis of Human Thyroid Carcinoma Cells through Suppression of EGFR/RAS/RAF/MEK/ERK Signaling Pathway. *Cancer Cell Int.* **2019**, *19*, 43. [CrossRef]
143. Lakshmi, A.; Subramanian, S.P. Tangeretin Ameliorates Oxidative Stress in the Renal Tissues of Rats with Experimental Breast Cancer Induced by 7,12-Dimethylbenz[a]anthracene. *Toxicol. Lett.* **2014**, *229*, 333–348. [CrossRef] [PubMed]
144. Braidy, N.; Behzad, S.; Habtemariam, S.; Ahmed, T.; Daglia, M.; Nabavi, S.M.; Sobarzo-Sanchez, E.; Nabavi, S.F. Neuroprotective Effects of Citrus Fruit-Derived Flavonoids, Nobiletin and Tangeretin in Alzheimer's and Parkinson's Disease. *CNS Neurol. Disord. Drug Targets* **2017**, *16*, 387–397. [CrossRef] [PubMed]
145. Chong, S.Y.; Wu, M.Y.; Lo, Y.C. Tangeretin Sensitizes SGS1-Deficient Cells by Inducing DNA Damage. *J. Agric. Food Chem.* **2013**, *61*, 6376–6382. [CrossRef] [PubMed]
146. Arafa, E.S.A.; Shurrab, N.T.; Buabeid, M.A. Therapeutic Implications of a Polymethoxylated Flavone, Tangeretin, in the Management of Cancer via Modulation of Different Molecular Pathways. *Adv. Pharmacol. Pharm. Sci.* **2021**, *2021*, 4709818. [CrossRef] [PubMed]
147. Koolaji, N.; Shammugasamy, B.; Schindeler, A.; Dong, Q.; Dehghani, F.; Valtchev, P. Citrus Peel Flavonoids as Potential Cancer Prevention Agents. *Curr. Dev. Nutr.* **2020**, *4*, nzaa025. [CrossRef] [PubMed]
148. Ortuno, A.; Benavente-Garcia, O.; Castillo, J.; Alcaraz, M.; Vicente, V.; Del Rio, J. Beneficial Action of Citrus Flavonoids on Multiple Cancer-Related Biological Pathways. *Curr. Cancer Drug Targets* **2007**, *7*, 795–809. [CrossRef] [PubMed]
149. Kandaswami, C.; Perkins, E.; Soloniuk, D.S.; Drzewiecki, G.; Middleton, E. Antiproliferative Effects of Citrus Flavonoids on a Human Squamous Cell Carcinoma in Vitro. *Cancer Lett.* **1991**, *56*, 147–152. [CrossRef]
150. Lin, J.J.; Huang, C.C.; Su, Y.L.; Luo, H.L.; Lee, N.L.; Sung, M.T.; Wu, Y.J. Proteomics Analysis of Tangeretin-Induced Apoptosis through Mitochondrial Dysfunction in Bladder Cancer Cells. *Int. J. Mol. Sci.* **2019**, *20*, 1017. [CrossRef]
151. Rooprai, H.K.; Christidou, M.; Murray, S.A.; Davies, D.; Selway, R.; Gullan, R.W.; Pilkington, G.J. Inhibition of Invasion by Polyphenols from Citrus Fruit and Berries in Human Malignant Glioma Cells In Vitro. *Anticancer Res.* **2021**, *41*, 619–633. [CrossRef]
152. Surichan, S.; Arroo, R.R.; Tsatsakis, A.M.; Androutsopoulos, V.P. Tangeretin Inhibits the Proliferation of Human Breast Cancer Cells via CYP1A1/CYP1B1 Enzyme Induction and CYP1A1/CYP1B1–Mediated Metabolism to the Product 4′ Hydroxy Tangeretin. *Toxicol. Vitr.* **2018**, *50*, 274–284. [CrossRef]
153. Weng, C.J.; Yen, G.C. Flavonoids, a Ubiquitous Dietary Phenolic Subclass, Exert Extensive In Vitro Anti-Invasive and in Vivo Anti-Metastatic Activities. *Cancer Metastasis Rev.* **2012**, *31*, 323–351. [CrossRef] [PubMed]
154. Yumnam, S.; Raha, S.; Kim, S.; Venkatarame Gowda Saralamma, V.; Lee, H.; Ha, S.; Heo, J.; Lee, S.; Kim, E.; Lee, W.; et al. Identification of a Novel Biomarker in Tangeretin-induced Cell Death in AGS Human Gastric Cancer Cells. *Oncol. Rep.* **2018**, *40*, 3249–3260. [CrossRef] [PubMed]
155. Rajesh, Y.; Pal, I.; Banik, P.; Chakraborty, S.; Borkar, S.A.; Dey, G.; Mukherjee, A.; Mandal, M. Insights into Molecular Therapy of Glioma: Current Challenges and next Generation Blueprint. *Acta Pharmacol. Sin.* **2017**, *38*, 591–613. [CrossRef] [PubMed]
156. Erices, J.I.; Torres, Á.; Niechi, I.; Bernales, I.; Quezada, C. Current Natural Therapies in the Treatment against Glioblastoma. *Phyther. Res.* **2018**, *32*, 2191–2201. [CrossRef] [PubMed]
157. Ma, L.L.; Wang, D.; Yu, X.D.; Zhou, Y.L. Tangeretin Induces Cell Cycle Arrest and Apoptosis through Upregulation of PTEN Expression in Glioma Cells. *Biomed. Pharmacother.* **2016**, *81*, 491–496. [CrossRef] [PubMed]
158. Arivazhagan, L.; Sorimuthu Pillai, S. Tangeretin, a citrus pentamethoxyflavone, exerts cytostatic effect via p53/p21 up-regulation and suppresses metastasis in 7,12-dimethylbenz(α)anthracene-induced rat mammary carcinoma. *J. Nutr. Biochem.* **2014**, *24*, 1140–1153. [CrossRef] [PubMed]
159. Sangavi, P.; Langeswaran, K. Anti-Tumorigenic Efficacy of Tangeretin in Liver Cancer—An in-Silico Approach. *Curr. Comput.-Aided. Drug Des.* **2020**, *17*, 337–343. [CrossRef]
160. Yoon, J.H.; Lim, T.G.; Lee, K.M.; Jeon, A.J.; Kim, S.Y.; Lee, K.W. Tangeretin Reduces Ultraviolet B (UVB)-Induced Cyclooxygenase-2 Expression in Mouse Epidermal Cells by Blocking Mitogen-Activated Protein Kinase (MAPK) Activation and Reactive Oxygen Species (ROS) Generation. *J. Agric. Food Chem.* **2011**, *59*, 222–228. [CrossRef]

161. Chen, Q.; Gu, Y.; Tan, C.; Sundararajan, B.; Li, Z.; Wang, D.; Zhou, Z. Comparative Effects of Five Polymethoxyflavones Purified from Citrus Tangerina on Inflammation and Cancer. *Front. Nutr.* **2022**, *9*, 963662. [CrossRef]
162. Zhu, G.; Lin, C.; Cheng, Z.; Wang, Q.; Hoffman, R.M.; Singh, S.R.; Huang, Y.; Zheng, W.; Yang, S.; Ye, J. TRAF6-Mediated Inflammatory Cytokines Secretion in LPS-Induced Colorectal Cancer Cells Is Regulated by MiR-140. *Cancer Genom. Proteom.* **2020**, *17*, 23–33. [CrossRef]
163. Jain, S.; Dash, P.; Minz, A.P.; Satpathi, S.; Samal, A.G.; Behera, P.K.; Satpathi, P.S.; Senapati, S. Lipopolysaccharide (LPS) Enhances Prostate Cancer Metastasis Potentially through NF-κB Activation and Recurrent Dexamethasone Administration Fails to Suppress It In Vivo. *Prostate* **2019**, *79*, 168–182. [CrossRef] [PubMed]
164. Li, J.; Yin, J.; Shen, W.; Gao, R.; Liu, Y.; Chen, Y.; Li, X.; Liu, C.; Xiang, R.; Luo, N. TLR4 Promotes Breast Cancer Metastasis via Akt/GSK3β/β-Catenin Pathway upon LPS Stimulation. *Anat. Rec.* **2017**, *300*, 1219–1229. [CrossRef] [PubMed]
165. Liu, J.; Xu, D.; Wang, Q.; Zheng, D.; Jiang, X.; Xu, L. LPS Induced miR-181a Promotes Pancreatic Cancer Cell Migration via Targeting PTEN and MAP2K4. *Dig. Dis. Sci.* **2014**, *59*, 1452–1460. [CrossRef] [PubMed]
166. Dey, D.K.; Chang, S.N.; Vadlamudi, Y.; Park, J.G.; Kang, S.C. Synergistic Therapy with Tangeretin and 5-Fluorouracil Accelerates the ROS/JNK Mediated Apoptotic Pathway in Human Colorectal Cancer Cell. *Food Chem. Toxicol.* **2020**, *143*, 111529. [CrossRef] [PubMed]
167. Wei, G.J.; Chao, Y.H.; Tung, Y.C.; Wu, T.Y.; Su, Z.Y. A Tangeretin Derivative Inhibits the Growth of Human Prostate Cancer LNCaP Cells by Epigenetically Restoring P21 Gene Expression and Inhibiting Cancer Stem-like Cell Proliferation. *AAPS J.* **2019**, *21*, 86. [CrossRef] [PubMed]
168. Miller, E.G.; Peacock, J.J.; Bourland, T.C.; Taylor, S.E.; Wright, J.M.; Patil, B.S.; Miller, E.G. Inhibition of Oral Carcinogenesis by Citrus Flavonoids. *Nutr. Cancer* **2007**, *60*, 69–74. [CrossRef] [PubMed]
169. Chen, K.-H.; Weng, M.-S.; Lin, J.-K. Tangeretin Suppresses IL-1β-Induced Cyclooxygenase (COX)-2 Expression through Inhibition of P38 MAPK, JNK, and AKT Activation in Human Lung Carcinoma Cells. *Biochem. Pharmacol.* **2007**, *73*, 215–227. [CrossRef]
170. Zhu, W.B.; Xiao, N.; Liu, X.J. Dietary Flavonoid Tangeretin Induces Reprogramming of Epithelial to Mesenchymal Transition in Prostate Cancer Cells by Targeting the PI3K/Akt/MTOR Signaling Pathway. *Oncol. Lett.* **2018**, *15*, 433–440. [CrossRef]
171. He, Z.; Li, B.; Rankin, G.O.; Rojanasakul, Y.; Chen, Y.C. Selecting Bioactive Phenolic Compounds as Potential Agents to Inhibit Proliferation and VEGF Expression in Human Ovarian Cancer Cells. *Oncol. Lett.* **2015**, *9*, 1444–1450. [CrossRef]
172. Jaboin, J.; Iii, W.A.V.; Banik, N.L.; Giglio, P. A Novel Component from Citrus, Ginger, and Mushroom Family Exhibits Antitumor Activity on Human Meningioma Cells through Suppressing the Wnt/β-Catenin Signaling Pathway. *Tumor Biol.* **2022**, *36*, 7027–7034. [CrossRef]
173. Li, Y.R.; Li, S.; Ho, C.T.; Chang, Y.H.; Tan, K.T.; Chung, T.W.; Wang, B.Y.; Chen, Y.K.; Lin, C.C. Tangeretin Derivative, 5-Acetyloxy-6,7,8,4′-Tetramethoxyflavone Induces G2/M Arrest, Apoptosis and Autophagy in Human Non-Small Cell Lung Cancer Cells In Vitro and In Vivo. *Cancer Biol. Ther.* **2016**, *17*, 48–64. [CrossRef]
174. Periyasamy, K.; Baskaran, K.; Ilakkia, A.; Vanitha, K.; Selvaraj, S.; Sakthisekaran, D. Antitumor Efficacy of Tangeretin by Targeting the Oxidative Stress Mediated on 7,12-Dimethylbenz(a) Anthracene-Induced Proliferative Breast Cancer in Sprague-Dawley Rats. *Cancer Chemother. Pharmacol.* **2015**, *75*, 263–272. [CrossRef]

Disclaimer/Publisher's Note: The statements, opinions and data contained in all publications are solely those of the individual author(s) and contributor(s) and not of MDPI and/or the editor(s). MDPI and/or the editor(s) disclaim responsibility for any injury to people or property resulting from any ideas, methods, instructions or products referred to in the content.

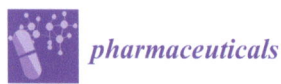

Review

Research Progress of Flavonoids Regulating Endothelial Function

Hao Li and Qi Zhang *

The Basic Medical College, Shaanxi University of Chinese Medicine, Xianyang 712046, China; 221010011697@sntcm.edu.cn
* Correspondence: zhangqi@sntcm.edu.cn

Abstract: The endothelium, as the guardian of vascular homeostasis, is closely related to the occurrence and development of cardiovascular diseases (CVDs). As an early marker of the development of a series of vascular diseases, endothelial dysfunction is often accompanied by oxidative stress and inflammatory response. Natural flavonoids in fruits, vegetables, and Chinese herbal medicines have been shown to induce and regulate endothelial cells and exert anti-inflammatory, anti-oxidative stress, and anti-aging effects in a large number of in vitro models and in vivo experiments so as to achieve the prevention and improvement of cardiovascular disease. Focusing on endothelial mediation, this paper introduces the signaling pathways involved in the improvement of endothelial dysfunction by common dietary and flavonoids in traditional Chinese medicine and describes them based on their metabolism in the human body and their relationship with the intestinal flora. The aim of this paper is to demonstrate the broad pharmacological activity and target development potential of flavonoids as food supplements and drug components in regulating endothelial function and thus in the prevention and treatment of cardiovascular diseases. This paper also introduces the application of some new nanoparticle carriers in order to improve their bioavailability in the human body and play a broader role in vascular protection.

Keywords: flavonoids; endothelial dysfunction; oxidative stress; NO; bioavailability

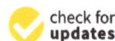

Citation: Li, H.; Zhang, Q. Research Progress of Flavonoids Regulating Endothelial Function. *Pharmaceuticals* **2023**, *16*, 1201. https://doi.org/10.3390/ph16091201

Academic Editors: Fernando Calzada, Miguel Valdes and Chung-Yi Chen

Received: 17 July 2023
Revised: 9 August 2023
Accepted: 20 August 2023
Published: 23 August 2023

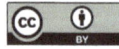

Copyright: © 2023 by the authors. Licensee MDPI, Basel, Switzerland. This article is an open access article distributed under the terms and conditions of the Creative Commons Attribution (CC BY) license (https:// creativecommons.org/licenses/by/ 4.0/).

1. Introduction

Cardiovascular disease (CVD), which includes coronary artery disease, stroke, hypertension, heart failure, rheumatic etiology/congenital heart disease, and peripheral vascular disease, is the leading cause of death worldwide, causing about 17.3 million deaths per year and showing a sustained growth trend [1]. Endothelial dysfunction in the vascular system interacts with the pathogenesis of CVDs and often becomes the initial stage of vascular disease [2].The disruption of the endothelium-dependent vasodilator–contractor balance directly or indirectly affects most CVDs, such as hypertension, coronary artery disease, chronic heart failure, peripheral artery disease, and diabetes mellitus [3].The arterial wall is composed of three layers from the outside to the inside, namely the adventitia, media, and intima. Vascular endothelial cells (VECs) are a layer of flat squamous cells that continuously cover the surface of the vascular lumen and form the intima layer together with connective tissue [4] (Figure 1). The endothelium is often in a metabolically active state. As the hub of the cell network, it is not only an important barrier between the blood and the vessel wall but also secretes a variety of vasoactive factors according to the local environment to affect the balance between vasodilation and contraction responses. Endothelium-dependent vasodilators mainly involve NO, endothelium-derived hyperpolarizing factor (EDFF), and prostacyclin (PGI2), while endothelium-dependent vasoconstrictor responses are mainly associated with endothelin-1 (ET-1), angiotensin II (Ang II), reactive oxygen species (ROS), and thromboxane A2 (TXA2) [5]. Of these, NO is a key active substance to maintain vascular homeostasis. The decrease of NO bioavailability, including the decrease of NO production and/or the increase of NO degradation by superoxide anion, marks the beginning of endothelial dysfunction. Oxidative stress induced by CVD-related events often inhibits the bioavailability of NO and induces chronic vascular inflammation, which aggravates endothelial damage.

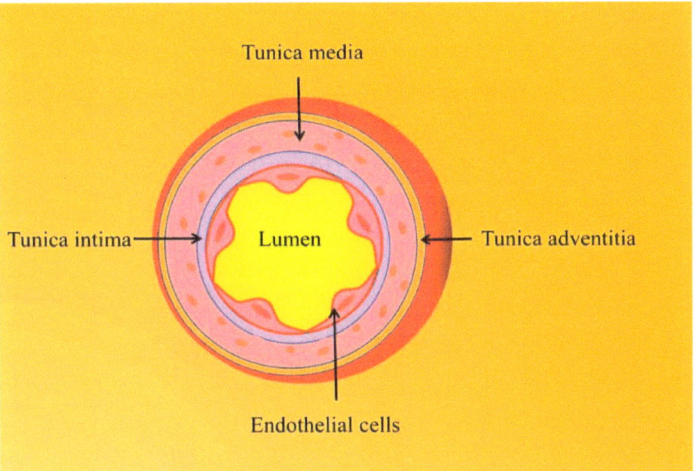

Figure 1. The arterial vessel wall is composed of three layers from outer to inner, namely the adventitia, media, and intima.

For a long time, people have gradually realized that diet plays an important role in the etiology of many chronic diseases, causing differences in the incidence and mortality of chronic diseases among populations in different countries and regions of the world. Therefore, it is crucial to prevent CVD by adjusting the diet. Based on this, the traditional Mediterranean diet (MedDiet), rich in vegetables, fruits, nuts, beans, etc., has been identified as one of the healthiest CVD-preventing diets [6]. One of its main active ingredients, polyphenols, is a secondary metabolite of plants and a major source of antioxidants in the diet. According to the molecular skeleton structure, it can be divided into flavonoids and non-flavonoids such as phenolic acids, stilbenes, phenolic alcohols, lignans, etc. [7]. Thus far, more than 8000 polyphenols have been known, of which more than 5000 are flavonoids [8]. Within each category, there is considerable heterogeneity in the number and position of substituents such as hydroxyl(OH), methoxy(OCH3) and sugar groups, which determine the physicochemical properties and biological activity of polyphenols. For example, the position and degree of hydroxylation significantly affect their antioxidant properties [9]. Numerous epidemiological studies have shown that moderate intake of dietary polyphenolic compounds may contribute to the prevention of atherosclerosis (AS), arterial hypertension, and coronary heart disease (CHD) [9]. Previous studies have shown that intake of foods with high dietary flavonoid content is negatively correlated with cardiovascular disease mortality, and its pharmacological activity may be related to food type, intake dose, and in vivo bioavailability [10]. In addition, as natural products widely found in nature, flavonoids are also extremely abundant in Chinese herbs and have been proven to achieve the function of preventing and controlling CVD through multi-targeting and multi-pathway effects [11,12].

Currently, traditional antihypertensive drugs and nitric oxide substitutes are commonly used to improve cardiovascular diseases. Considering the inevitable side effects and drug tolerance, new anti-inflammatory agents and antioxidants based on phytochemicals have attracted increasing scientific interest [13]. Among many natural active molecules, flavonoids have received special attention due to their wide range of biological activities. However, the detailed mechanism of protecting endothelial cells (ECs) is still unknown. This review focuses on the literature in recent years and preliminarily summarizes the performance and potential mechanism of flavonoids and polyphenols in improving endothelial dysfunction and cardiovascular health and discusses their bioavailability after metabolism in the human body.

1.1. Endothelial Function and Vascular Homeostasis

Known as the gatekeeper of vascular biology due to their location at the critical interface between circulating blood and the cellular environment, the ECs' surface is covered with a polysaccharide calyx, formed by negatively charged glycoproteins, proteoglycans, and glycosaminoglycans, which can inhibit platelet and leukocyte adhesion and promote vascular barrier permeability. It can also mediate shear-stress-induced NO release and exert vascular protection [14]. NO is produced by the oxidation of L-arginine by endothelial nitric oxide synthase (eNOS) with the help of the cofactor tetrahydrobiopterin (BH4) [15]. It then diffuses into subcutaneous vascular smooth muscle cells and triggers cyclic guanosine monophosphate (cGMP)-dependent vasodilation through activation of guanylate cyclase (SGC) [16]. Cyclooxygenase (COX)-derived PGI2 stimulates the prostacyclin receptor and activates adenylate cyclase (AC) in smooth muscle cells and then activates the cyclic adenosine monophosphate/protein kinase A (cAMP/PKA) signaling pathway to reduce Ca2+-mediated vascular tone (Figure 2). Several vasoconstrictor molecules produced by the endothelium, such as ET-1, Ang-II, and TxA2, tend to be released to regulate platelet activity, coagulation cascade reactions, and the fibrinolytic system under physiological conditions. Under physiological conditions, ECs constitute a non-adhesive surface that prevents platelet activation and coagulation cascade reactions. After vascular injury, endothelial activation is involved in all subsequent major hemostatic events and restricts clot formation to specific areas where hemostasis is required as well as restoration of vascular integrity [17]. There are also mechanosensors/mechanosensitive complexes on the surface of ECs that sense shear stresses generated by blood flow and convert them into biochemical signals that regulate vascular tone and homeostasis in vivo and intervene in NO production to achieve vascular homeostasis through a variety of mechanisms [18]. ECs also have metabolic activity, maintaining their proliferation and vasodilation functions through amino acid (AA) metabolism. Endothelial glutaminase can catalyze the metabolism of glutamine to α-ketoglutarate, induce endothelial senescence, and inhibit endothelial cell proliferation through pharmacological effects [19]. The functions of healthy endothelium, such as dynamic maintenance of vascular tension, anti-oxidation, anti-thrombosis, anti-inflammation, and participation in vascular metabolism, are of great significance to the homeostasis of cardiovascular system and have great reference value for the preclinical testing of new drugs (Figure 3).

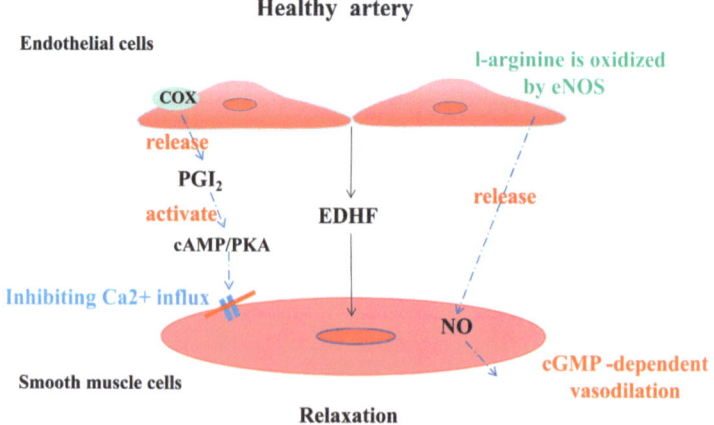

Figure 2. Endothelial-derived vasoactive factors regulate vascular tone in healthy arterial vessels.

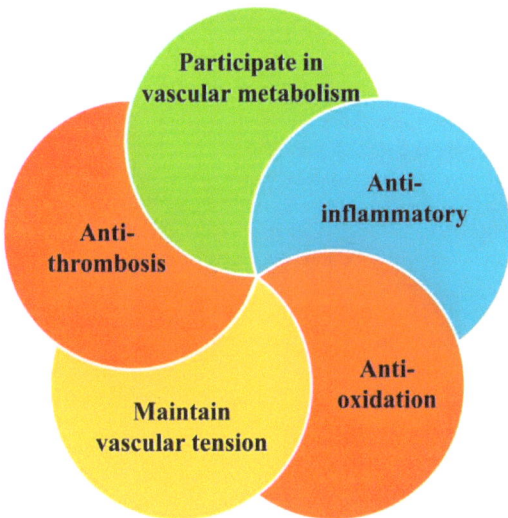

Figure 3. Regulation of vascular homeostasis by healthy endothelium.

1.2. Endothelial Dysfunction

1.2.1. Oxidative Stress and eNOS Uncoupling

A healthy endothelium enables the regulation and maintenance of vascular homeostasis, and any disturbance to this delicate and valuable balance can lead to the development of endothelial dysfunction. As mentioned earlier, NO is an endothelium-derived relaxing factor that, in addition to regulating vasodilatation, affects vascular homeostasis through a variety of pathways, such as inhibition of smooth muscle cell proliferation, platelet aggregation, adhesion of platelets and monocytes to endothelial cells, LDL oxidation, expression of adhesion molecules, and endothelin production. However, increased oxidative stress or reduced antioxidant enzyme activity, for example, can lead to reduced NO bioavailability [20,21].

Oxidative stress may be caused by the excessive production or accumulation of free-radical-reactive substances such as reactive oxygen species (ROS), reactive nitrogen species (RNS), and reactive sulfur species (RSS) [22]. Among them, ROS includes molecules such as H_2O_2, superoxide anion ($O_2^{\bullet-}$) and hydroxyl radical (•OH), which are key molecules in maintaining the redox state of cells and physiological signaling [23]. Oxidative stress is usually defined as a pathological state caused by the imbalance between prooxidants and antioxidants. The pro-oxidants that have been found include NADPH oxidase (NOX), xanthine oxidase (XO), mitochondrial respiratory chain enzymes, and dysfunctional eNOS. The antioxidant enzyme system includes superoxide dismutase (SOD), catalase (CAT), glutathione peroxidase (GPx), heme oxygenase (HO), thioredoxin reductase (Trx), and paraoxonase (PONs) [15]. There is evidence that oxidative stress induced by a large amount of ROS in the vascular wall will aggravate endothelial dysfunction, and CVD-related events such as diabetes, hypertension, dyslipidemia, smoking, or obesity are often important inducing factors [24].

Under oxidative stress conditions, eNOS removes an electron from NADPH and donates it to O_2 to generate $O_2^{\bullet-}$ rather than NO, and this process is known as eNOS uncoupling [25]. BH4 has an important auxiliary role for efficient electron transfer in the eNOS-catalyzed cycle. In the process of oxidative stress, $O_2^{\bullet-}$ reacts with NO to produce peroxynitrite (ONOO-), which can rapidly oxidize BH4 to BH2. The decrease in the BH4/BH2 ratio leads to the fact that electrons cannot be transferred to the N-terminal oxygenase domain of other eNOS monomers, thus exacerbating eNOS uncoupling [26]. Studies have shown that NOX-derived H_2O_2 in endothelial cells down-regulates the expression of DHFR in response to angiotensin II, which also leads to the lack of BH4 and the decoupling of eNOS [27]. In addition, oxidative stress has been shown to promote the synthesis of asymmetric dimethyl-l-arginine (ADMA), which competes with the eNOS substrate l-arginine [28], thereby inhibiting eNOS synthesis of NO. Oxidative stress can also promote the S-glutathionylation of eNOS to reversibly reduce the production of NO and increase the production of O^{2-} [29].

The substrates and cofactors in the process of NO synthesis by eNOS are affected by oxidative stress, and the products of eNOS uncoupling promote the production of ROS, resulting in a vicious circle that drastically reduces NO bioavailability, severely disrupts the endothelial environmental homeostasis, and leads to a cascade of cardiovascular diseases.

1.2.2. Inflammation

Inflammation has been reported to play an important role in all stages of the AS process, with vascular inflammation being the process that leads to alterations in the vascular wall and subsequently to endothelial dysfunction [30]. Chronic inflammation may be caused by a variety of stimuli, such as oxidative stress, pro-inflammatory cytokines, hypercholesterolemia, hypertension, and shear stress [31]. When damaged, ECs are activated and produce inflammatory factors such as interleukin-8 (IL-8), chemokines, colony-stimulating factors, interferons, monocyte chemotactic protein-1 (MCP-1), intercellular adhesion molecule-1 (ICAM-1), p-selectin, e-selectin, and vascular adhesion molecule-1 (VCAM-1). These substances attract monocytes and neutrophils, which attach to activated ECs and penetrate the arterial wall, thereby triggering inflammation [32].

O^{2-} and other ROS generated by oxidative stress stimulate nuclear factor kappa B (NF-κB), which in turn activates various pro-inflammatory cytokines such as tumor necrosis factor-α (TNF-α) and IL-1. TNF-a and IL-1β can stimulate endothelial cells to secrete other pro-inflammatory cytokines (IL-6), which in turn stimulate hepatocytes to produce and release a variety of acute phase reactants, including fibrinogen and C-reactive protein, regulating chronic inflammation and acute-phase response [33]. The circulating inflammatory markers C-reactive protein and IL-6 are able to up-regulate the production of tissue factor (TF) and vascular hemophilic factor (vWF), while inhibition of the expression of thrombomodulin, NO, and PGI2 allows for a shift in the endothelial milieu from an antithrombotic to a prothrombotic state [17]. Endothelial dysfunction can also be induced directly via oxidative low-density lipoprotein (LDL) receptor-1 [34]. At the same time, TNF-α in turn activates NF-κB to increase the expression of cell adhesion molecules [35]. In addition, TNF-α was found to up-regulate NOX activity in endothelial cells and increase O^{2-} levels in the vessel wall [36]. Such a positive feedback accelerates monocyte adhesion to the endothelium, leading to chronic inflammation of the vessel wall. Other factors such as oxidized low-density lipoprotein (ox-LDL) can stimulate the secretion of adhesion molecules by ECs and trigger the formation of vascular lesions. Ang II, a key effector of RAS, activates NF-κB, which up-regulates the expression of inflammatory cytokines and adhesion molecules exerting inflammatory effects and promoting the development of AS plaques [37]. It also activates their vascular G-protein-coupled receptors, leading to NOX activation and increased ROS production [38]. Lipopolysaccharide (LPS) can activate immune cells (such as macrophages) to secrete inflammation-mediated cytokines to catalyze inflammation. It can also activate ERK1/2, JNK, and p38 MAP kinases (MAPKs), which ultimately regulate the activity of transcription factor NF-kB and regulate the expression of inflammatory mediators such as inducible nitric oxide synthase (iNOS), cyclooxygenase-2 (COX-2), TNF-α, IL-1α, IL-1β, and IL-6 [39,40]. Vascular inflammation is one of the major disruptors of the vascular homeostatic environment and endothelial normal physiology, and the NF-B and MAPK pathways are closely related to the secretion of pro-inflammatory cytokines, which deserves to be further explored in the exploration of anti-inflammatory therapeutic strategies in the future.

In addition to the typical endothelial dysfunction-causing factors described above, disruption of vascular homeostatic balance by other pathways is of equal interest, for example, the endothelial-to-mesenchymal transition (EndoMT) by TGF-β signaling, in which ECs lose endothelial features but acquire mesenchymal-like morphology and gene expression patterns [41]. In addition, in the development of AS, endothelial-dependent permeability and vasodilation are often inhibited by VECs death, especially the regulatory death of endothelial cells, such as ferroptosis and autophagy [42]. As one of the initial inducing factors of AS, ferroptosis promotes the collapse of cell membrane and mitochondrial membrane, resulting in endothelial injury and death. It can also induce intravascular plaque formation, and the resulting vascular remodeling is a key factor in the stability of plaque in advanced AS [43]. Excessive autophagy caused by severe oxidative stress or inflammatory stimulation causes autophagy-dependent cell death and destroys plaque stability [44]. Autophagy of endothelial cells causes VCAM-1, ICAM-1, and other levels to shift down, while the infiltration of macrophages and foam cells increases, which also promotes arterial thrombosis [45] (Figure 4).

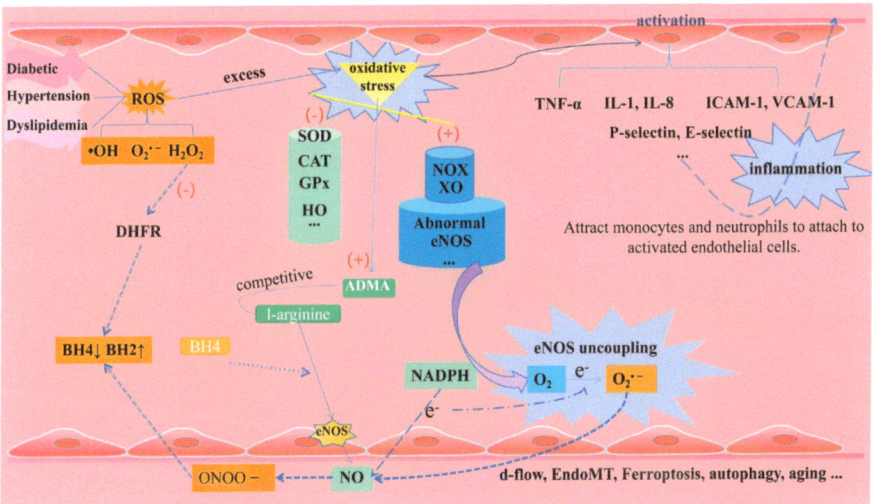

Figure 4. Endothelial dysfunction (including oxidative stress, eNOS uncoupling, inflammation, and other factors).

In fact, there are often synergistic or promoting effects between many factors that cause endothelial dysfunction, which have a superposition effect on disrupting vascular homeostasis and accelerating the occurrence and development of CVDs. Through the in-depth study of the mechanism of endothelial function/disorder, we can accelerate the discovery of new therapeutic drugs and implement effective targeted therapy.

2. Flavonoids

2.1. Sources, Classification, and Chemical Properties of Flavonoids

Flavonoids are the most abundant and widely studied natural phenolic compounds, which are commonly found in fruits, vegetables, wine, tea, and Chinese herbal medicine [46]. Flavonoids have a basic C6-C3-C6 15-carbon skeleton consisting of two aromatic rings and a pyran ring. They are classified into six subclasses based on their carbon structure and oxidation level, namely flavones, flavonols, flavanones, flavan-3-ols (flavanols), isoflavones, and anthocyanins [47] (Figures 5 and 6). Dietary flavonoids in nature exist in the form of glycosides such as glucosides, galactosides, arabinosides, rhamnosides, and rutinosides [48]. All dietary flavonoids except flavanols exist in glycosylated forms [49], and deglycosylation is a key step in the absorption and metabolism of flavonoid glycosides [50]. In nature, flavonoids usually do not exist alone. Oral intake of dietary flavonoids can also interact with other compounds, such as carbohydrates, fats, proteins, acids, etc., and their physiological activity may also change [51]. When flavonoids derived from Chinese herbal medicines are administered orally, their effectiveness as therapeutic drugs is seriously reduced due to their poor solubility, low permeability, and poor stability. For example, the 2,3-position double bonds of flavonoids and flavonols easily form a planar structure, resulting in tight molecular arrangement, so it is difficult for solvent molecules to penetrate their molecular structure [52]. Despite this, flavonoids have been shown to exert a wide range of pharmacological activities and involve multiple signaling pathways to achieve antioxidant, anti-inflammatory, anti-hyperlipidemic, and cardioprotective effects [53] (Table 1).

Table 1. Endothelial-protective mechanisms of flavonoids in vivo and in vitro. ↑ for up-regulation, and ↓ for suppression.

Model	Components	Dose	Function	Signal Passage	Ref.
Hypoxia-induced pulmonary hypertension in rats	Luteolin	10–100 μmol/L, 28 days	Aortic ring relaxation; Mean pulmonary arterial hypertension ↓;	HIF-2α-Arg-NO axis ↓ and PI3K-AKT-eNOS-NO ↑	[54]
H_2O_2-induced injury of HUVECs	Luteolin	2.5–20 μM, pretreatment 2 h	Anti-oxidative stress; improves mitochondrial function	AMPK/PKC ↑; P38 MAPK/NF-κB ↓	[55,56]
TNF-α-induced adhesion of human EA.hy 926 ECs	Luteolin	0.5–20 μM, pretreatment 1 h	(MCP-1, ICAM-1, VCAM-1) ↓	IKBα/NF-κB ↓	[57]
TNF-α-induced C57BL/6 mice	Luteolin	Modified diet containing 93.93% luteolin	Anti-inflammatory	IKBα/NF-κB ↓	[57]
HUVECs	Luteolin-7-O-Glucoside	20 μL, treatment for 48 h	Anti-oxidative stress; Anti-inflammatory; Anti-proliferation	JAK/STAT3↓; Nox4/ROS-NF-κB↓; MAPK ↓	[58]
AngII-induced injury of HUVECs	Baicalin	6.25–50 μM	Anti-oxidative stress; Anti-apoptosis	Activation of the ACE2/Ang-(1-7)/Mas axis; PI3K/AKT/eNOS ↑	[59]
Norbascine-induced pulmonary hypertension in rats	Baicalein	10 mg/kg/day, 28 days	Anti-oxidative stress; Mean pulmonary arterial hypertension ↓	Akt/ERK1/2/GSK3β/β-catenin ↓; ET-1/ETAR ↓; ROS ↓	[60]
LPS-induced rats	Baicalin	50, 100 mg/kg/day, 3 days	Inhibited platelet hyperactivation; Anti-inflammatory; TSP1 ↓	Furin/TGFβ1/Smad3/TSP-1 ↓	[61]
TNF-α-induced injury of HUVECs	Baicalin	/	Anti-platelet adhesion; TSP1, ICAM-1 ↓	AKT/Ca2+/ROS ↓	[61]
TNF-α-induced injury of HUVECs	Quercetin	10 μM; 30 μg/mL	Anti-inflammatory; anti-apoptosis E-selectin, VCAM-1, ICAM-1, IL-6, IL-8 ↓	Activator protein 1 (AP-1) ↓ NF-κB ↓	[62–64]
DF-induced inflammation of HUVECs	Quercetin	5 μM	Anti-inflammatory	NRP2 -VEGFC complex ↓	[65]
H_2O_2-induced injury of HUVECs	Quercetin–lycopene combination (molar ratio 5:1)	8 μM, 12 h	Anti-oxidative stress; Anti-inflammatory	SIRT1-Nox4-ROS ↓	[66]
High-fat diet (HFD)-fed ApoE$^{-/-}$ mice	Quercetin	4 mg/day, 8 weeks	Anti-oxidative stress	NOX ↓; HO-1 ↑	[67]
H/R-induced injury of HBMECs	Quercetin	0.1–1 μmol/L, 8 h	Anti-oxidative stress; Enhance cell viability; Anti-apoptosis; ICAM-1, VCAM-1 ↓	Keap1/Nrf2 ↑	[68]

Table 1. Cont.

Model	Components	Dose	Function	Signal Passage	Ref.
AngII-infused hypertensive mice	EGCG	50 mg/kg/day	Anti-oxidative stress; Systolic blood pressure ↓	NOX ↓; BH4-eNOS-NO ↑	[69]
Homocysteine-induced injury of HUVECs	EGCG	Pretreatment 2 h	Anti-oxidative stress; Anti-apoptosis	SIRT1/AMPK ↑; Akt/eNOS ↑	[70]
H_2O_2-induced injury of HUVECs	EGCG	1–10 μmol/L, pretreatment 24 h	Anti-oxidative stress; Induced autophagy	PI3K-AKT-mTOR ↓	[71]
TNF-α-induced injury of human coronary artery endothelial cells (HCAECs)	EGCG	/	Anti-inflammatory	NF-κB ↓	[72]
ox-LDL-induced injury of HUVECs	Naringin	50, 100 μM, pretreatment 2 h	Anti-inflammatory; Anti-apoptosis; Anti-EndMT	Hippo-YAP ↓	[73]
Homocysteine-induced injury of HUVECs	Naringenin	200 μM, treatment for 24 h	Anti-oxidative stress; Reduced eNOS uncoupling	AMPKα/Sirt1 ↑	[74]
High glucose (HG)- or free fatty acids (FFA)-induced apoptosis in HUVECs	Naringenin	0–100 μM	Anti-apoptosis	PI3K/Akt and JNK1 ↑; Nrf2 ↑; HO-1 ↑	[75]
HUVECs	Hesperidin	1 μM, 2 h	Promoted NO production and expression of MasR	TRPV1-CaMKII/p38 MAPK/MasR ↑; TRPV1-CaMKII/eNOS/NO ↑	[76,77]
Ox-LDL-induced senescence of HUVECs	Genistein	1 μM, pretreatment 30 min	Induced autophagy; Anti-aging	SIRT1/LKB1/AMPK ↑	[78]
H_2O_2-induced senescence of HUVECs	Genistein	40, 80 μg/mL, 24 h	Anti-apoptosis; Anti-aging	TXNIP/NLRP3 ↓	[79]
LPS-induced chronic vascular inflammatory response in mice	Genistein	10 mg/kg/day, 20 weeks	Anti-inflammatory	miR-21/NF-κB p65 ↓	[80]
Vascular endothelial cells (VECs)	Genistein	10 μM, pretreatment 2 h	Anti-inflammatory	miR-21/NF-κB p65 ↓	[80]
High glucose (HG)-induced injury of HUVECs	Blueberry anthocyanins	5 μg/mL, pretreatment 24 h	Anti-oxidative stress; Induced vasodilation	PI3K/Akt ↑; PKCζ ↓	[81]
Aged SD rats	Mulberry extract	300 mg/kg	Anti-oxidative stress; Anti-aging; Reduced eNOS uncoupling	SIRT1 ↑;	[82]
PA-treated SV 40 transfected aortic rat endothelial cells (SVAREC)	Anthocyanin from red radish	50, 100, 200, 400 μg/mL, 24 h	Anti-apoptosis	p38 MAPK ↓	[83]
HUVECs	Crocetin	10, 20, 40 μM	Inhibited cell migration and angiogenesis	VEGFR2/SRC/FAK ↓	[84]
HUVECs	Crocin	100, 200, 400 μM	Inhibited cell migration and angiogenesis	VEGFR2/MEK/ERK ↓	[84]

Table 1. Cont.

Model	Components	Dose	Function	Signal Passage	Ref.
LPS-stimulated brain microvascular endothelial cells	Hydroxysafflor Yellow A	/	Prevented ZO-1 degradation and protected the blood–brain barrier	HIF-1α/NOX2 ↓	[85]
U-46,619- and PE-inhibited rat MAs	Hydroxysafflor Yellow A	$10^{-7}, 10^{-6}, 10^{-5}, 10^{-4}$ M	Increased Ca2+ influx and expanded blood vessels	TRPV4-coupled Ca2+/PKA/eNOS ↑	[86]

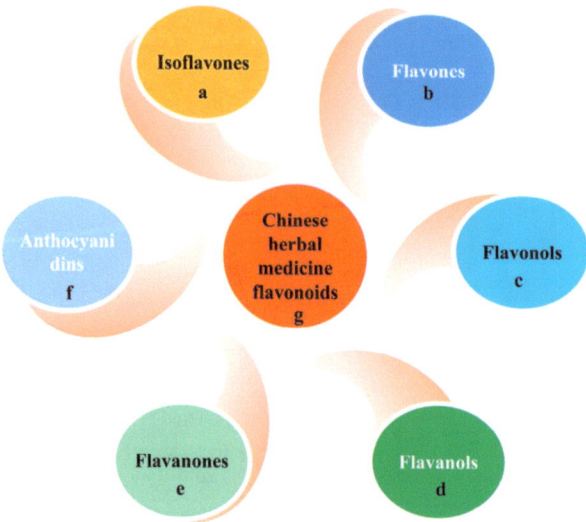

Figure 5. Flavonoids in dietary and herbal medicines.

2.2. Bioavailability of Flavonoids

As mentioned earlier, although epidemiological studies have demonstrated the ability of long-term, high intake of flavonoid-rich foods to reduce the incidence of CVD events, their bioavailability in the human body is actually very low due to differences in composition, subclasses, glycosylation, molecular weight, and esterification [87]. After oral ingestion, dietary flavonoids are first metabolized through the detoxification pathways of exogenous substances and drugs; however, the ability of saliva and gastric acid to modify the structure of the compounds in a primary way is limited and minor [50]. Due to the relatively small area of the gastric mucosa, it also limits its absorption capacity. Several types of flavonoids known to be absorbed by the human body through the stomach are quercetin, genistein, and daidzein [88]. The small intestine is a key part of drug absorption and metabolism. Flavonoid aglycones are hydrophobic and have a small molecular structure. They can be directly absorbed by villous epithelial cells on the small intestine wall through passive diffusion [89]. The absorption rate of flavonoids is different due to the influence of structure and pH. Studies have shown that acidic media are more conducive to the passage of flavonoids through the Caco-2 cell model [90]. There are two main pathways known for the absorption of flavonoid glycosides in the small intestine. One is that flavonoid glycosides can be hydrolyzed to glycosides by lactase-phlorizin hydrolase (LPH) at the edge of the mammalian small intestine [91]. The other pathway is that flavonoid glycosides hydrolyzed to glycosides by broad-spectrum β-glycosidases (e.g., cytosolic β-glucosidase (CBG)) are able to exert deglycosylation to convert sugar-bound polyphenols to glycosidic ketones, which are then transported via the sodium-glucose co-transporter type 1 (SGLT1) to intestinal epithelial cells, where the phase II enzyme produces the corresponding affixed metabolites, which finally enter the circulatory system as glycosides or couplers. [92,93]. Three types of phase II enzymes that have been reported to be present in intestinal epithelial cells are uridine-5′-diphosphate-glucuronosyltransferase (UGT), sulfotransferase (SULT), and catechol-O-methyltransferase (COMT). In humans, both UGT and SULT are thought to contribute to monoglucuronide and sulfate production [94,95].

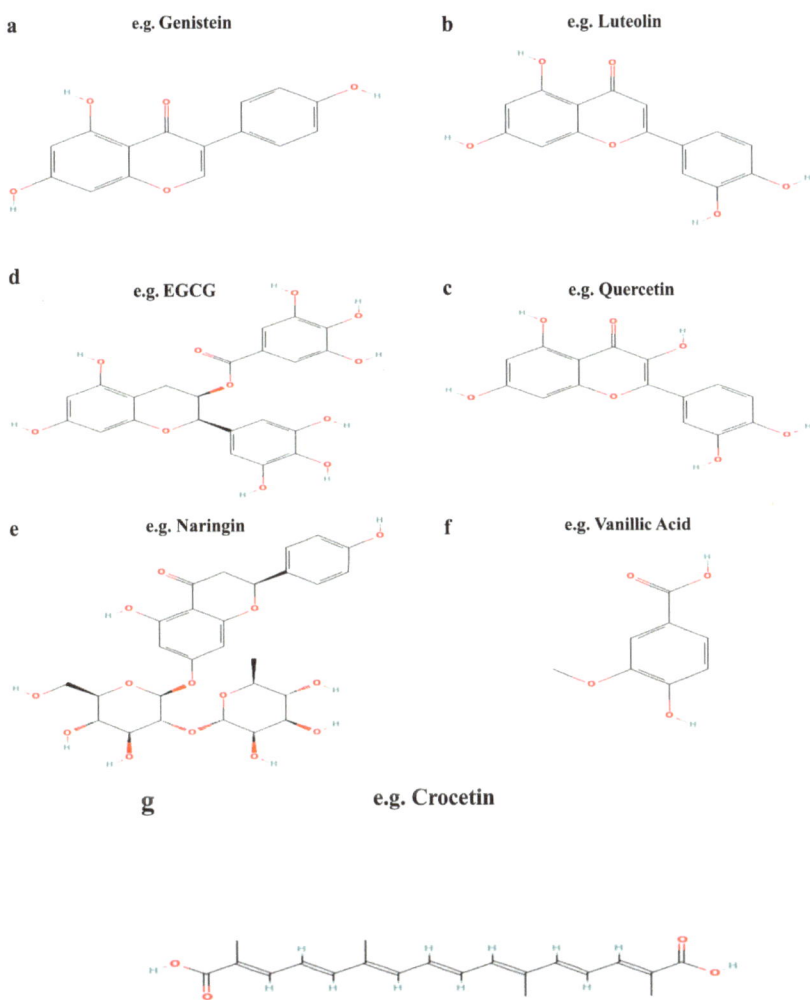

Figure 6. Molecular structure of typical flavonoids in dietary and herbal medicines.

The liver is another important site for the phase II metabolism of flavonoids, where there are two main forms of metabolism: oxidation and conjugation reactions. Oxidation reaction mainly relies on cytochrome P450 enzymes in the liver to metabolize flavonoids [96]. The binding reaction mainly refers to the action of various catalysis enzymes, prompting the phase I metabolites containing some polar functional groups (such as hydroxyl) and some endogenous substances coupled or combined to produce a variety of binding products [97]. The conjugates are further metabolized by sulphation and methylation, after which they either enter the blood circulation or return to the digestive tract via the hepatic–intestinal circulation [98]. Although this enterohepatic circulation contributes to higher plasma levels and half-lives of flavonoids, the total intake of dietary polyphenols in the small intestine is only approximately 10% [99], with the remaining metabolites being transported to the large intestine.

The gut microbiota is able to deconstruct the original compounds into more readily absorbed flavonoid metabolites through several intertwined steps of ester and glycoside hydrolysis, demethylation, dehydroxylation, and decarboxylation. Metabolites produced in the large intestine are reabsorbed for further phase II metabolism at the local and/or liver levels and eventually excreted in large quantities into the urine [100]. Indeed, polyphenols, including flavonoids, are able to exert a prebiotic effect on the intestinal flora, and proanthocyanidins in particular have an inhibitory effect on the progression of lifestyle-related diseases such as diabetes by altering the pattern of the intestinal microbiota [101] (Figure 7).

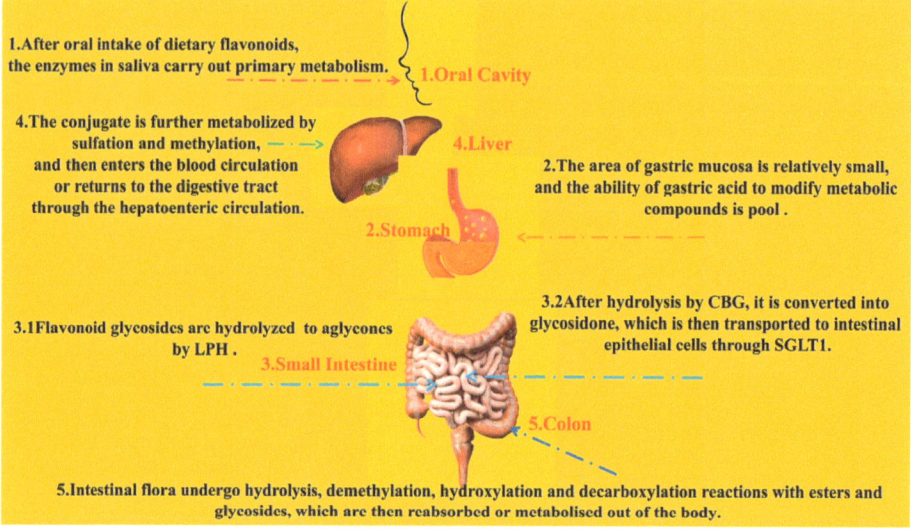

Figure 7. Metabolic pathways of flavonoids in the human body.

The ability of dietary flavonoids to actually exert vasoprotective effects after in vivo metabolism is limited, and further exploration of the dependency relationship with gut flora may be a new idea to improve their bioavailability.

3. Protective Effects of Flavonoids on Endothelial Cells
3.1. Flavones (Luteolin and Baicalin)

Flavones are widely distributed in the plant kingdom, including in parsley, celery, red peppers, and various herbs. In contrast to other subunits, they have a double bond between C2 and C3 in the flavonoid backbone, are not substituted at the C3 position, and are oxidized at the C4 position [102]. We next discuss two well-studied flavones: luteolin and baicalin.

Luteolins are widely found in a variety of food and medicinal plants, including artichoke (*Cynara cardunculus*), which is one of the world's best-known "medicinal" plants, with a long history of medicinal therapeutic use [103]. In terms of vascular relaxation, studies have shown that luteolin can directly act on vascular ECs in a dose-dependent manner (10–100 µmol/L), leading to rapid activation of eNOS and production of NO, resulting in relaxation of vascular tension in rat aortic rings and playing the same mechanism in primary human aortic endothelial cells (HAEC) [54]. By down-regulating the HIF-2α-Arg-NO axis and promoting the PI3K-AKT-eNOS-NO signaling pathway, luteolin regulates the NO content in the lungs of hypoxic pulmonary hypertension (HPH) rats and the supernatant of pulmonary artery endothelial cells (PAECs), thereby improving hypoxia-induced pulmonary hypertension [54]. In H_2O_2-induced injury of human umbilical vein endothelial cells (HUVECs), luteolin (2.5–20 mM) was able to regulate the AMPK/PKC pathway [55] and inhibit the ROS-mediated activation of the P38 MAPK/NF-kB signaling pathway [56], respectively, thereby exerting anti-oxidative stress properties. Literature studies in recent years have shown that luteolins also possess significant anti-inflammatory properties. In vitro experiments have shown that physiologically achievable concentrations (0.5µM–2 µM) of luteolin can effectively inhibit TNF-α-induced expression of MCP-1, ICAM-1, and VCAM-1; block monocyte adhesion to ECs; and ameliorate vascular endothelial inflammation through inhibition of the IKBα/NF-κB signaling pathway [57]. For microvascular ECs, it increases cAMP levels and inhibits ERK phosphorylation, thereby inhibiting lymphocyte function-associated antigen-1 (LFA-1) expression in neutrophils and exerting an anti-inflammatory effect by attenuating adhesion to the endothelium [104]. Luteolin-7-O-glucoside (LUT-7G), a glycosylated form of luteolin, has been shown to exert anti-inflammatory, antioxidant, and antiproliferative properties by targeting the JAK/STAT3 pathway to inhibit STAT3 and down-regulating the expression of IL-1β, a target gene involved in inflammation and ROS production in ECs [58]. Other studies have also shown that luteolin inhibit the Gas6/Axl (growth-arrest-specific protein 6/tyrosine protein kinase receptor) pathway to resist angiogenesis [105] and may also activate the large conductance calcium-regulated potassium channel (mitoBKCa) to exert cardioprotective effects [106].

Baicalin is the most abundant flavonoid in the Chinese herb *Scutellaria baicalensis*, and baicalin is metabolized to baicalein by β-glucuronidase in the intestines, a metabolic process that is a key stage in the absorption of baicalin [107]. In terms of ameliorating vasodilatory dysfunction, baicalein (6.25–50 µmol/L) was able to activate the angiotensin-converting enzyme ACE2/Ang-(1-7)/Mas axis to reduce AngII levels, causing concentration-dependent vasodilation in Ang II-pretreated endothelium-intact aortic rings [59]. Notably, the vasodilatory function of baicalein may act directly on vascular smooth muscle through different Ca^{2+} channels as well as activated KATP channels rather than endothelium-dependently [108]. In terms of anti-oxidative stress, several studies have shown that baicalein attenuates NOX activity, down-regulates ROS levels, and up-regulates eNOS expression to increase NO production, which is often associated with activation of the PI3K/AKT/eNOS pathway [108–110]. Malondialdehyde (MDA), superoxide dismutase (SOD), and glutathione peroxidase (GSH-Px) are important indicators for assessing oxidation, and ROS in vivo can be catalytically inactivated and scavenged by SOD and GSH-Px [111]. Baicalein has been found to be effective in reducing MDA levels and increasing SOD and GSH-Px activities in rat lung tissues [112]. The endothelin-1/endothelin A receptor (ET-1/ETAR) cascade has been suggested to be an important source of ROS, and the antioxidant activity of baicalein may be at least partly due to its inhibition of the ET-1/ET product, namely ROS formation [60]. Inflammatory coagulation dysfunction is based on inflammatory responses and platelet overactivation in endothelial dysfunction. Recent studies have shown that baicalein was able to inhibit both the Furin/TGFβ1/Smad3/thrombospondin-1 (TSP-1) pathway in ECs and the AKT/Ca2+/ROS pathway in platelets to ameliorate inflammatory coagulopathy [61]. It exerts anti-inflammatory effects by significantly inhibiting the expression of NF-κB, TNF-α, IL-6, and IL-1β [113,114]. In vitro experiments, baicalin was found to enhance AMPK-TFEB activity activating autophagy. Meanwhile, it was also able to increase the expression of the anti-apoptotic protein B-cell lymphoma 2 (Bcl2) and down-regulate the expression of the pro-apoptotic proteins BCL2-Associated X (Bax) and C-caspase3 to exert endothelial protective effects [115]. The protective effect of baicalin on the endothelium may also be reflected in the regulation of lnRNA NEAT1 as well as miRNA-205-5p [116]. In addition to medical experiments, baicalein has been applied to surface engineering of vascular scaffolds, and scaffolds with appropriate fixation densities of approximately 2.03 μg/cm^2 successfully supported the growth of ECs and also modulated oxidative stress, inflammation, and hyperlipidemia in the pathological microenvironment, thereby inhibiting endothelial dysfunction [117].

Taken together, both luteolin and baicalin, which belong to the same family of flavonoids, exhibited pharmacological effects in terms of anti-inflammatory, antioxidant, and improvement of exogenously induced vasodilatory dysfunction.

3.2. Flavonols (Quercetin)

Among flavonoids, flavonols (together with flavanols) are by far the most abundant and widely distributed in nature, the typical flavonol being quercetin. Quercetin rapidly binds to glucuronic acid and/or sulphate during first-pass metabolism (entero-hepatic) so that the important metabolites of quercetin in human plasma are quercetin-3-glucuronide, quercetin-3-sulphate, and isorhamnetin-3-glucuronide. Quercitin's bioavailability depends on the properties of the attached sugars and the food matrix composition (ethanol, fat, and emulsifiers), which may affect its solubility [118]. Interestingly, the bioavailability of quercetin glucoside from onions or processed onions is much higher than that of pure quercetin glycosides in capsules or tablets [119]. In in vitro assays involving HUVECs, quercetin exerted a wide range of anti-inflammatory properties. These include inhibition of the NFκB signaling pathway and down-regulation of the gene expression of inflammatory cytokines (e.g., IL-1β, IL-6, IL-8, and TNF-α) [62,63]. It is also able to inhibit the expression of E-selectin, MCP-1, VCAM-1, and ICAM-1 to prevent monocyte adhesion to endothelial cells [64]. It is important to note that in the large intestine, the catabolic metabolite of quercetin by the microbiota, 3-(3-hydroxyphenyl)propionic acid, exerts an anti-inflammatory effect through inhibition of TNFα-induced adhesion of monocytes to HAEC and inhibition of the up-regulation of E-selectin but is not involved in the regulation of ICAM-1/VCAM-1 [120]. However, in a novel in vitro multicellular model mimicking the intestinal-endothelial-monocyte/macrophage axis, quercetin intervention was able to reduce soluble vascular cell adhesion molecule-1 (sVCAM-1) levels, thereby improving the pro-inflammatory cellular environment [62]. In addition, it protects endothelial function from inflammation induced by local perturbation of blood flow, such as disturbed flow (DF), through inhibition of the NRP2-VEGFC (neuropilin 2–vascular endothelial growth factor C) complex [65]. Recent studies have shown that quercetin–lycopene combination (molar ratio 5:1) prevents oxidative stress in HUVEC cells by inhibiting the SIRT1-Nox4-ROS axis, reducing ROS production [66]. Its antioxidant effect is also manifested in enhancing the expression and activity of the antioxidant enzyme heme oxygenase-1 (HO-1), which has been confirmed in vivo/in vitro experiments [67]. In a human brain microvascular endothelial cells (HBMECs) injury model established by hypoxia/reoxygenation (H/R), quercetin (0.5–1μmol/L) can up-regulate the levels of Kelch-like ECH-associated protein 1 (Keap1) and nuclear factor erythroid-2 related factor 2 (Nrf2) to enhance antioxidant capacity [68]. The improvement of quercetin on diabetes-induced endothelial dysfunction is reflected in many aspects, including inhibition of endoplasmic reticulum stress-mediated oxidative stress [68,121,122], differential regulation of glucose uptake/metabolism in endothelial cells [123], and activation of autophagy [124]. The mechanisms of quercetin in alleviating endothelial senescence [125] and inhibiting EndoMT have been continuously excavated in recent years, the latter being mainly reflected in the inhibitory effects on mediators of EndoMT, such as TGF-β, Caveolin-1, NFκB, and ET-1 [126].

3.3. Flavanols (EGCG)

Flavanols are commonly found in fruits, green tea, red wine, chocolate, and other foods. The most common type of flavanols in nature is flavan-3-ols, which have a monomer form (catechin) and polymer form (proanthocyanidins) and other derivative compounds (such as theaflavins and thearubigins) [127]. Among green tea polyphenols, epigallocatechin gallate (EGCG) is considered to be the most abundant and active compound and has a wide range of therapeutic properties in cardiovascular and metabolic diseases, including anti-atherosclerosis, anti-diabetes, anti-inflammation, and antioxidants [128]. In an Ang II-induced hypertensive mouse model, EGCG (50 mg/kg/day) attenuates oxidative stress by down-regulating NOX expression and inhibits eNOS uncoupling to increase NO utilization, thereby exerting antihypertensive effects [69]. In vitro, EGCG can prevent homocysteine-induced oxidative stress and endothelial cell apoptosis by enhancing SIRT1/AMPK and Akt/eNOS signaling pathways [70]. Activated AMPK may also down-regulate the PI3K-AKT-mTOR pathway to induce autophagy, thereby achieving a protective effect on the endothelium [71]. Inhibition of inflammation by EGCG is mainly achieved by down-regulation of multiple components of the TNF-α-induced NF-κB signaling pathway, achieving inhibition of inflammatory gene transcription and protein expression [72]. In addition, the inhibitory effect of EGCG on EndMT has been confirmed, providing more possibilities for the prevention and treatment of cardiovascular diseases in the future [129]. The multi-type nanoparticle carriers developed for EGCG have been tested in simulated gastric and intestinal fluid environments to enhance their stability in acid–base and enzymatic hydrolysis environments, which is conducive to improving bioavailability in the human body [130,131].

3.4. Flavanones (Hesperidin and Naringin)

Flavanones, including hesperidin (hesperetin) and naringin (naringenin), are polyphenolic compounds highly and almost exclusively found in citrus. The protective effects of flavanones on the endothelium are mainly in terms of anti-inflammatory, antioxidant, and vasorelaxant properties, which are clinically important for vascular diseases such as hypertension and atherosclerosis [132]. Studies have shown that naringin (50, 100 μM) attenuated oxygenated low-density lipoprotein-induced inflammatory injury in HUVECs by down-regulating IL-1β, IL-6, and IL-18 levels. Meanwhile, VE-calmodulin, a specific dermatocyte marker for EndMT, was significantly attenuated, and serial evidence suggests that this may act by inhibiting the Hippo-YAP pathway [73]. Li et al. [74] confirmed that naringenin could activate AMPKα/Sirt1 signaling pathway, restore mitochondrial Ca2+ balance, reduce eNOS uncoupling, and increase NO bioavailability to improve damaged ECs by new transcriptomics technology. Its up-regulation of heat-shock protein 70 in endothelial cells has potential implications for the amelioration of endothelial damage in diabetes and related diseases [133]. Naringenin attenuates high-glucose-induced apoptosis in HUVECs, which may play a role in increasing HO-1 expression in HUVECs through up-regulation of PI3K/Akt or JNK pathways [75]. The vasodilatory effect of naringenin mainly involves the inhibition of multiple Ca2+ channels, whereas hesperidin stimulates a transient receptor potential vanilloid 1 (TRPV1)-mediated cascade reaction that activates the expression of both the CaMKII/p38 MAPK/MasR and the CaMKII/eNOS/NO signaling axes in HUVEC to promote NO production and vasorelaxant Mas receptor (MasR) expression [76,77]. Multiple nanodelivery systems increase the oral availability and targeting of compounds. For example, naringin/indocyanine green-loaded lipid nano-emulsions can effectively target VCAM-1 in the vascular endothelium to exert anti-inflammatory effects [134].

3.5. Isoflavones (Genistein and Daidzein)

The main plant source of dietary isoflavones is the soybean, with genistein (GE) and daidzein (DE) being the most abundant soy isoflavones, the latter being metabolized to estragole by intestinal flora [135]. Preliminary in vitro experiments have shown that Ge and De are able to be taken up by ECs and metabolized by phase II enzymes to methoxylated and glucuronide- and sulphate-conjugated compounds. However, the metabolite estragole was only taken up by ECs and not metabolized [136]. In an animal experiment, GE (40, 80 mg/kg) was used to treat two-kidney-one-clip (2k1c) hypertensive rats, which showed that GE inhibited ACE activity; attenuated Ang II, MDA, and SOD levels; and alleviated nephrogenic vasculopathy mediated by the RAS system [137]. In in vitro experiments, GE (1 μM) can enhance the autophagy flux mediated by SIRT1/LKB1/AMPK pathway to prevent oxLDL-induced HUVECs senescence [78]. In another H_2O_2-mediated HUVECs senescence, GE (40, 80 μg/mL) exerted its anti-aging effect by inhibiting the TXNIP/NLRP3 (thioredoxin-interacting protein) axis [79]. In addition, GE was found to inhibit chronic vascular inflammatory responses in mice, which may be related to the inhibition of VEC inflammatory injury through the miR-21/NF-κB p65 pathway [138]. In previous studies, DE and estragole were found to have anti-oxidative stress effects, both involving inhibition of NF-κB proteins, with the latter further inhibiting endoplasmic reticulum stress, thereby attenuating atherosclerosis in ApoE-deficient mice [80,138,139].

3.6. Anthocyanins

Anthocyanins, as a natural pigment, are water-soluble and often abundant in fruits and vegetables such as blueberries, grapes, dragon fruit, purple sweet potatoes, and purple kale and are extremely important secondary metabolites in plants [140]. Anthocyanins are metabolized by the enterohepatic metabolism, where they are degraded to glucuronic acid and methylated and sulphated metabolites, i.e., phase II metabolites, and thereafter peak in plasma (<5 μM) in 1–3 h [141]. Unabsorbed anthocyanins are extensively metabolized to phenolic acids in the colon by the intestinal flora. Phenolic acids after methylation, such as vanillic acid (VA) or ferulic acid (FA), can be detected in plasma within 1 h after intake at peak concentration (2–15 μM) [142]. Various anthocyanins (usually in glycoside form) have been shown to increase cell viability by reducing ROS and NOX4 expression through a PI3K/Akt calcium-independent pathway in ECs. It has also been shown to promote catabolism of the protein kinase C zeta (PKCζ) pathway, increase eNOS and NO biomass levels, and reduce xanthine oxidase-1 (XO-1) and LDL levels to exert vasodilatory effects [81]. In a related study in aged rats, anthocyanins were found to modulate ROS formation and down-regulate SIRT1 to reduce eNOS uncoupling and prevent endothelial senescence by enhancing NO bioavailability [82]. It should be noted that the anthocyanin cornflower-3-glucoside (C3G), after 4 h of co-cultivation with epithelial cells, resulted in a loss of up to 96% due to an increase in the content of its metabolite protocatechuic acid (PCA) [82]. In addition, the C3G metabolite, i.e., PCA, with vanillic acid (VA) only caused a decrease in superoxide production and did not up-regulate eNOS levels, so it can be predicted that phenolic metabolites only increase the bioavailability of NO without increasing its production [143]. In terms of anti-inflammation, individual anthocyanins and their phenolic metabolites were able to attenuate monocyte adhesion to TNF-α-activated ECs at physiological concentrations (0.1–2 μM); however, this is not mediated by adhesion molecules such as VCAM-1 [144]. In addition, the mixture of various anthocyanins and metabolites (0.1 μM) can regulate the expression of EC permeability-related miRNAs, thereby reducing monocyte adhesion and transendothelial cell migration [145]. Studies have shown that anthocyanins can up-regulate antioxidant defenses such as HO-1 and SOD (in a concentration-dependent manner) through direct activation of the Nrf2 signaling pathway, which may prevent oxidative damage [146]. Transcriptomic and further analyses demonstrated that carrot-derived anthocyanins also inhibit palmitate-induced endothelial cell apoptosis via the p38 MAPK pathway [83]. In recent studies, genetic manipulation techniques have been applied to increase the anthocyanin content of plant-derived diets, mainly by up-regulating the expression of genes in metabolic pathways, which may also help to counteract the reduced bioavailability in vivo [147].

3.7. Chinese Herbal Medicine Flavonoids (Crocetin and Crocin)

For thousands of years, the wide application of Chinese herbal medicine, especially the compound decoction of multiple herbs, has played a great role in the prevention and treatment of cardiovascular diseases. With the development of medical information technology, flavonoids derived from Chinese herbal medicine have attracted more and more attention from researchers due to their significant clinical efficacy and relatively low drug toxicity.

Crocetin and its glycoside crocin are two important carotenoids isolated from the dried stigma of saffron. In the HUVEC model, crocetin (10, 20, and 40 µM) and crocetin (100, 200, and 400 µM) inhibited cell migration and angiogenesis and inhibited phosphorylation of vascular endothelial growth factor receptor 2 (VEGFR2) and its downstream pathway molecules (e.g., p-SRC, p-FAK, p-MEK, and p-ERK) [84]. Among them, molecular docking studies showed that crocetin showed stronger ability to bind to VEGFR2. In addition, a pharmacokinetic study showed that crocin is hydrolyzed into crocetin through the gastrointestinal tract and then absorbed and detected in plasma [148]. Occlusive zone-1 (ZO-1) is a scaffold protein in cerebrovascular endothelium, which is related to the function of blood–brain barrier. Loss of ZO-1 and disruption of the permeability of the blood–brain barrier (BBB) are easily observed in cerebral ischemia cases associated with oxidative stress and inflammatory response [149]. Hydroxy saffron yellow A (HYSA) is the main active ingredient of safflower. Studies have shown that HSYA protects ZO-1 from proteasome degradation by inhibiting the HIF-1α/NOX2 signaling cascade, thereby protecting cerebrovascular integrity and reducing brain damage [85]. In a study on the dilation activity of mesenteric artery rings (MAs) in rats, HYSA reversed the contraction of MAs induced by phenylephrine (PE, 1 µM) and U 46,619 (10 µM) in a dose-dependent manner. This function is related to the TRPV4-coupled Ca^{2+}/PKA/eNOS signaling pathway, which achieves vasodilation by increasing Ca^{2+} influx [86]. In addition, flavonoids from other traditional Chinese medicines (TCM), such as ginkgolide B, have been found to stimulate SOD activity and increase SOD1 expression in diabetic aortas, thereby activating the Akt/eNOS signaling pathway and causing endothelium-dependent relaxation [150]. Since the application of herbs in TCM is often in the form of compounded soups and often in certain ratios, future pharmacological studies on flavonoid compounds in Chinese herbs may try to combine them in anticipation of obtaining higher efficacy and developing a wider range of drug targets.

4. Conclusions and Perspectives

The endothelium can secrete a variety of vasoactive factors, and it is not only the guardian of the cardiovascular environment but also the victim of cardiovascular disease. Traditional endothelial dysfunction involves inflammatory responses, oxidative stress, and its induction of platelet aggregation, autophagy, and apoptosis. Iron death [151], d-flow [152], and its associated EndMT [153] are considered as some of the key drivers of vascular inflammation and AS, which have been on the rise in recent years. As described in the text, natural flavonoid compounds or their metabolic components have been shown to target the endothelium through multiple pathways to exert regulatory effects and thereby ameliorate cardiovascular-related diseases. It is worth noting that TCM often applies herbs in disease treatment by combining multiple types of herbs in different dosages and preparing them according to specific methods, which may be informative for the exploration of enhanced pharmacological activities of flavonoids. In addition, improving the bioavailability of dietary flavonoids in vivo should still be a hotspot for future research, especially the further metabolism of intestinal flora and the further development of modern technological tools such as nanoparticles and vascular scaffold surface engineering.

Author Contributions: Q.Z. conceived and designed the study; H.L. wrote the manuscript. All authors have read and agreed to the published version of the manuscript.

Funding: This research was supported by the National Natural Science Foundation of China (82074380) under the name of Professor Qi Zhang.

Institutional Review Board Statement: Not applicable.

Informed Consent Statement: Not applicable.

Data Availability Statement: Data sharing not applicable.

Conflicts of Interest: The authors declare no conflict of interest.

References

1. Sacks, F.M.; Lichtenstein, A.H.; Wu, J.H.Y.; Appel, L.J.; Creager, M.A.; Kris-Etherton, P.M.; Miller, M.; Rimm, E.B.; Rudel, L.L.; Robinson, J.G.; et al. Dietary Fats and Cardiovascular Disease: A Presidential Advisory from the American Heart Association. *Circulation* **2017**, *136*, e1–e23. [CrossRef]
2. Incalza, M.A.; D'Oria, R.; Natalicchio, A.; Perrini, S.; Laviola, L.; Giorgino, F. Oxidative Stress and Reactive Oxygen Species in Endothelial Dysfunction Associated with Cardiovascular and Metabolic Diseases. *Vasc. Pharmacol.* **2018**, *100*, 1–19. [CrossRef] [PubMed]
3. Endemann, D.H.; Schiffrin, E.L. Endothelial Dysfunction. *J. Am. Soc. Nephrol.* **2004**, *15*, 1983–1992. [CrossRef] [PubMed]
4. Konukoglu, D.; Uzun, H. Endothelial Dysfunction and Hypertension. *Adv. Exp. Med. Biol.* **2017**, *956*, 511–540. [CrossRef] [PubMed]
5. Vanhoutte, P.M.; Shimokawa, H.; Feletou, M.; Tang, E.H.C. Endothelial Dysfunction and Vascular Disease—A 30th Anniversary Update. *Acta Physiol.* **2017**, *219*, 22–96. [CrossRef] [PubMed]
6. Salas-Salvadó, J.; Becerra-Tomás, N.; García-Gavilán, J.F.; Bulló, M.; Barrubés, L. Mediterranean Diet and Cardiovascular Disease Prevention: What Do We Know? *Prog. Cardiovasc. Dis.* **2018**, *61*, 62–67. [CrossRef] [PubMed]
7. Dai, J.; Mumper, R.J. Plant Phenolics: Extraction, Analysis and Their Antioxidant and Anticancer Properties. *Molecules* **2010**, *15*, 7313–7352. [CrossRef]
8. Durazzo, A.; Lucarini, M.; Souto, E.B.; Cicala, C.; Caiazzo, E.; Izzo, A.A.; Novellino, E.; Santini, A. Polyphenols: A Concise Overview on the Chemistry, Occurrence, and Human Health. *Phytother. Res.* **2019**, *33*, 2221–2243. [CrossRef]
9. Middleton, E.; Kandaswami, C.; Theoharides, T.C. The Effects of Plant Flavonoids on Mammalian Cells: Implications for Inflammation, Heart Disease, and Cancer. *Pharmacol. Rev.* **2000**, *52*, 673–751.
10. Bohn, T. Dietary Factors Affecting Polyphenol Bioavailability. *Nutr. Rev.* **2014**, *72*, 429–452. [CrossRef]
11. Gao, J.; Hou, T. Cardiovascular Disease Treatment Using Traditional Chinese Medicine: Mitochondria as the Achilles' Heel. *Biomed. Pharmacother.* **2023**, *164*, 114999. [CrossRef] [PubMed]
12. Jiang, Y.; Zhao, Q.; Li, L.; Huang, S.; Yi, S.; Hu, Z. Effect of Traditional Chinese Medicine on the Cardiovascular Diseases. *Front. Pharmacol.* **2022**, *13*, 806300. [CrossRef] [PubMed]
13. Xiao, J.; Bai, W. Bioactive Phytochemicals. *Crit. Rev. Food Sci. Nutr.* **2019**, *59*, 827–829. [CrossRef]
14. Gouverneur, M.; Van Den Berg, B.; Nieuwdorp, M.; Stroes, E.; Vink, H. Vasculoprotective Properties of the Endothelial Glycocalyx: Effects of Fluid Shear Stress. *J. Intern. Med.* **2006**, *259*, 393–400. [CrossRef] [PubMed]
15. Förstermann, U.; Xia, N.; Li, H. Roles of Vascular Oxidative Stress and Nitric Oxide in the Pathogenesis of Atherosclerosis. *Circ. Res.* **2017**, *120*, 713–735. [CrossRef] [PubMed]
16. Zhao, Y.; Vanhoutte, P.M.; Leung, S.W.S. Vascular Nitric Oxide: Beyond ENOS. *J. Pharmacol. Sci.* **2015**, *129*, 83–94. [CrossRef]
17. Versteeg, H.H.; Heemskerk, J.W.M.; Levi, M.; Reitsma, P.H.; Middleton, E.A.; Weyrich, A.S.; Zimmerman, G.A.; Bevers, E.M.; Williamson, P.L.; Wu, X.; et al. New Fundamentals in Hemostasis. *Physiol. Rev.* **2013**, *93*, 327–358. [CrossRef] [PubMed]
18. Chatterjee, S. Endothelial Mechanotransduction, Redox Signaling and the Regulation of Vascular Inflammatory Pathways. *Front. Physiol.* **2018**, *9*, 524. [CrossRef]
19. Huang, H.; Vandekeere, S.; Kalucka, J.; Bierhansl, L.; Zecchin, A.; Brüning, U.; Visnagri, A.; Yuldasheva, N.; Goveia, J.; Cruys, B.; et al. Role of Glutamine and Interlinked Asparagine Metabolism in Vessel Formation. *EMBO J.* **2017**, *36*, 2334–2352. [CrossRef]
20. Yetik-Anacak, G.; Catravas, J.D. Nitric Oxide and the Endothelium: History and Impact on Cardiovascular Disease. *Vasc. Pharmacol.* **2006**, *45*, 268–276. [CrossRef]
21. Puddu, G.M.; Cravero, E.; Arnone, G.; Muscari, A.; Puddu, P. Molecular Aspects of Atherogenesis: New Insights and Unsolved Questions. *J. Biomed. Sci.* **2005**, *12*, 839–853. [CrossRef] [PubMed]
22. Di Meo, S.; Venditti, P. Evolution of the Knowledge of Free Radicals and Other Oxidants. *Oxid. Med. Cell. Longev.* **2020**, *2020*, 9829176. [CrossRef] [PubMed]
23. Shaito, A.; Aramouni, K.; Assaf, R.; Parenti, A.; Orekhov, A.; Yazbi, A.E.; Pintus, G.; Eid, A.H. Oxidative Stress-Induced Endothelial Dysfunction in Cardiovascular Diseases. *Front. Biosci.* **2022**, *27*, 105. [CrossRef] [PubMed]
24. Cai, H.; Harrison, D.G. Endothelial Dysfunction in Cardiovascular Diseases: The Role of Oxidant Stress. *Circ. Res.* **2000**, *87*, 840–844. [CrossRef]
25. Daiber, A.; Xia, N.; Steven, S.; Oelze, M.; Hanf, A.; Kröller-Schön, S.; Münzel, T.; Li, H. New Therapeutic Implications of Endothelial Nitric Oxide Synthase (ENOS) Function/Dysfunction in Cardiovascular Disease. *Int. J. Mol. Sci.* **2019**, *20*, 187. [CrossRef] [PubMed]
26. Milstien, S.; Katusic, Z. Oxidation of Tetrahydrobiopterin by Peroxynitrite: Implications for Vascular Endothelial Function. *Biochem. Biophys. Res. Commun.* **1999**, *263*, 681–684. [CrossRef]
27. Chalupsky, K.; Cai, H. Endothelial Dihydrofolate Reductase: Critical for Nitric Oxide Bioavailability and Role in Angiotensin II Uncoupling of Endothelial Nitric Oxide Synthase. *Proc. Natl. Acad. Sci. USA* **2005**, *102*, 9056–9061. [CrossRef]

28. Böger, R.H.; Sydow, K.; Borlak, J.; Thum, T.; Lenzen, H.; Schubert, B.; Tsikas, D.; Bode-Böger, S.M. LDL Cholesterol Upregulates Synthesis of Asymmetrical Dimethylarginine in Human Endothelial Cells: Involvement of S-Adenosylmethionine-Dependent Methyltransferases. *Circ. Res.* **2000**, *87*, 99–105. [CrossRef]
29. Chen, C.A.; Wang, T.Y.; Varadharaj, S.; Reyes, L.A.; Hemann, C.; Talukder, M.A.H.; Chen, Y.R.; Druhan, L.J.; Zweier, J.L. S-Glutathionylation Uncouples ENOS and Regulates Its Cellular and Vascular Function. *Nature* **2010**, *468*, 1115–1120. [CrossRef]
30. Ali, L.; Schnitzler, J.G.; Kroon, J. Metabolism: The Road to Inflammation and Atherosclerosis. *Curr. Opin. Lipidol.* **2018**, *29*, 474–480. [CrossRef]
31. Tabas, I.; García-Cardeña, G.; Owens, G.K. Recent Insights into the Cellular Biology of Atherosclerosis. *J. Cell Biol.* **2015**, *209*, 13–22. [CrossRef]
32. Zhu, Y.; Xian, X.; Wang, Z.; Bi, Y.; Chen, Q.; Han, X.; Tang, D.; Chen, R. Research Progress on the Relationship between Atherosclerosis and Inflammation. *Biomolecules* **2018**, *8*, 80. [CrossRef] [PubMed]
33. Libby, P. Interleukin-1 Beta as a Target for Atherosclerosis Therapy: Biological Basis of CANTOS and Beyond. *J. Am. Coll. Cardiol.* **2017**, *70*, 2278–2289. [CrossRef] [PubMed]
34. Li, L.; Roumeliotis, N.; Sawamura, T.; Renier, G. C-Reactive Protein Enhances LOX-1 Expression in Human Aortic Endothelial Cells: Relevance of LOX-1 to C-Reactive Protein-Induced Endothelial Dysfunction. *Circ. Res.* **2004**, *95*, 877–883. [CrossRef] [PubMed]
35. Binesh, A.; Devaraj, S.N.; Halagowder, D. Molecular Interaction of NFκB and NICD in Monocyte-Macrophage Differentiation Is a Target for Intervention in Atherosclerosis. *J. Cell. Physiol.* **2019**, *234*, 7040–7050. [CrossRef]
36. Kleinbongard, P.; Heusch, G.; Schulz, R. TNFalpha in Atherosclerosis, Myocardial Ischemia/Reperfusion and Heart Failure. *Pharmacol. Ther.* **2010**, *127*, 295–314. [CrossRef]
37. Trojanowicz, B.; Ulrich, C.; Seibert, E.; Fiedler, R.; Girndt, M. Uremic Conditions Drive Human Monocytes to Pro-Atherogenic Differentiation via an Angiotensin-Dependent Mechanism. *PLoS ONE* **2014**, *9*, e102137. [CrossRef]
38. Das, S.; Zhang, E.; Senapati, P.; Amaram, V.; Reddy, M.A.; Stapleton, K.; Leung, A.; Lanting, L.; Wang, M.; Chen, Z.; et al. A Novel Angiotensin II-Induced Long Noncoding RNA Giver Regulates Oxidative Stress, Inflammation, and Proliferation in Vascular Smooth Muscle Cells. *Circ. Res.* **2018**, *123*, 1298–1312. [CrossRef]
39. Park, M.Y.; Ha, S.E.; Kim, H.H.; Bhosale, P.B.; Abusaliya, A.; Jeong, S.H.; Park, J.S.; Heo, J.D.; Kim, G.S. Scutellarein Inhibits LPS-Induced Inflammation through NF-κB/MAPKs Signaling Pathway in RAW264.7 Cells. *Molecules* **2022**, *27*, 3782. [CrossRef]
40. Dhingra, S.; Sharma, A.K.; Singla, D.K.; Singal, P.K. P38 and ERK1/2 MAPKs Mediate the Interplay of TNF-Alpha and IL-10 in Regulating Oxidative Stress and Cardiac Myocyte Apoptosis. *Am. J. Physiol. Heart Circ. Physiol.* **2007**, *293*, H3524–H3531. [CrossRef]
41. Souilhol, C.; Harmsen, M.C.; Evans, P.C.; Krenning, G. Endothelial-Mesenchymal Transition in Atherosclerosis. *Cardiovasc. Res.* **2018**, *114*, 565–577. [CrossRef] [PubMed]
42. Zheng, D.; Liu, J.; Piao, H.; Zhu, Z.; Wei, R.; Liu, K. ROS-Triggered Endothelial Cell Death Mechanisms: Focus on Pyroptosis, Parthanatos, and Ferroptosis. *Front. Immunol.* **2022**, *13*, 1039241. [CrossRef] [PubMed]
43. Ouyang, S.; You, J.; Zhi, C.; Li, P.; Lin, X.; Tan, X.; Ma, W.; Li, L.; Xie, W. Ferroptosis: The Potential Value Target in Atherosclerosis. *Cell Death Dis.* **2021**, *12*, 782. [CrossRef]
44. Bravo-San Pedro, J.M.; Kroemer, G.; Galluzzi, L. Autophagy and Mitophagy in Cardiovascular Disease. *Circ. Res.* **2017**, *120*, 1812–1824. [CrossRef] [PubMed]
45. Mameli, E.; Martello, A.; Caporali, A. Autophagy at the Interface of Endothelial Cell Homeostasis and Vascular Disease. *FEBS J.* **2022**, *289*, 2976–2991. [CrossRef]
46. Khan, H.; Belwal, T.; Efferth, T.; Farooqi, A.A.; Sanches-Silva, A.; Vacca, R.A.; Nabavi, S.F.; Khan, F.; Prasad Devkota, H.; Barreca, D.; et al. Targeting Epigenetics in Cancer: Therapeutic Potential of Flavonoids. *Crit. Rev. Food Sci. Nutr.* **2021**, *61*, 1616–1639. [CrossRef] [PubMed]
47. Mulvihill, E.E.; Huff, M.W. Antiatherogenic Properties of Flavonoids. Implications for Cardiovascular Health. *Can. J. Cardiol.* **2010**, *26* (Suppl. A), 17A–21A. [CrossRef]
48. Xiao, J.; Capanoglu, E.; Jassbi, A.R.; Miron, A. Advance on the Flavonoid C-Glycosides and Health Benefits. *Crit. Rev. Food Sci. Nutr.* **2016**, *56* (Suppl. 1), S29–S45. [CrossRef]
49. Manach, C.; Scalbert, A.; Morand, C.; Rémésy, C.; Jiménez, L. Polyphenols: Food Sources and Bioavailability. *Am. J. Clin. Nutr.* **2004**, *79*, 727–747. [CrossRef]
50. Walle, T.; Browning, A.M.; Steed, L.L.; Reed, S.G.; Walle, U.K. Flavonoid Glucosides Are Hydrolyzed and Thus Activated in the Oral Cavity in Humans. *J. Nutr.* **2005**, *135*, 48–52. [CrossRef]
51. Chen, L.; Cao, H.; Huang, Q.; Xiao, J.; Teng, H. Absorption, Metabolism and Bioavailability of Flavonoids: A Review. *Crit. Rev. Food Sci. Nutr.* **2022**, *62*, 7730–7742. [CrossRef] [PubMed]
52. Chuang, S.Y.; Lin, Y.K.; Lin, C.F.; Wang, P.W.; Chen, E.L.; Fang, J.Y. Elucidating the Skin Delivery of Aglycone and Glycoside Flavonoids: How the Structures Affect Cutaneous Absorption. *Nutrients* **2017**, *9*, 1304. [CrossRef] [PubMed]
53. Wen, K.; Fang, X.; Yang, J.; Yao, Y.; Nandakumar, K.S.; Salem, M.L.; Cheng, K. Recent Research on Flavonoids and Their Biomedical Applications. *Curr. Med. Chem.* **2021**, *28*, 1042–1066. [CrossRef] [PubMed]
54. Ji, L.; Su, S.; Xin, M.; Zhang, Z.; Nan, X.; Li, Z.; Lu, D. Luteolin Ameliorates Hypoxia-Induced Pulmonary Hypertension via Regulating HIF-2α-Arg-NO Axis and PI3K-AKT-ENOS-NO Signaling Pathway. *Phytomedicine* **2022**, *104*, 154329. [CrossRef]

55. Ou, H.C.; Pandey, S.; Hung, M.Y.; Huang, S.H.; Hsu, P.T.; Day, C.H.; Pai, P.; Viswanadha, V.P.; Kuo, W.W.; Huang, C.Y. Luteolin: A Natural Flavonoid Enhances the Survival of HUVECs against Oxidative Stress by Modulating AMPK/PKC Pathway. *Am. J. Chin. Med.* **2019**, *47*, 541–557. [CrossRef]
56. Chen, H.I.; Hu, W.S.; Hung, M.Y.; Ou, H.C.; Huang, S.H.; Hsu, P.T.; Day, C.H.; Lin, K.H.; Viswanadha, V.P.; Kuo, W.W.; et al. Protective Effects of Luteolin against Oxidative Stress and Mitochondrial Dysfunction in Endothelial Cells. *Nutr. Metab. Cardiovasc. Dis.* **2020**, *30*, 1032–1043. [CrossRef]
57. Jia, Z.; Nallasamy, P.; Liu, D.; Shah, H.; Li, J.Z.; Chitrakar, R.; Si, H.; McCormick, J.; Zhu, H.; Zhen, W.; et al. Luteolin Protects against Vascular Inflammation in Mice and TNF-Alpha-Induced Monocyte Adhesion to Endothelial Cells via Suppressing IKBα/NF-KB Signaling Pathway. *J. Nutr. Biochem.* **2015**, *26*, 293–302. [CrossRef]
58. De Stefano, A.; Caporali, S.; Di Daniele, N.; Rovella, V.; Cardillo, C.; Schinzari, F.; Minieri, M.; Pieri, M.; Candi, E.; Bernardini, S.; et al. Anti-Inflammatory and Proliferative Properties of Luteolin-7-O-Glucoside. *Int. J. Mol. Sci.* **2021**, *22*, 1321. [CrossRef]
59. Wei, X.; Zhu, X.; Hu, N.; Zhang, X.; Sun, T.; Xu, J.; Bian, X. Baicalin Attenuates Angiotensin II-Induced Endothelial Dysfunction. *Biochem. Biophys. Res. Commun.* **2015**, *465*, 101–107. [CrossRef]
60. Hsu, W.L.; Lin, Y.C.; Jeng, J.R.; Chang, H.Y.; Chou, T.C. Baicalein Ameliorates Pulmonary Arterial Hypertension Caused by Monocrotaline through Downregulation of ET-1 and ETAR in Pneumonectomized Rats. *Am. J. Chin. Med.* **2018**, *46*, 769–783. [CrossRef]
61. Wang, P.; Wu, J.; Wang, Q.; Zhuang, S.; Zhao, J.; Yu, Y.; Zhang, W.; Zheng, Y.; Liu, X. Baicalin Inhibited Both the Furin/TGFβ1/Smad3/TSP-1 Pathway in Endothelial Cells and the AKT/Ca2+/ROS Pathway in Platelets to Ameliorate Inflammatory Coagulopathy. *Eur. J. Pharmacol.* **2023**, *949*, 175674. [CrossRef] [PubMed]
62. Vissenaekens, H.; Grootaert, C.; Raes, K.; De Munck, J.; Smagghe, G.; Boon, N.; Van Camp, J. Quercetin Mitigates Endothelial Activation in a Novel Intestinal-Endothelial-Monocyte/Macrophage Coculture Setup. *Inflammation* **2022**, *45*, 1600–1611. [CrossRef] [PubMed]
63. Ozyel, B.; Le Gall, G.; Needs, P.W.; Kroon, P.A. Anti-Inflammatory Effects of Quercetin on High-Glucose and Pro-Inflammatory Cytokine Challenged Vascular Endothelial Cell Metabolism. *Mol. Nutr. Food Res.* **2021**, *65*, e2000777. [CrossRef]
64. Chen, T.; Zhang, X.; Zhu, G.; Liu, H.; Chen, J.; Wang, Y.; He, X. Quercetin Inhibits TNF-α Induced HUVECs Apoptosis and Inflammation via Downregulating NF-KB and AP-1 Signaling Pathway in Vitro. *Medicine* **2020**, *99*, E22241. [CrossRef]
65. Zhou, W.; Wang, F.; Qian, X.; Luo, S.; Wang, Z.; Gao, X.; Kong, X.; Zhang, J.; Chen, S. Quercetin Protects Endothelial Function from Inflammation Induced by Localized Disturbed Flow by Inhibiting NRP2 -VEGFC Complex. *Int. Immunopharmacol.* **2023**, *116*, 109842. [CrossRef] [PubMed]
66. Chen, X.; Zheng, L.; Zhang, B.; Deng, Z.; Li, H. Synergistic Protection of Quercetin and Lycopene against Oxidative Stress via SIRT1-Nox4-ROS Axis in HUVEC Cells. *Curr. Res. food Sci.* **2022**, *5*, 1985–1993. [CrossRef] [PubMed]
67. Luo, M.; Tian, R.; Lu, N. Quercetin Inhibited Endothelial Dysfunction and Atherosclerosis in Apolipoprotein E-Deficient Mice: Critical Roles for NADPH Oxidase and Heme Oxygenase-1. *J. Agric. Food Chem.* **2020**, *68*, 10875–10883. [CrossRef]
68. Li, M.T.; Ke, J.; Guo, S.F.; Wu, Y.; Bian, Y.F.; Shan, L.L.; Liu, Q.Y.; Huo, Y.J.; Guo, C.; Liu, M.Y.; et al. The Protective Effect of Quercetin on Endothelial Cells Injured by Hypoxia and Reoxygenation. *Front. Pharmacol.* **2021**, *12*, 732874. [CrossRef]
69. Mohd Sabri, N.A.; Lee, S.K.; Murugan, D.D.; Ling, W.C. Epigallocatechin Gallate (EGCG) Alleviates Vascular Dysfunction in Angiotensin II-Infused Hypertensive Mice by Modulating Oxidative Stress and ENOS. *Sci. Rep.* **2022**, *12*, 17633. [CrossRef]
70. Pai, P.Y.; Chou, W.C.; Chan, S.H.; Wu, S.Y.; Chen, H.I.; Li, C.W.; Hsieh, P.L.; Chu, P.M.; Chen, Y.A.; Ou, H.C.; et al. Epigallocatechin Gallate Reduces Homocysteine-Caused Oxidative Damages through Modulation SIRT1/AMPK Pathway in Endothelial Cells. *Am. J. Chin. Med.* **2021**, *49*, 113–129. [CrossRef]
71. Meng, J.; Chen, Y.; Wang, J.; Qiu, J.; Chang, C.; Bi, F.; Wu, X.; Liu, W. EGCG Protects Vascular Endothelial Cells from Oxidative Stress-Induced Damage by Targeting the Autophagy-Dependent PI3K-AKT-MTOR Pathway. *Ann. Transl. Med.* **2020**, *8*, 200. [CrossRef] [PubMed]
72. Reddy, A.T.; Lakshmi, S.P.; Maruthi Prasad, E.; Varadacharyulu, N.C.; Kodidhela, L.D. Epigallocatechin Gallate Suppresses Inflammation in Human Coronary Artery Endothelial Cells by Inhibiting NF-KB. *Life Sci.* **2020**, *258*, 118136. [CrossRef] [PubMed]
73. Zhao, H.; Liu, M.; Liu, H.; Suo, R.; Lu, C. Naringin Protects Endothelial Cells from Apoptosis and Inflammation by Regulating the Hippo-YAP Pathway. *Biosci. Rep.* **2020**, *40*, BSR20193431. [CrossRef] [PubMed]
74. Li, H.; Liu, L.; Cao, Z.; Li, W.; Liu, R.; Chen, Y.; Li, C.; Song, Y.; Liu, G.; Hu, J.; et al. Naringenin Ameliorates Homocysteine Induced Endothelial Damage via the AMPKα/Sirt1 Pathway. *J. Adv. Res.* **2021**, *34*, 137–147. [CrossRef]
75. Feng, J.; Luo, J.; Deng, L.; Zhong, Y.; Wen, X.; Cai, Y.; Li, J. Naringenin-Induced HO-1 Ameliorates High Glucose or Free Fatty Acids-Associated Apoptosis via PI3K and JNK/Nrf2 Pathways in Human Umbilical Vein Endothelial Cells. *Int. Immunopharmacol.* **2019**, *75*, 105769. [CrossRef] [PubMed]
76. Tan, C.S.; Tew, W.Y.; Jingying, C.; Yam, M.F. Vasorelaxant Effect of 5,7,4'- Trihydroxyflavanone (Naringenin) via Endothelium Dependent, Potassium and Calcium Channels in Sprague Dawley Rats: Aortic Ring Model. *Chem. Biol. Interact.* **2021**, *348*, 109620. [CrossRef]
77. Gao, G.; Nakamura, S.; Asaba, S.; Miyata, Y.; Nakayama, H.; Matsui, T. Hesperidin Preferentially Stimulates Transient Receptor Potential Vanilloid 1, Leading to NO Production and Mas Receptor Expression in Human Umbilical Vein Endothelial Cells. *J. Agric. Food Chem.* **2022**, *70*, 11290–11300. [CrossRef]

78. Zhang, H.; Yang, X.; Pang, X.; Zhao, Z.; Yu, H.; Zhou, H. Genistein Protects against Ox-LDL-Induced Senescence through Enhancing SIRT1/LKB1/AMPK-Mediated Autophagy Flux in HUVECs. *Mol. Cell. Biochem.* **2019**, *455*, 127–134. [CrossRef]
79. Wu, G.; Li, S.; Qu, G.; Hua, J.; Zong, J.; Li, X.; Xu, F. Genistein Alleviates H2O2-Induced Senescence of Human Umbilical Vein Endothelial Cells via Regulating the TXNIP/NLRP3 Axis. *Pharm. Biol.* **2021**, *59*, 1388–1401. [CrossRef]
80. XIE, X.; CONG, L.; LIU, S.; XIANG, L.; FU, X. Genistein Alleviates Chronic Vascular Inflammatory Response via the MiR-21/NF-κB P65 Axis in Lipopolysaccharide-treated Mice. *Mol. Med. Rep.* **2021**, *23*, 11831. [CrossRef]
81. Huang, W.; Hutabarat, R.P.; Chai, Z.; Zheng, T.; Zhang, W.; Li, D. Antioxidant Blueberry Anthocyanins Induce Vasodilation via PI3K/Akt Signaling Pathway in High-Glucose-Induced Human Umbilical Vein Endothelial Cells. *Int. J. Mol. Sci.* **2020**, *21*, 1575. [CrossRef]
82. Lee, G.H.; Hoang, T.H.; Jung, E.S.; Jung, S.J.; Han, S.K.; Chung, M.J.; Chae, S.W.; Chae, H.J. Anthocyanins Attenuate Endothelial Dysfunction through Regulation of Uncoupling of Nitric Oxide Synthase in Aged Rats. *Aging Cell* **2020**, *19*, e13279. [CrossRef]
83. Li, W.; Zhang, G.; Tan, S.; Gong, C.; Yang, Y.; Gu, M.; Mi, Z.; Yang, H.Y. Polyacylated Anthocyanins Derived from Red Radishes Protect Vascular Endothelial Cells Against Palmitic Acid-Induced Apoptosis via the P38 MAPK Pathway. *Plant Foods Hum. Nutr.* **2022**, *77*, 412–420. [CrossRef] [PubMed]
84. Zhao, C.; Kam, H.T.; Chen, Y.; Gong, G.; Hoi, M.P.M.; Skalicka-Woźniak, K.; Dias, A.C.P.; Lee, S.M.Y. Crocetin and Its Glycoside Crocin, Two Bioactive Constituents from *Crocus sativus* L. (Saffron), Differentially Inhibit Angiogenesis by Inhibiting Endothelial Cytoskeleton Organization and Cell Migration Through VEGFR2/SRC/FAK and VEGFR2/MEK/ERK Signaling Pathways. *Front. Pharmacol.* **2021**, *12*, 675359. [CrossRef]
85. Li, Y.; Liu, X.T.; Zhang, P.L.; Li, Y.C.; Sun, M.R.; Wang, Y.T.; Wang, S.P.; Yang, H.; Liu, B.L.; Wang, M.; et al. Hydroxysafflor Yellow A Blocks HIF-1 α Induction of NOX2 and Protects ZO-1 Protein in Cerebral Microvascular Endothelium. *Antioxidants* **2022**, *11*, 728. [CrossRef]
86. Yang, J.; Wang, R.; Cheng, X.; Qu, H.C.; Qi, J.; Li, D.; Xing, Y.; Bai, Y.; Zheng, X. The Vascular Dilatation Induced by Hydroxysafflor Yellow A (HSYA) on Rat Mesenteric Artery through TRPV4-Dependent Calcium Influx in Endothelial Cells. *J. Ethnopharmacol.* **2020**, *256*, 112790. [CrossRef] [PubMed]
87. Naeem, A.; Ming, Y.; Pengyi, H.; Jie, K.Y.; Yali, L.; Haiyan, Z.; Shuai, X.; Wenjing, L.; Ling, W.; Xia, Z.M.; et al. The Fate of Flavonoids after Oral Administration: A Comprehensive Overview of Its Bioavailability. *Crit. Rev. Food Sci. Nutr.* **2022**, *62*, 6169–6186. [CrossRef] [PubMed]
88. Takahama, U.; Yamauchi, R.; Hirota, S. Antioxidative Flavonoids in Adzuki-Meshi (Rice Boiled with Adzuki Bean) React with Nitrite under Simulated Stomach Conditions. *J. Funct. Foods* **2016**, *26*, 657–666. [CrossRef]
89. Babadi, D.; Dadashzadeh, S.; Osouli, M.; Daryabari, M.S.; Haeri, A. Nanoformulation Strategies for Improving Intestinal Permeability of Drugs: A More Precise Look at Permeability Assessment Methods and Pharmacokinetic Properties Changes. *J. Control. Release* **2020**, *321*, 669–709. [CrossRef]
90. Wang, S.; Mateos, R.; Goya, L.; Amigo-Benavent, M.; Sarriá, B.; Bravo, L. A Phenolic Extract from Grape By-Products and Its Main Hydroxybenzoic Acids Protect Caco-2 Cells against pro-Oxidant Induced Toxicity. *Food Chem. Toxicol.* **2016**, *88*, 65–74. [CrossRef]
91. Day, A.J.; Gee, J.M.; DuPont, M.S.; Johnson, I.T.; Williamson, G. Absorption of Quercetin-3-Glucoside and Quercetin-4'-Glucoside in the Rat Small Intestine: The Role of Lactase Phlorizin Hydrolase and the Sodium-Dependent Glucose Transporter. *Biochem. Pharmacol.* **2003**, *65*, 1199–1206. [CrossRef] [PubMed]
92. Németh, K.; Plumb, G.W.; Berrin, J.G.; Juge, N.; Jacob, R.; Naim, H.Y.; Williamson, G.; Swallow, D.M.; Kroon, P.A. Deglycosylation by Small Intestinal Epithelial Cell Beta-Glucosidases Is a Critical Step in the Absorption and Metabolism of Dietary Flavonoid Glycosides in Humans. *Eur. J. Nutr.* **2003**, *42*, 29–42. [CrossRef] [PubMed]
93. Kottra, G.; Daniel, H. Flavonold Glycosides Are Not Transported by the Human Na+/Glucose Transporter When Expressed in Xenopus Laevis Oocytes, but Effectively Inhibit Electrogenic Glucose Uptake. *J. Pharmacol. Exp. Ther.* **2007**, *322*, 829–835. [CrossRef] [PubMed]
94. Van Der Woude, H.; Boersma, M.G.; Vervoort, J.; Rietjens, I.M.C.M. Identification of 14 Quercetin Phase II Mono- and Mixed Conjugates and Their Formation by Rat and Human Phase II in Vitro Model Systems. *Chem. Res. Toxicol.* **2004**, *17*, 1520–1530. [CrossRef]
95. Mullen, W.; Edwards, C.A.; Crozier, A. Absorption, Excretion and Metabolite Profiling of Methyl-, Glucuronyl-, Glucosyl- and Sulpho-Conjugates of Quercetin in Human Plasma and Urine after Ingestion of Onions. *Br. J. Nutr.* **2006**, *96*, 107. [CrossRef]
96. Hollman, P.C.H. Absorption, Bioavailability, and Metabolism of Flavonoids. *Pharm. Biol.* **2004**, *42*, 74–83. [CrossRef]
97. Steed, A.L.; Christophi, G.P.; Kaiko, G.E.; Sun, L.; Goodwin, V.M.; Jain, U.; Esaulova, E.; Artyomov, M.N.; Morales, D.J.; Holtzman, M.J.; et al. The Microbial Metabolite Desaminotyrosine Protects from Influenza through Type I Interferon. *Science* **2017**, *357*, 498–502. [CrossRef]
98. Williamson, G.; Clifford, M.N. Role of the Small Intestine, Colon and Microbiota in Determining the Metabolic Fate of Polyphenols. *Biochem. Pharmacol.* **2017**, *139*, 24–39. [CrossRef]
99. Clifford, M.N. Diet-Derived Phenols in Plasma and Tissues and Their Implications for Health. *Planta Med.* **2004**, *70*, 1103–1114. [CrossRef]
100. Crozier, A.; Del Rio, D.; Clifford, M.N. Bioavailability of Dietary Flavonoids and Phenolic Compounds. *Mol. Asp. Med.* **2010**, *31*, 446–467. [CrossRef]

101. Kawabata, K.; Yoshioka, Y.; Terao, J. Role of Intestinal Microbiota in the Bioavailability and Physiological Functions of Dietary Polyphenols. *Molecules* **2019**, *24*, 370. [CrossRef] [PubMed]
102. Hostetler, G.L.; Ralston, R.A.; Schwartz, S.J. Flavones: Food Sources, Bioavailability, Metabolism, and Bioactivity. *Adv. Nutr.* **2017**, *8*, 423–435. [CrossRef] [PubMed]
103. Miean, K.H.; Mohamed, S. Flavonoid (Myricetin, Quercetin, Kaempferol, Luteolin, and Apigenin) Content of Edible Tropical Plants. *J. Agric. Food Chem.* **2001**, *49*, 3106–3112. [CrossRef] [PubMed]
104. Wang, Y.; Kong, X.; Wang, M.; Li, J.; Chen, W.; Jiang, D. Luteolin Partially Inhibits LFA-1 Expression in Neutrophils Through the ERK Pathway. *Inflammation* **2019**, *42*, 365–374. [CrossRef] [PubMed]
105. Li, X.; Chen, M.; Lei, X.; Huang, M.; Ye, W.; Zhang, R.; Zhang, D. Luteolin Inhibits Angiogenesis by Blocking Gas6/Axl Signaling Pathway. *Int. J. Oncol.* **2017**, *51*, 677–685. [CrossRef]
106. Kampa, R.P.; Flori, L.; Sęk, A.; Spezzini, J.; Brogi, S.; Szewczyk, A.; Calderone, V.; Bednarczyk, P.; Testai, L. Luteolin-Induced Activation of Mitochondrial BKCa Channels: Undisclosed Mechanism of Cytoprotection. *Antioxidants* **2022**, *11*, 1892. [CrossRef]
107. Kang, M.J.; Ko, G.S.; Oh, D.G.; Kim, J.S.; Noh, K.; Kang, W.; Yoon, W.K.; Kim, H.C.; Jeong, H.G.; Jeong, T.C. Role of Metabolism by Intestinal Microbiota in Pharmacokinetics of Oral Baicalin. *Arch. Pharmacal Res.* **2014**, *37*, 371–378. [CrossRef]
108. Ding, L.; Jia, C.; Zhang, Y.; Wang, W.; Zhu, W.; Chen, Y.; Zhang, T. Baicalin Relaxes Vascular Smooth Muscle and Lowers Blood Pressure in Spontaneously Hypertensive Rats. *Biomed. Pharmacother.* **2019**, *111*, 325–330. [CrossRef]
109. Bai, J.; Wang, Q.; Qi, J.; Yu, H.; Wang, C.; Wang, X.; Ren, Y.; Yang, F. Promoting Effect of Baicalin on Nitric Oxide Production in CMECs via Activating the PI3K-AKT-ENOS Pathway Attenuates Myocardial Ischemia-Reperfusion Injury. *Phytomedicine* **2019**, *63*, 153035. [CrossRef]
110. Tsai, C.L.; Tsai, C.W.; Chang, W.S.; Lin, J.C.; Hsia, T.C.; Bau, D.T. Protective Effects of Baicalin on Arsenic Trioxide-Induced Oxidative Damage and Apoptosis in Human Umbilical Vein Endothelial Cells. *In Vivo* **2021**, *35*, 155–162. [CrossRef]
111. Forrester, S.J.; Kikuchi, D.S.; Hernandes, M.S.; Xu, Q.; Griendling, K.K. Reactive Oxygen Species in Metabolic and Inflammatory Signaling. *Circ. Res.* **2018**, *122*, 877–902. [CrossRef]
112. Shi, R.; Wei, Z.; Zhu, D.; Fu, N.; Wang, C.; Yin, S.; Liang, Y.; Xing, J.; Wang, X.; Wang, Y. Baicalein Attenuates Monocrotaline-Induced Pulmonary Arterial Hypertension by Inhibiting Vascular Remodeling in Rats. *Pulm. Pharmacol. Ther.* **2018**, *48*, 124–135. [CrossRef] [PubMed]
113. Hao, Z.; Zhang, Z.; Zhao, Y.; Wang, D. Baicalin Reduces Immune Cell Infiltration by Inhibiting Inflammation and Protecting Tight Junctions in Ischemic Stroke Injury. *Am. J. Chin. Med.* **2023**, *51*, 355–372. [CrossRef] [PubMed]
114. Lee, W.; Ku, S.K.; Bae, J.S. Antiplatelet, Anticoagulant, and Profibrinolytic Activities of Baicalin. *Arch. Pharmacal Res.* **2015**, *38*, 893–903. [CrossRef] [PubMed]
115. Zhang, L.; Yu, G.; Yu, Q.; Wang, L.; Wu, L.; Tao, Z.; Ding, J.; Lin, D. Baicalin Promotes Random-Pattern Skin Flap Survival by Inducing Autophagy via AMPK-Regulated TFEB Nuclear Transcription. *Phytother. Res.* **2023**. [CrossRef]
116. Zhao, L.; Xiong, M.; Liu, Y. Baicalin Enhances the Proliferation and Invasion of Trophoblasts and Suppresses Vascular Endothelial Damage by Modulating Long Non-Coding RNA NEAT1/MiRNA-205-5p in Hypertensive Disorder Complicating Pregnancy. *J. Obstet. Gynaecol. Res.* **2021**, *47*, 3060–3070. [CrossRef]
117. Liu, L.; Lan, X.; Chen, X.; Dai, S.; Wang, Z.; Zhao, A.; Lu, L.; Huang, N.; Chen, J.; Yang, P.; et al. Multi-Functional Plant Flavonoids Regulate Pathological Microenvironments for Vascular Stent Surface Engineering. *Acta Biomater.* **2023**, *157*, 655–669. [CrossRef] [PubMed]
118. Perez-Vizcaino, F.; Duarte, J. Flavonols and Cardiovascular Disease. *Mol. Asp. Med.* **2010**, *31*, 478–494. [CrossRef]
119. Terao, J. Potential Role of Quercetin Glycosides as Anti-Atherosclerotic Food-Derived Factors for Human Health. *Antioxidants* **2023**, *12*, 258. [CrossRef] [PubMed]
120. Feng, J.; Ge, C.; Li, W.; Li, R. 3-(3-Hydroxyphenyl)Propionic Acid, a Microbial Metabolite of Quercetin, Inhibits Monocyte Binding to Endothelial Cells via Modulating E-Selectin Expression. *Fitoterapia* **2022**, *156*, 105071. [CrossRef] [PubMed]
121. Suganya, N.; Mani, K.P.; Sireesh, D.; Rajaguru, P.; Vairamani, M.; Suresh, T.; Suzuki, T.; Chatterjee, S.; Ramkumar, K.M. Establishment of Pancreatic Microenvironment Model of ER Stress: Quercetin Attenuates β-Cell Apoptosis by Invoking Nitric Oxide-CGMP Signaling in Endothelial Cells. *J. Nutr. Biochem.* **2018**, *55*, 142–156. [CrossRef] [PubMed]
122. Suganya, N.; Dornadula, S.; Chatterjee, S.; Mohanram, R.K. Quercetin Improves Endothelial Function in Diabetic Rats through Inhibition of Endoplasmic Reticulum Stress-Mediated Oxidative Stress. *Eur. J. Pharmacol.* **2018**, *819*, 80–88. [CrossRef] [PubMed]
123. Tumova, S.; Kerimi, A.; Williamson, G. Long Term Treatment with Quercetin in Contrast to the Sulfate and Glucuronide Conjugates Affects HIF1α Stability and Nrf2 Signaling in Endothelial Cells and Leads to Changes in Glucose Metabolism. *Free Radic. Biol. Med.* **2019**, *137*, 158–168. [CrossRef] [PubMed]
124. Rezabakhsh, A.; Rahbarghazi, R.; Malekinejad, H.; Fathi, F.; Montaseri, A.; Garjani, A. Quercetin Alleviates High Glucose-Induced Damage on Human Umbilical Vein Endothelial Cells by Promoting Autophagy. *Phytomedicine* **2019**, *56*, 183–193. [CrossRef] [PubMed]
125. Fan, T.; Du, Y.; Zhang, M.; Zhu, A.R.; Zhang, J. Senolytics Cocktail Dasatinib and Quercetin Alleviate Human Umbilical Vein Endothelial Cell Senescence via the TRAF6-MAPK-NF-KB Axis in a YTHDF2-Dependent Manner. *Gerontology* **2022**, *68*, 920–934. [CrossRef] [PubMed]
126. Dagher, O.; Mury, P.; Thorin-Trescases, N.; Noly, P.E.; Thorin, E.; Carrier, M. Therapeutic Potential of Quercetin to Alleviate Endothelial Dysfunction in Age-Related Cardiovascular Diseases. *Front. Cardiovasc. Med.* **2021**, *8*, 658400. [CrossRef]

127. Márquez Campos, E.; Jakobs, L.; Simon, M.C. Antidiabetic Effects of Flavan-3-Ols and Their Microbial Metabolites. *Nutrients* **2020**, *12*, 1592. [CrossRef]
128. Eng, Q.Y.; Thanikachalam, P.V.; Ramamurthy, S. Molecular Understanding of Epigallocatechin Gallate (EGCG) in Cardiovascular and Metabolic Diseases. *J. Ethnopharmacol.* **2018**, *210*, 296–310. [CrossRef]
129. Kim, S.; Lee, H.; Moon, H.; Kim, R.; Kim, M.; Jeong, S.; Kim, H.; Kim, S.H.; Hwang, S.S.; Lee, M.Y.; et al. Epigallocatechin-3-Gallate Attenuates Myocardial Dysfunction via Inhibition of Endothelial-to-Mesenchymal Transition. *Antioxidants* **2023**, *12*, 1059. [CrossRef]
130. Zhang, J.; Cui, H.; Qiu, J.; Wang, X.; Zhong, Y.; Yao, C.; Yao, L.; Zheng, Q.; Xiong, C.H. Stability of Glycosylated Complexes Loaded with Epigallocatechin 3-Gallate (EGCG). *Food Chem.* **2023**, *410*, 135364. [CrossRef]
131. Zhang, W.; Shen, H.; Li, Y.; Yang, K.; Lei, P.; Gu, Y.; Sun, L.; Xu, H.; Wang, R. Preparation of Type-A Gelatin/Poly-γ-Glutamic Acid Nanoparticles for Enhancing the Stability and Bioavailability of (-)-Epigallocatechin Gallate. *Foods* **2023**, *12*, 1748. [CrossRef] [PubMed]
132. Imperatrice, M.; Cuijpers, I.; Troost, F.J.; Sthijns, M.M.J.P.E. Hesperidin Functions as an Ergogenic Aid by Increasing Endothelial Function and Decreasing Exercise-Induced Oxidative Stress and Inflammation, Thereby Contributing to Improved Exercise Performance. *Nutrients* **2022**, *14*, 2955. [CrossRef] [PubMed]
133. Zhang, Z.; Liu, H.; Hu, X.; He, Y.; Li, L.; Yang, X.; Wang, C.; Hu, M.; Tao, S. Heat Shock Protein 70 Mediates the Protective Effect of Naringenin on High-Glucose-Induced Alterations of Endothelial Function. *Int. J. Endocrinol.* **2022**, *2022*, 7275765. [CrossRef] [PubMed]
134. Fuior, E.V.; Mocanu, C.A.; Deleanu, M.; Voicu, G.; Anghelache, M.; Rebleanu, D.; Simionescu, M.; Calin, M. Evaluation of VCAM-1 Targeted Naringenin/Indocyanine Green-Loaded Lipid Nanoemulsions as Theranostic Nanoplatforms in Inflammation. *Pharmaceutics* **2020**, *12*, 1066. [CrossRef]
135. Zaheer, K.; Humayoun Akhtar, M. An Updated Review of Dietary Isoflavones: Nutrition, Processing, Bioavailability and Impacts on Human Health. *Crit. Rev. Food Sci. Nutr.* **2017**, *57*, 1280–1293. [CrossRef] [PubMed]
136. Toro-Funes, N.; Morales-Gutiérrez, F.J.; Veciana-Nogués, M.T.; Vidal-Carou, M.C.; Spencer, J.P.E.; Rodriguez-Mateos, A. The Intracellular Metabolism of Isoflavones in Endothelial Cells. *Food Funct.* **2015**, *6*, 98–108. [CrossRef] [PubMed]
137. Poasakate, A.; Maneesai, P.; Potue, P.; Bunbupha, S.; Tong-Un, T.; Settheetham-Ishida, W.; Khamseekaew, J.; Pakdeechote, P. Genistein Alleviates Renin-Angiotensin System Mediated Vascular and Kidney Alterations in Renovascular Hypertensive Rats. *Biomed. Pharmacother.* **2022**, *146*, 112601. [CrossRef]
138. Zhang, T.; Hu, Q.; Shi, L.; Qin, L.; Zhang, Q.; Mi, M. Equol Attenuates Atherosclerosis in Apolipoprotein E-Deficient Mice by Inhibiting Endoplasmic Reticulum Stress via Activation of Nrf2 in Endothelial Cells. *PLoS ONE* **2016**, *11*, e0167020. [CrossRef]
139. Park, M.H.; Ju, J.W.; Kim, M.; Han, J.S. The Protective Effect of Daidzein on High Glucose-Induced Oxidative Stress in Human Umbilical Vein Endothelial Cells. *Z. Naturforsch. C.* **2016**, *71*, 21–28. [CrossRef]
140. Dong, Y.; Wu, X.; Han, L.; Bian, J.; He, C.; El-Omar, E.; Gong, L.; Wang, M. The Potential Roles of Dietary Anthocyanins in Inhibiting Vascular Endothelial Cell Senescence and Preventing Cardiovascular Diseases. *Nutrients* **2022**, *14*, 2836. [CrossRef]
141. De Ferrars, R.M.; Czank, C.; Zhang, Q.; Botting, N.P.; Kroon, P.A.; Cassidy, A.; Kay, C.D. The Pharmacokinetics of Anthocyanins and Their Metabolites in Humans. *Br. J. Pharmacol.* **2014**, *171*, 3268–3282. [CrossRef] [PubMed]
142. Czank, C.; Cassidy, A.; Zhang, Q.; Morrison, D.J.; Preston, T.; Kroon, P.A.; Botting, N.P.; Kay, C.D. Human Metabolism and Elimination of the Anthocyanin, Cyanidin-3-Glucoside: A (13)C-Tracer Study. *Am. J. Clin. Nutr.* **2013**, *97*, 995–1003. [CrossRef] [PubMed]
143. Edwards, M.; Czank, C.; Woodward, G.M.; Cassidy, A.; Kay, C.D. Phenolic Metabolites of Anthocyanins Modulate Mechanisms of Endothelial Function. *J. Agric. Food Chem.* **2015**, *63*, 2423–2431. [CrossRef] [PubMed]
144. Krga, I.; Monfoulet, L.E.; Konic-Ristic, A.; Mercier, S.; Glibetic, M.; Morand, C.; Milenkovic, D. Anthocyanins and Their Gut Metabolites Reduce the Adhesion of Monocyte to TNFα-Activated Endothelial Cells at Physiologically Relevant Concentrations. *Arch. Biochem. Biophys.* **2016**, *599*, 51–59. [CrossRef] [PubMed]
145. Krga, I.; Tamaian, R.; Mercier, S.; Boby, C.; Monfoulet, L.E.; Glibetic, M.; Morand, C.; Milenkovic, D. Anthocyanins and Their Gut Metabolites Attenuate Monocyte Adhesion and Transendothelial Migration through Nutrigenomic Mechanisms Regulating Endothelial Cell Permeability. *Free Radic. Biol. Med.* **2018**, *124*, 364–379. [CrossRef]
146. Herrera-Bravo, J.; Beltrán, J.F.; Huard, N.; Saavedra, K.; Saavedra, N.; Alvear, M.; Lanas, F.; Salazar, L.A. Anthocyanins Found in Pinot Noir Waste Induce Target Genes Related to the Nrf2 Signalling in Endothelial Cells. *Antioxidants* **2022**, *11*, 1239. [CrossRef]
147. Chen, B.H.; Inbaraj, B.S. Nanoemulsion and Nanoliposome Based Strategies for Improving Anthocyanin Stability and Bioavailability. *Nutrients* **2019**, *11*, 1052. [CrossRef]
148. Xi, L.; Qian, Z.; Du, P.; Fu, J. Pharmacokinetic Properties of Crocin (Crocetin Digentiobiose Ester) Following Oral Administration in Rats. *Phytomedicine* **2007**, *14*, 633–636. [CrossRef]
149. Sweeney, M.D.; Zhao, Z.; Montagne, A.; Nelson, A.R.; Zlokovic, B.V. Blood-Brain Barrier: From Physiology to Disease and Back. *Physiol. Rev.* **2019**, *99*, 21–78. [CrossRef]
150. Taguchi, K.; Okudaira, K.; Matsumoto, T.; Kobayashi, T. Ginkgolide B Caused the Activation of the Akt/ENOS Pathway through the Antioxidant Effect of SOD1 in the Diabetic Aorta. *Pflugers Arch.* **2023**, *475*, 453–463. [CrossRef]
151. Jiang, X.; Stockwell, B.R.; Conrad, M. Ferroptosis: Mechanisms, Biology and Role in Disease. *Nat. Rev. Mol. Cell Biol.* **2021**, *22*, 266–282. [CrossRef] [PubMed]

152. Williams, D.; Mahmoud, M.; Liu, R.; Andueza, A.; Kumar, S.; Kang, D.W.; Zhang, J.; Tamargo, I.; Villa-Roel, N.; Baek, K.I.; et al. Stable Flow-Induced Expression of KLK10 Inhibits Endothelial Inflammation and Atherosclerosis. *Elife* **2022**, *11*, e72579. [CrossRef] [PubMed]
153. Liang, G.; Wang, S.; Shao, J.; Jin, Y.J.; Xu, L.; Yan, Y.; Günther, S.; Wang, L.; Offermanns, S. Tenascin-X Mediates Flow-Induced Suppression of EndMT and Atherosclerosis. *Circ. Res.* **2022**, *130*, 1647–1659. [CrossRef] [PubMed]

Disclaimer/Publisher's Note: The statements, opinions and data contained in all publications are solely those of the individual author(s) and contributor(s) and not of MDPI and/or the editor(s). MDPI and/or the editor(s) disclaim responsibility for any injury to people or property resulting from any ideas, methods, instructions or products referred to in the content.

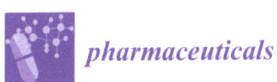

Article

Rutin Gel with Bone Graft Accelerates Bone Formation in a Rabbit Model by Inhibiting MMPs and Enhancing Collagen Activities

Fahad F. Albaqami [1,*], Hassan N. Althurwi [2], Khalid M. Alharthy [2], Abubaker M. Hamad [3] and Fatin A. Awartani [4,*]

1. Postgraduate Doctorate Program, Periodontics and Community Dentistry Department, College of Dentistry, King Saud University, Riyadh 11545, Saudi Arabia
2. Pharmacology and Toxicology Department, College of Pharmacy, Prince Sattam bin Abdulaziz University, Al-Kharj 11942, Saudi Arabia; h.althurwi@psau.edu.sa (H.N.A.); k.alharthy@psau.edu.sa (K.M.A.)
3. Department of Nursing, College of Health Sciences and Nursing, Al-Rayan Colleges, Al-Madeena Al-Munowara 41411, Saudi Arabia; abkr.hamad@gmail.com
4. Periodontics and Community Dentistry Department, College of Dentistry, King Saud University, Riyadh 11563, Saudi Arabia
* Correspondence: albaqami.bsd@gmail.com (F.F.A.); fawartani@live.com (F.A.A.); Tel.: +966-114784524 (ext. 331) (F.A.A.)

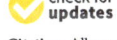

Citation: Albaqami, F.F.; Althurwi, H.N.; Alharthy, K.M.; Hamad, A.M.; Awartani, F.A. Rutin Gel with Bone Graft Accelerates Bone Formation in a Rabbit Model by Inhibiting MMPs and Enhancing Collagen Activities. *Pharmaceuticals* 2023, 16, 774. https://doi.org/10.3390/ph16050774

Academic Editor: Chung-Yi Chen

Received: 27 April 2023
Revised: 18 May 2023
Accepted: 19 May 2023
Published: 22 May 2023

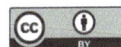

Copyright: © 2023 by the authors. Licensee MDPI, Basel, Switzerland. This article is an open access article distributed under the terms and conditions of the Creative Commons Attribution (CC BY) license (https:// creativecommons.org/licenses/by/ 4.0/).

Abstract: Bone graft techniques are used to compensate for bone loss in areas with deficient regeneration. However, matrix metalloproteases (MMPs) can limit bone formation by degrading extracellular matrices, which are required for bone regrowth. Noteworthily, rutin is a natural flavonoid compound that inhibits the genetic expression of various MMPs. Therefore, rutin may serve as an inexpensive and stable alternative to the growth factors used to accelerate dental bone graft healing. This study aimed to evaluate the potential of mixing rutin gel with allograft bone to accelerate the healing of bone defects in an in vivo rabbit model. Bone defects were surgically induced in New Zealand rabbits (*n* = 3 per group) and subsequently treated with bone grafts along with rutin or control gel. Overall, treatment with rutin significantly prevented the expression of several MMPs and increased type III collagen in the gingiva around the surgical site. Additionally, rutin-treated animals showed enhanced bone formation with higher bone marrow content in the jawbone defect area compared with the control group. Taken together, these findings demonstrate that rutin gel, when added to bone grafts, quickly enhances bone formation and may serve as a suitable alternative to expensive growth factors for the same purpose.

Keywords: rutin; matrix metalloprotease (MMP); extracellular matrix (ECM); bone graft; collagen; natural product; flavonoid; in vivo; rabbit

1. Introduction

In periodontics, bone graft materials are used to encourage bone formation at defective sites, a process that increases the potential and predictability of bone regeneration. After the bone graft is placed at the planned site, bone formation is affected by the particle size of the bone graft, its physical and chemical properties, and the grafting procedure used [1]. Moreover, various types of growth factors can be added to the bone graft to trigger healing processes, resulting in accelerated bone formation and enhanced healing, which occurs through the induction of chemotaxis, as well as osteoblast proliferation and differentiation. Indeed, multiple studies showed that growth factors used in bone graft procedures have positive effects on bone formation [2–4].

Bone healing is a complex process in which diverse cell types, signaling pathways, and extracellular matrix (ECM) components interact [5]. In particular, matrix metalloproteases (MMPs) are a family of zinc-dependent endopeptidases that are responsible for the breakdown of the organic matrix [6]. MMPs control various biological activities, including cell migration, angiogenesis, wound healing, and tissue remodeling, by cleaving ECM proteins [7]; thus, they are associated with bone healing [8]. Moreover, extracellular matrices, such as type I collagen, are responsible for bone elasticity and toughness. In turn, type III collagen is a reconstituted collagen that plays a critical role in tissue damage repair, being highly expressed during injured tissue remodeling, promoting angiogenesis, and maintaining capillary function [9]. As vascularization can help accelerate the bone graft-mediated healing process [10], the MMP and ECM levels need to be reduced and enhanced, respectively, to support and increase the bone graft success rate.

Various methods have been investigated for controlling MMP activity and expression, including the application of small-molecule inhibitors, gene therapy, and alteration of native MMP inhibitors [11]. Noteworthily, some bioactive molecules present in natural products can inhibit the MMP downstream pathways; thus, these molecules can represent valuable therapeutic tools for pathological conditions, including inflammatory processes and autoimmune diseases (such as osteoarthritis, periodontitis, and fibrotic disorders) [12]. Several studies have shown that rutin (Figure 1), a polyphenolic flavonoid found in fruits and vegetables, has several pharmacological benefits which are similar to other flavonoid compounds for treating different diseases, such as osteoporosis, cancer, diabetes, hypertension, viral infections, bacterial infections, and depression. Furthermore, rutin exerts powerful anti-inflammatory effects, decreases MMP expression, inhibits osteoclast formation, and promotes the proliferation and differentiation of osteoblasts. Unlike other flavonoids, rutin is non-toxic and non-oxidizable [13–16]. Hence, the safety, stability, and cost-effectiveness of rutin make it a suitable replacement for currently used growth factors.

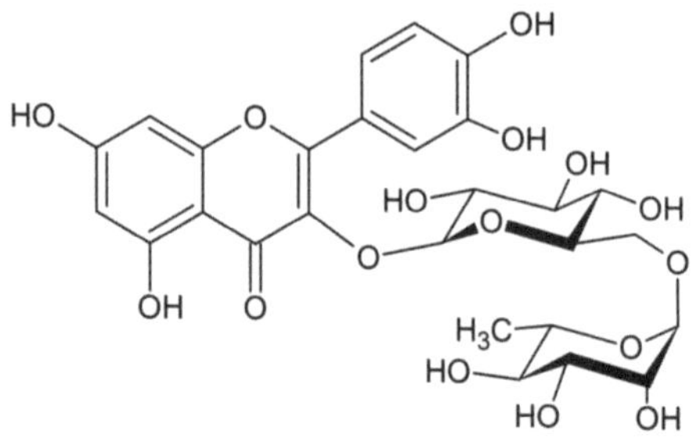

Figure 1. Chemical structure of rutin.

Rutin is poorly soluble in aqueous solvents, which hinders its application in clinical settings due to reduced bioavailability. Therefore, we used the proniosomal gel to improve rutin solubility and bioavailability. In addition, using gel will aid in extending rutin's pharmacological effects due to the controlled release properties of gel formulations. A further advantage of using proniosomal gel is that it can penetrate physiological barriers [17]. Thus, adding rutin gel to the defect area may inhibit the release of MMPs from the surrounding tissue into the defect area containing the bone graft.

The present study aims to provide an easy, simple, and rapid pathway to achieve desired results through bone grafting in vivo using rutin as a replacement for growth factors. Our study findings are expected to pave the way for the methodological development of practical dentistry, which will ultimately reduce the economic burden of the treatments and improve patient outcomes.

2. Results

The pilot study revealed that at the end of the sixth week, the bone healing process was still incomplete, whereas the healing process and new bone formation were almost completed 12 weeks after just tooth extraction (without intervention).

2.1. Gene Expression

Briefly, six New Zealand rabbits (n = 3) were randomly divided into two groups following unilateral lower first premolar tooth extraction: the control group received vehicle gel (without rutin) and the treated group received rutin gel, which was mixed with bone graft to fill the bone defect. As described in Section 4, the animals were euthanized after six weeks of treatment, and specimens were collected for analysis of gene expression and histomorphometry.

Application of the rutin gel at the grafted bone site resulted in reduced expression of *MMP1* (12.69 ± 10.73 vs. 100 ± 20.44; Figure 2a), *MMP3* (22.94 ± 11.78 vs. 100 ± 29.23; Figure 2b), *MMP9* (40.27 ± 23.02 vs. 100 ± 19.75; Figure 2c), and *MMP13* (17.26 ± 14.13 vs. 100 ± 33.85; Figure 2d) in the gingiva of the animals as compared with the control group. Indeed, rutin treatment significantly decreased the levels of *MMP1*, *MMP3*, *MMP9*, and *MMP13* by 87%, 77%, 60%, and 83%, respectively, as compared with those in the control group. In contrast, *COL3A1* levels were significantly increased in the gingiva upon rutin treatment as compared with the non-treated control group (2230.09 ± 714.31 vs. 100 ± 20.67; Figure 2e).

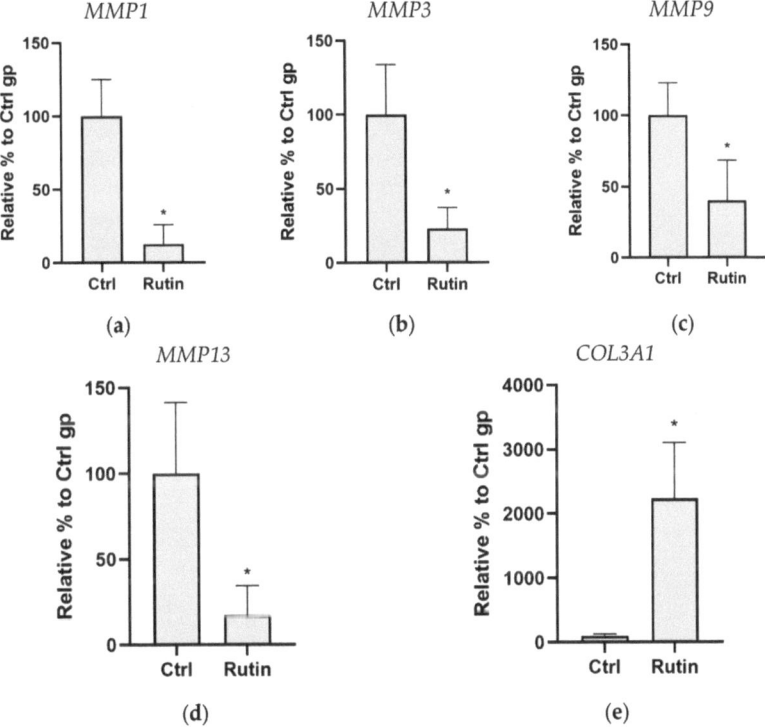

Figure 2. Effect of rutin gel treatment on *MMP* and *COL3A1* expression in the gingiva. The expression levels of *MMP1* (**a**), *MMP3* (**b**), *MMP9* (**c**), *MMP13* (**d**), and *COL3A1* (**e**) were determined by quantitative real-time polymerase chain reaction. Data are presented as mean ± standard deviation of three independent experiments. * $p < 0.05$ compared with control (Ctrl).

2.2. Histomorphometry

A detailed analysis of the histological features of the bone deficit site revealed that the apical width, bone formation area, and bone marrow region were significantly increased in animals treated with rutin gel (Table 1). The remaining histological parameters analyzed showed a trend of improved outcome upon rutin treatment ($p > 0.05$). In the control and rutin treatment groups, there was no significant difference in connective regions (%). Noteworthily, the amount of connective tissue was reduced at the bone deficit site in rutin-treated animals as compared with the control group, but this difference was not statistically significant.

Table 1. Characterization of the histological parameters of the grafted bone site.

Histological Parameters	Control Group	Rutin-Treated Group
Coronal width (mm)	1.7 ± 0.2	1.2 ± 0.3
Middle width (mm)	0.8 ± 0.32	1.3 ± 0.05
Apical width (mm)	4.5 ± 0.4	6.3 ± 0.4 *
Bone formation area diameter (mm)	2.8 ± 0.5	4.5 ± 0.4 *
Mineralized bone region (%)	26.6 ± 6.4	34.2 ± 4.5
Bone marrow region (%)	11 ± 3.9	32.3 ± 12.1 *
Connective tissue region (%)	46.9 ± 10.9	33.0 ± 8.7

Data are presented as mean ± standard deviation ($n = 3$ per group). * $p < 0.05$ compared with the control group as determined by Student's t-test.

Histological analysis of sliced tissue samples of the grafted bone area was performed to determine the amount of newly formed bone (Figure 3a) and bone marrow (Figure 3b) in the two experimental groups. In line with the above-described results, newly formed bone was significantly less in the control group than in the rutin-treated group, whereas the bone marrow levels were significantly higher upon rutin treatment (Figure 3a,b).

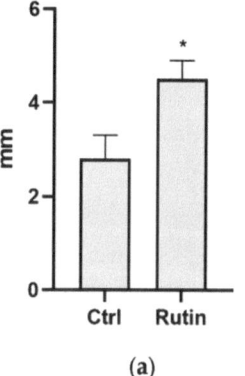
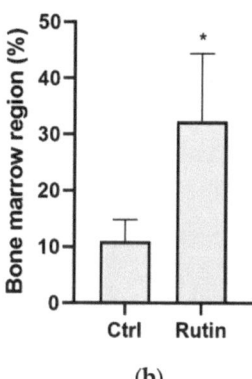

(a) (b)

Figure 3. Effect of rutin gel treatment on bone formation and bone marrow at the grafted bone area. The area of newly formed bone (**a**) and percentage of bone marrow (**b**) were determined in the sliced bone sample of the grafted bone area using histological analysis techniques. Data are presented as mean ± standard deviation of three independent experiments. * $p < 0.05$ compared with control (Ctrl).

Further histological analyses showed improved bone formation and distribution and higher levels of collagen fibers as well as improved angiogenesis upon rutin treatment (Figure 4b,d,f) as compared with the control group (Figure 4a,c,e).

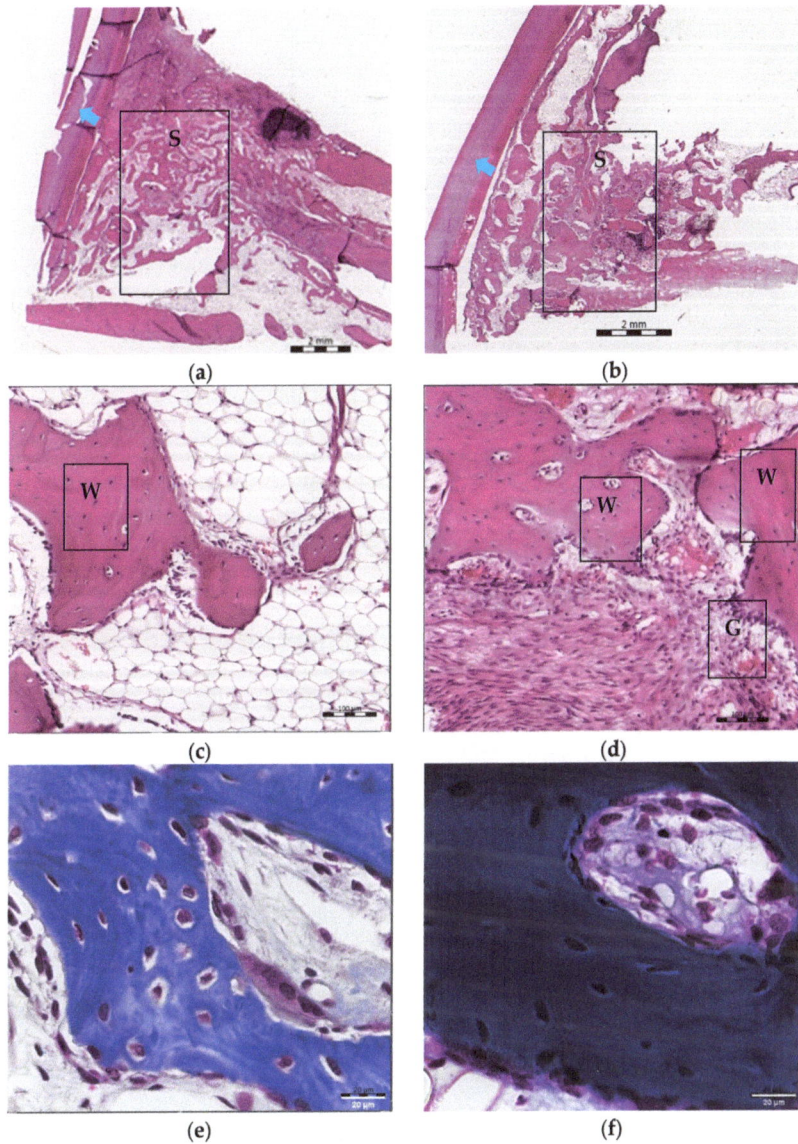

Figure 4. Effect of rutin gel treatment on bone formation, angiogenesis, bone marrow, and collagen fibers at the grafted bone site. Hematoxylin–eosin and Masson's trichrome staining of jawbone samples from control (**a,c,e**) and rutin-treated (**b,d,f**) animals, respectively. In (**a,b**) samples, the letter S refers to the area of study where bone formation and bone marrow were measured in the lower first premolar tooth socket; additionally, the blue arrow shows the lower second premolar tooth (magnification 40×, scale bar is 2 mm). In (**c,d**) samples, the area of bone formation is indicated by the letter W and the area of angiogenesis is indicated by the letter G at the place of blood cell collection (magnification 100×, scale bar is 100 μm). In (**e,f**) samples, collagen area is indicated by blue color staining (magnification 400×, scale bar is 20 μm).

3. Discussion

This study showed that treatment with rutin can significantly reduce the levels of *MMP1*, *MMP3*, *MMP9*, and *MMP13* at bone formation sites, which agrees with previous reports. Consequently, rutin could significantly improve the desired functional outcomes [18–20]. A previous study reported that both MMP-1 and MMP-13 are expressed in osteoarthritic cartilage; thus, the collagenolytic activity observed in osteoarthritic cartilage is likely due to the combined activity of these two enzymes [21]. Moreover, it is believed that MMP-9 and MMP-13 play critical roles in periodontal and alveolar bone homeostasis in both health and disease conditions. In particular, MMP-9 and MMP-13 are present in inflamed areas around necrotic bones and within the epithelium [22]. According to several studies, MMP-3 is involved in the production of inflammatory cytokines and in osteoporosis and regulates bone destruction; therefore, MMP-3 may be responsible for delayed fracture healing [23].

In the present study, the rutin-treated group showed a significant increase in *COL3A1* expression, which agrees with the results of a previous study [20]. Type III collagen plays a crucial role in granulation tissue formation during tissue regeneration and repairs the damage. Additionally, it maintains the structural support required for blood vessel growth, thereby contributing to angiogenesis [24]. Moreover, type III collagen can bind to cytokines, chemokines, and growth factor receptors on the cell surface, thereby stimulating cellular activity during wound healing. Given its proprieties, type III collagen has been used to promote cell growth and differentiation during constructive remodeling. In general, this ECM component enhances the communication and interaction between cells and accelerates bone defect repair by interacting with various growth factors [9].

Histological findings showed that rutin treatment can enhance bone formation in the buccal region, which is most likely due to an interaction between the anti-inflammatory and osteogenic properties of rutin. This finding is consistent with previously published studies which showed that rutin administration to a rat model of osteoporosis in mandibular alveolar bone significantly increases bone formation [25]. Additional research also showed that rutin facilitates osteoblast differentiation and bone formation [26]. This was attributed to the upregulation of osteogenic markers and the downregulation of inflammatory cytokines [27]. Hence, rutin may be an effective treatment for bone disorders.

Herein, our histomorphometry results revealed a significant increase in the bone marrow area upon rutin treatment. In accordance with our findings, a previous in vivo study confirmed that rutin can promote the differentiation of marrow mesenchymal stem cells into osteoblasts [28]. During osteogenesis stages, osteoblasts deposit collagen rapidly without mineralizing it. Afterward, the mineralization rate increases to equal the collagen synthesis rate. As collagen synthesis decreases, mineralization continues until the produced collagen is fully mineralized [29]. Notably, the bone marrow was reported to play an important role in bone formation by producing osteoblasts and periosteum elements, which facilitate the connection with the surrounding tissues [30,31]. The present findings suggested that MMPs could play a role in the integration of the grafted bone with the host bone. Therefore, rutin's potential to promote bone healing could be mediated by increasing type III collagen and decreasing MMP levels, which are known to impair tissue repair and degrade extracellular matrix components (Figure 5). Therefore, rutin can work as a suitable adjuvant agent for bone grafts to be added at the bone defect site to accelerate the grafted bone success.

Further evaluation of rutin as an adjuvant agent for bone grafts is still required to optimize the bone regeneration process. In particular, future studies should explore the most appropriate rutin dosage to use in the clinical setting and the precise molecular mechanisms underlying its therapeutic effects. The study was limited by the fact that it was conducted on healthy laboratory animals, which differed from humans in health status, diet, and environment. Therefore, clinical translation of these laboratory findings requires extensive preclinical research.

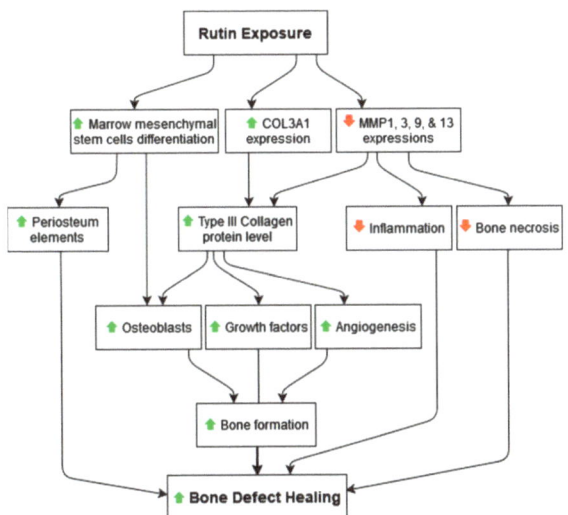

Figure 5. Proposed therapeutic mechanism of rutin for the acceleration and high success rates of bone grafts.

4. Materials and Methods

4.1. Preparation of the Rutin Gel

The rutin gel was prepared as previously described, but with some modifications [17]. Rutin and vehicle (without rutin) gels were prepared using the required components, which were safe and approved by the Food and Drug Administration. Briefly, ethanol (1 mL; Sigma-Aldrich, St. Louis, MO, USA) was used to solubilize the rutin powder (2.5 mg; APExBio, Houston, TX, USA), lipophilic surfactant "Span 60" (600 mg), soy lecithin (300 mg), and cholesterol (100 mg) (all from SRL, Mumbai, India). The mixture was warmed for approximately 5 min in a water bath at 70 °C with agitation. Pre-warmed distilled water (0.33 mL) was then added to the mixture and kept at the same temperature for approximately 3 min. After the solution was cooled to room temperature, the gel was stored in the dark until further use. A vehicle gel without rutin (used for the control group) was prepared by following all steps except for the addition of rutin. As part of the surgical procedure, 900 mg of bone graft was mixed with 100 mg of vehicle or rutin gel. The rutin dose used in this study was selected based on the safety margin previously reported [32,33].

4.2. In Vivo Experiments

In this study, six male New Zealand rabbits aged 10 months weighing between 2.75 and 3.5 kg were randomly divided into two groups: the control group received the vehicle gel, and the treated group received the rutin gel, which was combined with a demineralized freeze-dried bone allograft (DFDBA) and pericardium membrane (both from Zimmer Biomet, Palm Beach Gardens, FL, USA). A sterile standard diet and free access to water were provided to all animals under pathogen-free conditions.

4.3. Surgical Procedure

For general anesthesia, 40 mcg/kg dexmedetomidine HCl (used as sedative agent; APExBio) was combined with continuous isoflurane (Baxter, Deerfield, IL, USA) inhalation. Lidocaine hydrochloride (9 mg/kg; Sigma-Aldrich, St. Louis, MO, USA) was used to induce local anesthesia. The experimental defects were created using an extraoral approach through skin incisions. The first premolar to first molar teeth were incised, and a sulcular incision was made from the distal side of the lower second premolar to the mesial side of the first premolar. A vertical incision was made on the mesial side of the first premolar to achieve primary closure. Once the alveolar bone was exposed by raising the flap, lower anterior pediatric forceps were used to extract (atraumatic extraction) the mandibular first premolar PM-1 (unilaterally) from the lower teeth. Subsequently, the granulation tissue in the socket was completely cured. Randomly selected defects were assigned to the control and rutin groups. The defects were filled with 80 mg DFDBA with or without rutin gel and then covered with a pericardium collagen membrane. Interrupted sutures (resorbable polyglycolic acid, Unimed, Riyadh, Saudi Arabia) were used to close the flaps.

Following surgery, all animals were provided with special food pellets. As part of their post-surgery care, the rabbits were intramuscularly administered analgesics (1 mg/kg ketoprofen; Vemedim Animal Health, Can Tho, Vietnam) and antibiotics (4 mg/kg enrofloxacin; Avico, Amman, Jordan) every 24 h for 5 days. Two weeks after surgery, the extraoral sutures were removed and the intraoral sutures were reabsorbed (Figure 6).

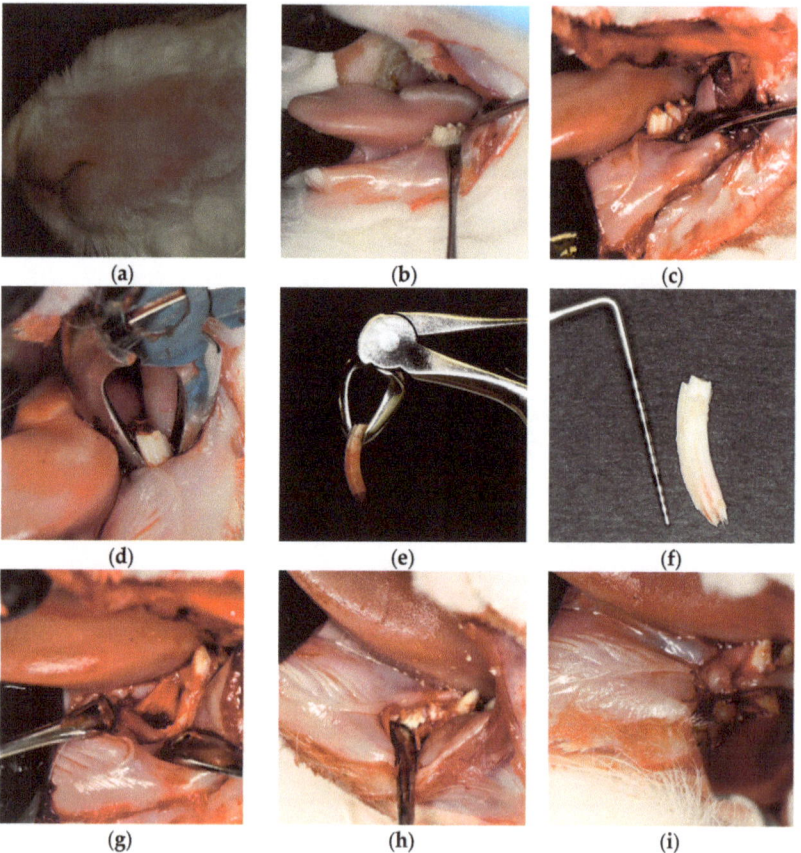

Figure 6. Cont.

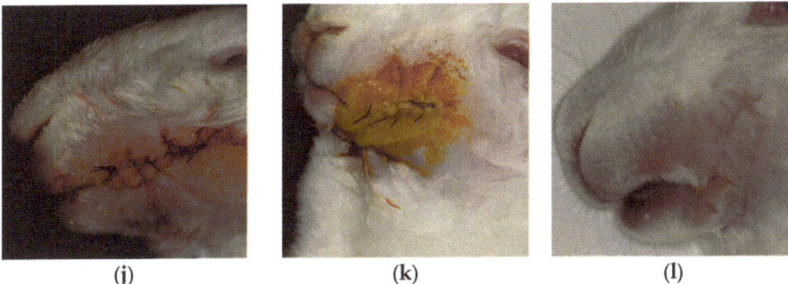

Figure 6. Surgical procedure. Hair was shaved after anesthesia (**a**); an external approach involves an incision in the skin exposing the surgical area (**b**); the alveolar bone was exposed around the first premolar (**c**); the extraction was performed with a lower anterior forceps (**d**); extracted lower first premolar (**e**); the lower first premolar was measured 15 mm long using the University of North Carolina-15 probe (**f**); first premolar socket (**g**); transplanted bone graft in the tooth socket and covered with a pericardium membrane (**h**); the surgical site was sutured with a resorbable type of polyglycolic acid sutures (**i**); the surgical site was sutured with extraoral sutures (**j**); an antiseptic and an antibiotic were applied to the skin after surgery (**k**); surgery site after 6 weeks (**l**).

4.4. Sample Collection

The experiment was terminated after 6 weeks based on the findings of our pilot study. In this pilot study, we examined bone formation without intervention (just tooth extraction) at different time points. At the end of the sixth week, we found that the bone healing process was still incomplete, whereas the healing process and new bone formation were almost completed 12 weeks after extraction. Therefore, we chose 6 weeks as a relevant time point for comparison as we were interested in studying whether adding rutin to the bone graft accelerates bone formation or not.

The animals were euthanized with carbon dioxide after 6 weeks. Then, the jawbones were extracted from sacrificed rabbits (Figure 7a,b). Bone specimens were obtained using surgical bone saw discs from the mesial aspect of the lower first molar to the mesial aspect of the lower first premolar (Figure 7c). The bone samples were fixed in 10% formalin for examination. In addition, soft tissue specimens around the surgical site were also collected from the area adjacent to the grafted bone and stored at $-80\,°C$. The groups were blindly assigned to independent examiners to prevent bias.

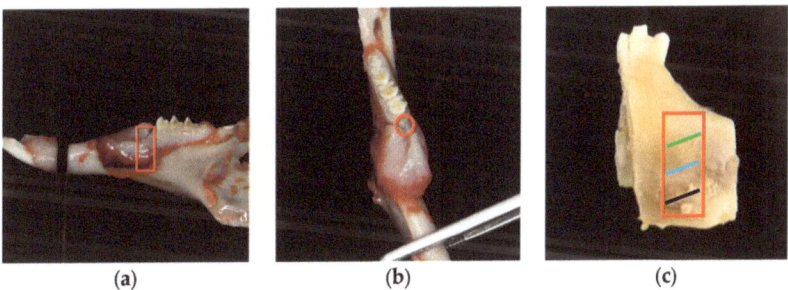

Figure 7. Preparation of the bone defect area for the sectioning procedure. Side view of extracted jawbone from a sacrificed rabbit with marked region of interest (**a**). Top view of extracted jawbone with marked region of interest (**b**). The area of interest was cut from the jawbone for histomorphometric analysis conducted in the marked red region. Green, blue, and black lines within the study area indicate coronal, middle, and apical widths, respectively (**c**).

4.5. RNA Extraction and cDNA Synthesis

Total RNA was extracted from tissue samples using Invitrogen TRIzol reagent (Thermo Fisher Scientific, Waltham, MA, USA), according to the manufacturer's instructions, and was quantified by measuring the absorbance at 260 nm using a Jenway Genova Nano Micro-Volume Life Science Spectrophotometer (Antylia Scientific, Vernon Hills, IL, USA). To determine the purity of the RNA, absorbance ratios of 260/280 nm (>1.8) were used. The respective cDNA was synthesized using High-Capacity cDNA Reverse Transcription Kit (Applied Biosystems, Waltham, MA, USA), in accordance with the manufacturer's instructions. Briefly, 1.5 µg of total RNA obtained from each sample was mixed with 2 µL 10× of reverse transcriptase buffer, 0.8 µL of 25× dNTP mix, 2 µL of 10× reverse transcriptase random primers (100 mM of each), 1 µL of MultiScribe reverse transcriptase, and 4.2 µL of nuclease-free water. The final reaction mixture was maintained at 25 °C for 10 min, then heated to 37 °C for 120 min, heated again to 85 °C for 5 min, and then cooled down to 4 °C.

4.6. Quantification of mRNA Expression

The quantitative expression of specific mRNAs was assessed by real-time polymerase chain reaction (PCR). Briefly, 1.4 µL of cDNA was added to 25 µL PCR reaction mixture, which also contained 0.25 µL of forward and reverse primers (100 nM final concentration of each primer), 10.6 µL nuclease-free water, and 12.5 µL SYBR Green Universal Master Mix (Applied Biosystems, Waltham, MA, USA). The primers used in the study (Table 2) were synthesized by Metabion (Planegg, Germany) and based on previously published studies [34–37]. The samples were analyzed in 96-well optical reaction plates using an ABI Prism 7500 System (Applied Biosystems, Waltham, MA, USA).

Table 2. Sequences of the primers used for real-time polymerase chain reaction analysis.

Gene	Forward Primer (5′–3′)	Reverse Primer (5′–3′)
MMP1	CCTGATGTGGCTCAGTTCGT	GTCCACATCTGCCCTTGACA
MMP3	TGGACCTGGAAATGTTTTGG	ATCAAAGTGGGCATCTCCAT
MMP9	ACGGCCGACTATGACACC	TTGCCGTCCTGGGTGTAG
MMP13	CCTCTTCTTCTCCGGAAACC	GGTAGTCTTGGTCCATGGTATGA
COL3A1	GCAGGGACTCCAGGTCTTAGAGG	CGTGTTCACCTCTCTCTCCCAGGG
GAPDH	CACAGTTTCCATCCCAGACC	TGGTTTCATGACAAGGTAGGG

As previously described [38], real-time PCR data were analyzed as relative gene expression using the $2^{-\Delta\Delta Ct}$ method. The target gene levels were normalized to those of *GAPDH* for comparing the fold change between the treated and untreated groups based on the following equation: fold change = $2^{-\Delta(\Delta Ct)}$, where $\Delta Ct = Ct_{target} - Ct_{GAPDH}$ and $\Delta(\Delta Ct) = \Delta Ct_{treated} - \Delta Ct_{untreated}$.

4.7. Histomorphometry

The measuring of histomorphometric parameters was described, specified, and accomplished according to the work of Okada et al. (2019) [39]. Approximately 3–5 mm thick bone samples were used from each group and immediately fixed in 10% formalin. A solution of 10% formalin and 12.5% EDTA was used for 6 weeks to decalcify the samples. Each sample was then submitted within a well-labeled cassette into an automatic tissue processing machine (ASP300s; Leica Biosystems, Wetzlar, Germany). Each sample was embedded in paraffin wax, and microtomy in the sagittal direction was performed using a rotary microtome (SHUR/Cut 4500; TBS, Durham, NC, USA) [40]. Two slides were produced from each block: one for hematoxylin–eosin staining for general purposes and the other for Masson's trichrome staining as a special staining method for connective tissue fibers [41,42]. Both stains were obtained from Nanjing Sen Beijing Jia Biological Technology Co. (Nanjing, China). To determine the most central part of the bone defect (extraction location) for histomorphometry analysis, digital periapical radiography using a hand-held

X-ray generator (Genoray America, Inc., Orange, CA, USA) was performed as shown in Figure 8. Five randomly selected microscopic fields were analyzed for each sample at 400× magnification.

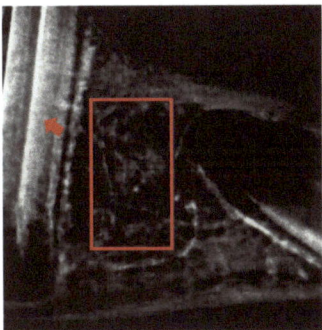

Figure 8. Periapical radiograph showing the most central area of the bone defect (rectangle shape) that was used for histomorphometry analysis of the lower first premolar tooth socket, in which randomly selected microscopic fields were analyzed.

Each bone sample came with a tooth, and the sample was oriented such that the tooth was posterior to the study area, apical width was measured in lower position of the study area, middle width was measured in the central position of the study area, coronal width was measured in the higher position of the study area, and bone formation area was the place where bone growth was observed within the study area.

4.8. Statistical Analysis

The collected data were analyzed using GraphPad Prism software version 9.4.0 (GraphPad Software, Boston, MA, USA). A total of six samples divided into two groups (n = 3 for each group) were analyzed. Unpaired t-tests were used to determine significant differences between the groups. $p < 0.05$ was deemed statistically significant.

5. Conclusions

Rutin gel and bone grafts can be locally applied to bone defects without the need for specialized instruments. This mixture, which contains biocompatible, readily available, inexpensive, and safe substances, supports rapid bone production and promotes good bone health. Hence, rutin gel and bone grafts can be used together to treat a wide range of dental and bone-related conditions. These findings provide new foundations for the periodontics and medical fields as they describe an easy, simple, and cost-effective approach for achieving the desired results in bone grafting procedures. In future studies, bending, axial compression, and torsion tests could be used to assess bone mechanical strength following rutin treatment with a bone graft mixture.

Author Contributions: Conceptualization, F.F.A., H.N.A., K.M.A. and F.A.A.; methodology, F.F.A., H.N.A., K.M.A. and F.A.A.; validation, F.F.A., H.N.A., K.M.A. and F.A.A.; formal analysis, F.F.A., H.N.A., K.M.A. and F.A.A.; investigation, F.F.A., H.N.A., K.M.A. and A.M.H.; writing—original draft preparation, F.F.A. and F.A.A.; writing—review and editing, F.F.A. and F.A.A.; visualization, F.F.A., H.N.A., K.M.A. and F.A.A.; supervision, F.F.A., H.N.A. and F.A.A.; project administration, F.F.A., H.N.A. and F.A.A. All authors have read and agreed to the published version of the manuscript.

Funding: This research received no external funding.

Institutional Review Board Statement: The University Research Ethics Committee in Health & Science Disciplines at Prince Sattam Bin Abdulaziz University (Alkharj, Saudi Arabia) approved the protocol (Approval No. 74/2021) for animal experiments in the College of Pharmacy, Pharmacology, and Toxicology laboratories.

Informed Consent Statement: Not applicable.

Data Availability Statement: All the data are given in the manuscript.

Acknowledgments: The authors thank Mohammed Nazam Ansari for technical assistance in monitoring animal health conditions.

Conflicts of Interest: The authors declare no conflict of interest.

References

1. Titsinides, S.; Agrogiannis, G.; Karatzas, T. Bone grafting materials in dentoalveolar reconstruction: A comprehensive review. *Jpn. Dent. Sci. Rev.* **2019**, *55*, 26–32. [CrossRef] [PubMed]
2. Bouxsein, M.L.; Turek, T.J.; Blake, C.A.; D'Augusta, D.; Li, X.; Stevens, M.; Seeherman, H.J.; Wozney, J.M. Recombinant Human Bone Morphogenetic Protein-2 Accelerates Healing in a Rabbit Ulnar Osteotomy Model. *J. Bone Joint Surg. Am.* **2001**, *83*, 1219–1230. [CrossRef]
3. El Bialy, I.; Jiskoot, W.; Reza Nejadnik, M. Formulation, Delivery and Stability of Bone Morphogenetic Proteins for Effective Bone Regeneration. *Pharm. Res.* **2017**, *34*, 1152–1170. [CrossRef] [PubMed]
4. Shimono, K.; Oshima, M.; Arakawa, H.; Kimura, A.; Nawachi, K.; Kuboki, T. The effect of growth factors for bone augmentation to enable dental implant placement: A systematic review. *Jpn. Dent. Sci. Rev.* **2010**, *46*, 43–53. [CrossRef]
5. Einhorn, T.A.; Gerstenfeld, L.C. Fracture healing: Mechanisms and interventions. *Nat. Rev. Rheumatol.* **2015**, *11*, 45–54. [CrossRef]
6. Kusano, K.; Miyaura, C.; Inada, M.; Tamura, T.; Ito, A.; Nagase, H.; Kamoi, K.; Suda, T. Regulation of Matrix Metalloproteinases (MMP-2, -3, -9, and -13) by Interleukin-1 and Interleukin-6 in Mouse Calvaria: Association of MMP Induction with Bone Resorption. *Endocrinology* **1998**, *139*, 1338–1345. [CrossRef]
7. Bonnans, C.; Chou, J.; Werb, Z. Remodelling the extracellular matrix in development and disease. *Nat. Rev. Mol. Cell Biol.* **2014**, *15*, 786–801. [CrossRef]
8. Elgezawi, M.; Haridy, R.; Almas, K.; Abdalla, M.A.; Omar, O.; Abuohashish, H.; Elembaby, A.; Christine Wölfle, U.; Siddiqui, Y.; Kaisarly, D. Matrix Metalloproteinases in Dental and Periodontal Tissues and Their Current Inhibitors: Developmental, Degradational and Pathological Aspects. *Int. J. Mol. Sci.* **2022**, *23*, 8929. [CrossRef]
9. Cheng, P.; Li, D.; Gao, Y.; Cao, T.; Jiang, H.; Wang, J.; Li, J.; Zhang, S.; Song, Y.; Liu, B.; et al. Prevascularization promotes endogenous cell-mediated angiogenesis by upregulating the expression of fibrinogen and connective tissue growth factor in tissue-engineered bone grafts. *Stem Cell. Res. Ther.* **2018**, *9*, 176–189. [CrossRef]
10. Li, S.; Li, Y.; Jiang, Z.; Hu, C.; Gao, Y.; Zhou, Q. Efficacy of total flavonoids of Rhizoma drynariae on the blood vessels and the bone graft in the induced membrane. *Phytomedicine* **2022**, *99*, 153995–154003. [CrossRef]
11. Benjamin, M.M.; Khalil, R.A. Matrix metalloproteinase inhibitors as investigative tools in the pathogenesis and management of vascular disease. *Exp. Suppl.* **2012**, *103*, 209–279. [CrossRef]
12. Kumar, G.B.; Nair, B.G.; Perry, J.J.P.; Martin, D.B.C. Recent insights into natural product inhibitors of matrix metalloproteinases. *Medchemcomm* **2019**, *10*, 2024–2037. [CrossRef]
13. Ganeshpurkar, A.; Saluja, A.K. The Pharmacological Potential of Rutin. *Saudi Pharm. J.* **2017**, *25*, 149–164. [CrossRef]
14. Sharma, S.; Ali, A.; Ali, J.; Sahni, J.K.; Baboota, S. Rutin: Therapeutic potential and recent advances in drug delivery. *Expert Opin. Investig. Drugs* **2013**, *22*, 1063–1079. [CrossRef]
15. Younis, T.; Jabeen, F.; Hussain, A.; Rasool, B.; Raza Ishaq, A.; Nawaz, A.; El-Nashar, H.A.S.; El-Shazly, M. Antioxidant and Pulmonary Protective Potential of Fraxinus xanthoxyloides Bark Extract against CCl4-Induced Toxicity in Rats. *Chem. Biodivers.* **2023**, *20*, e202200755. [CrossRef]
16. Abdelghffar, E.A.R.; Mostafa, N.M.; El-Nashar, H.A.S.; Eldahshan, O.A.; Singab, A.N.B. Chilean pepper (*Schinus polygamus*) ameliorates the adverse effects of hyperglycaemia/dyslipidaemia in high fat diet/streptozotocin-induced type 2 diabetic rat model. *Ind. Crops Prod.* **2022**, *183*, 114953. [CrossRef]
17. Pinzaru, I.; Tanase, A.; Enatescu, V.; Coricovac, D.; Bociort, F.; Marcovici, I.; Watz, C.; Vlaia, L.; Soica, C.; Dehelean, C. Proniosomal Gel for Topical Delivery of Rutin: Preparation, Physicochemical Characterization and In Vitro Toxicological Profile Using 3D Reconstructed Human Epidermis Tissue and 2D Cells. *Antioxidants* **2021**, *10*, 85. [CrossRef]
18. Liu, L.L.; Zhang, Y.; Zhang, X.F.; Li, F.H. Influence of rutin on the effects of neonatal cigarette smoke exposure-induced exacerbated MMP-9 expression, Th17 cytokines and NF-κB/iNOS-mediated inflammatory responses in asthmatic mice model. *Korean J. Physiol. Pharmacol.* **2018**, *22*, 481–491. [CrossRef]
19. Chen, X.; Yu, M.; Xu, W.; Zou, L.; Ye, J.; Liu, Y.; Xiao, Y.; Luo, J. Rutin inhibited the advanced glycation end products-stimulated inflammatory response and extra-cellular matrix degeneration via targeting TRAF-6 and BCL-2 proteins in mouse model of osteoarthritis. *Aging* **2021**, *13*, 22134–22147. [CrossRef]
20. Her, Y.; Lee, T.K.; Kim, J.D.; Kim, B.; Sim, H.; Lee, J.C.; Ahn, J.H.; Park, J.H.; Lee, J.W.; Hong, J.; et al. Topical Application of Aronia melanocarpa Extract Rich in Chlorogenic Acid and Rutin Reduces UVB-Induced Skin Damage via Attenuating Collagen Disruption in Mice. *Molecules* **2020**, *25*, 4577. [CrossRef]

21. Mitchell, P.G.; Magna, H.A.; Reeves, L.M.; Lopresti-Morrow, L.L.; Yocum, S.A.; Rosner, P.J.; Geoghegan, K.F.; Hambor, J.E. Cloning, expression, and type II collagenolytic activity of matrix metalloproteinase-13 from human osteoarthritic cartilage. *J. Clin. Investig.* **1996**, *97*, 761–768. [CrossRef]
22. Soundia, A.; Hadaya, D.; Esfandi, N.; Gkouveris, I.; Christensen, R.; Dry, S.M.; Bezouglaia, O.; Pirih, F.; Nikitakis, N.; Aghaloo, T.; et al. Zoledronate Impairs Socket Healing after Extraction of Teeth with Experimental Periodontitis. *J. Dent. Res.* **2018**, *97*, 312–320. [CrossRef] [PubMed]
23. Hu, Y.; Zhang, T.; Huang, H.; Cheng, W.; Lai, Y.; Bai, X.; Chen, J.; Yue, Y.; Zheng, Z.; Guo, C.; et al. Fracture healing in a collagen-induced arthritis rat model: Radiology and histology evidence. *J. Orthop. Res.* **2018**, *36*, 2876–2885. [CrossRef] [PubMed]
24. Garnero, P. The Role of Collagen Organization on the Properties of Bone. *Calcif. Tissue Int.* **2015**, *97*, 229–240. [CrossRef] [PubMed]
25. Abdul-Fattah Baraka, N.; Fathallah Ahmed, N.; Ismail Hussein, S. The effect of Rutin hydrate on Glucocorticoids induced osteoporosis in mandibular alveolar bone in Albino rats (Radiological, histological and histochemical study). *Saudi Dent. J.* **2022**, *34*, 464–472. [CrossRef]
26. Lee, H.-H.; Jang, J.-W.; Lee, J.-K.; Park, C.-K. Rutin Improves Bone Histomorphometric Values by Reduction of Osteoclastic Activity in Osteoporosis Mouse Model Induced by Bilateral Ovariectomy. *J. Korean Neurosurg. Soc.* **2020**, *63*, 433–443. [CrossRef]
27. Chen, X.; Hu, C.; Wang, G.; Li, L.; Kong, X.; Ding, Y.; Jin, Y. Nuclear factor-κB modulates osteogenesis of periodontal ligament stem cells through competition with β-catenin signaling in inflammatory microenvironments. *Cell Death Dis.* **2013**, *4*, 510–518. [CrossRef]
28. Xiao, Y.; Wei, R.; Yuan, Z.; Lan, X.; Kuang, J.; Hu, D.; Song, Y.; Luo, J. Rutin suppresses FNDC1 expression in bone marrow mesenchymal stem cells to inhibit postmenopausal osteoporosis. *Am. J. Transl. Res.* **2019**, *11*, 6680–6690.
29. Moreira, C.A.; Dempster, D.W.; Baron, R. Anatomy and ultrastructure of bone–histogenesis, growth and remodeling. In *Endotext*; Feingold, K.R., Anawalt, B., Blackman, M.R., Boyce, A., Chrousos, G., Corpas, E., de Herder, W.W., Dhatariya, K., Dungan, K., Hofland, J., et al., Eds.; MDText.com, Inc.: South Dartmouth, MA, USA, 2000.
30. Colnot, C. Skeletal cell fate decisions within periosteum and bone marrow during bone regeneration. *J. Bone Miner. Res.* **2009**, *24*, 274–282. [CrossRef]
31. Petrescu, H.P.; Dinu, G.; Nodiți, G.; Berceanu-Văduva, M.; Bratu, D.C.; Vermeșan, D. Experimental morphologic and radiologic study of the integration of bone grafts into the host tissue and of the dynamics of the graft-receptor interface. *Rom. J. Morphol. Embryol.* **2014**, *55*, 607–612.
32. da Silva, J.; Herrmann, S.M.; Heuser, V.; Peres, W.; Possa Marroni, N.; González-Gallego, J.; Erdtmann, B. Evaluation of the genotoxic effect of rutin and quercetin by comet assay and micronucleus test. *Food Chem. Toxicol.* **2002**, *40*, 941–947. [CrossRef]
33. Cristina Marcarini, J.; Ferreira Tsuboy, M.S.; Cabral Luiz, R.; Regina Ribeiro, L.; Beatriz Hoffmann-Campo, C.; Ségio Mantovani, M. Investigation of cytotoxic, apoptosis-inducing, genotoxic and protective effects of the flavonoid rutin in HTC hepatic cells. *Exp. Toxicol. Pathol.* **2011**, *63*, 459–465. [CrossRef]
34. Saulnier, N.; Viguier, E.; Perrier-Groult, E.; Chenu, C.; Pillet, E.; Roger, T.; Maddens, S.; Boulocher, C. Intra-articular administration of xenogeneic neonatal Mesenchymal Stromal Cells early after meniscal injury down-regulates metalloproteinase gene expression in synovium and prevents cartilage degradation in a rabbit model of osteoarthritis. *Osteoarthr. Cartil.* **2015**, *23*, 122–133. [CrossRef]
35. Inoue, H.; Arai, Y.; Kishida, T.; Terauchi, R.; Honjo, K.; Nakagawa, S.; Tsuchida, S.; Matsuki, T.; Ueshima, K.; Fujiwara, H.; et al. Hydrostatic pressure influences HIF-2 alpha expression in chondrocytes. *Int. J. Mol. Sci.* **2015**, *16*, 1043–1050. [CrossRef]
36. Ishibashi, H.; Tonomura, H.; Ikeda, T.; Nagae, M.; Sakata, M.; Fujiwara, H.; Tanida, T.; Mastuda, K.-I.; Kawata, M.; Kubo, T. Hepatocyte growth factor/c-met promotes proliferation, suppresses apoptosis, and improves matrix metabolism in rabbit nucleus pulposus cells in vitro. *J. Orthop. Res.* **2016**, *34*, 709–716. [CrossRef]
37. González, J.C.; López, C.; Álvarez, M.E.; Pérez, J.E.; Carmona, J.U. Autologous leukocyte-reduced platelet-rich plasma therapy for Achilles tendinopathy induced by collagenase in a rabbit model. *Sci. Rep.* **2016**, *6*, 19623–19633. [CrossRef]
38. Livak, K.J.; Schmittgen, T.D. Analysis of relative gene expression data using real-time quantitative PCR and the 2−ΔΔCT method. *Methods* **2001**, *25*, 402–408. [CrossRef]
39. Okada, M.; Matsuura, T.; Akizuki, T.; Hoshi, S.; Shujaa Addin, A.; Fukuba, S.; Izumi, Y. Ridge preservation of extraction sockets with buccal bone deficiency using poly lactide-co-glycolide coated β-tricalcium phosphate bone grafts: An experimental study in dogs. *J. Periodontol.* **2019**, *90*, 1014–1022. [CrossRef]
40. Hamad, A.M.; Ahmed, H.G. Association of some carbohydrates with estrogen expression in breast lesions among Sudanese females. *J. Histotechnol.* **2018**, *41*, 2–9. [CrossRef]
41. Hamad, A.; Ahmed, H. Association of connective tissue fibers with estrogen expression in breast lesions among Sudanese females. *Int. Clin. Pathol. J* **2016**, *2*, 97–102. [CrossRef]
42. Suvarna, S.K.; Layton, C.; Bancroft, J.D. *Theory and Practice of Histological Techniqueseighth*; Elsevier: Amsterdam, The Netherlands, 2019.

Disclaimer/Publisher's Note: The statements, opinions and data contained in all publications are solely those of the individual author(s) and contributor(s) and not of MDPI and/or the editor(s). MDPI and/or the editor(s) disclaim responsibility for any injury to people or property resulting from any ideas, methods, instructions or products referred to in the content.

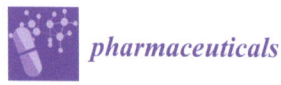

Article

Annona cherimola Miller and Its Flavonoids, an Important Source of Products for the Treatment of Diabetes Mellitus: In Vivo and In Silico Evaluations

Fernando Calzada [1,*], Miguel Valdes [2,*], Jesús Martínez-Solís [2], Claudia Velázquez [3] and Elizabeth Barbosa [2]

1 Unidad de Investigación Médica en Farmacología, UMAE Hospital de Especialidades 2° Piso CORSE, Centro Médico Nacional Siglo XXI, Instituto Mexicano del Seguro Social, Av. Cuauhtémoc 330, Col. Doctores, Mexico City CP 06720, Mexico
2 Instituto Politécnico Nacional, Sección de Estudios de Posgrado e Investigación, Escuela Superior de Medicina, Plan de San Luis y Salvador Díaz Mirón S/N, Col. Casco de Santo Tomás, Miguel Hidalgo, Mexico City CP 11340, Mexico; jarimarts27@gmail.com (J.M.-S.); rebc78@yahoo.com.mx (E.B.)
3 Área Académica de Farmacia, Instituto de Ciencias de la Salud, Universidad Autonoma del Estado de Hidalgo, Circuito exHacienda La Concepcion s/n, Carretera Pachuca-Atocpan, San Agustin Tlaxiaca CP 42076, Mexico; cvg09@yahoo.com
* Correspondence: fercalber10@gmail.com (F.C.); valdesguevaramiguel@gmail.com (M.V.); Tel.: +52-5627-6900 (ext. 21367) (F.C. & M.V.)

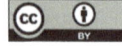

Citation: Calzada, F.; Valdes, M.; Martínez-Solís, J.; Velázquez, C.; Barbosa, E. *Annona cherimola* Miller and Its Flavonoids, an Important Source of Products for the Treatment of Diabetes Mellitus: In Vivo and In Silico Evaluations. *Pharmaceuticals* 2023, *16*, 724. https://doi.org/10.3390/ph16050724

Academic Editor: Patrícia Rijo

Received: 7 April 2023
Revised: 29 April 2023
Accepted: 3 May 2023
Published: 10 May 2023

Copyright: © 2023 by the authors. Licensee MDPI, Basel, Switzerland. This article is an open access article distributed under the terms and conditions of the Creative Commons Attribution (CC BY) license (https://creativecommons.org/licenses/by/4.0/).

Abstract: The antihyperglycemic activity of ethanolic extract from *Annona cherimola* Miller (EEAch) and its products were evaluated using in vivo and in silico assays. An α-glucosidase inhibition was evaluated with oral sucrose tolerance tests (OSTT) and molecular docking studies using acarbose as the control. SGLT1 inhibition was evaluated with an oral glucose tolerance test (OGTT) and molecular docking studies using canagliflozin as the control. Among all products tested, EEAc, the aqueous residual fraction (AcRFr), rutin, and myricetin reduced the hyperglycemia in DM2 mice. During the carbohydrate tolerance tests, all the treatments reduced the postprandial peak such as the control drugs. In the molecular docking studies, rutin showed more affinity in inhibiting α-glucosidase enzymes and myricetin in inhibiting the SGLT1 cotransporter, showing ∆G values of −6.03 and −3.32 kcal/mol^{-1}, respectively, in α-glucosidase enzymes. In the case of the SGLT1 cotransporter, molecular docking showed ∆G values of 22.82 and −7.89 in rutin and myricetin, respectively. This research sorts in vivo and in silico pharmacological studies regarding the use of *A. cherimola* leaves as a source for the development of new potential antidiabetic agents for T2D control, such as flavonoids rutin and myricetin.

Keywords: *Annona cherimola* Miller; antihyperglycemic activity; flavonoids; in vivo assays; in silico assays

1. Introduction

Diabetes Mellitus (DM) type 2 is characterized by polydipsia, polyphagia, polyuria, and weight loss and accounts for 90 to 95% of all diabetes cases [1]. According to the International Federation of Diabetes, there are over 537 million people worldwide living whit in 2021 [2]. Further, the WHO estimates that DM caused 1.6 million deaths in 2016; therefore, it is considered one of the main causes of deaths globally [3].

In addition to lack of insulin secretion or resistance in skeletal muscle tissue, this chronic disease has a polygenic origin that includes another factor called ominous octet [4], which leads to an increase in blood glucose levels that is the main characteristic and cause of micro- and macrovascular consequences [5].

Generally, for the therapeutic management of diabetes, drugs with varying chemical structures are used to normalize blood glucose levels through different mechanisms of action [6]. These treatments are administered orally or in the parenteral way for life, which often represents a high financial cost. Moreover, the appearance of adverse effects or hypersensitivity reactions are situations that make it necessary to suspend the treatment or change it constantly [7]. These reasons make the development of new agents with antidiabetic properties important. One of the main targets for the search for new antidiabetic drugs is the inhibition of intestinal glucosidases. Iminosugars synthesized and sugar derivatives are potential antidiabetic drugs, showing a favorable impact in glycosidase inhibition, improving their activity through inhibitor synthesis and design of conformational preorganization [8,9]. On the other hand, medicinal plants are an excellent alternative to finding complementary treatments to achieve improved control of hyperglycemia [10].

More than 400 plant species have been registered for the control of diabetes [11]; however, only a few of these have received scientific and chemical evaluations to prove their effectiveness [12]. Compounds in medicinal plants have antidiabetic potential through several mechanisms [13], including the inhibition of glucose uptake in the gut, stimulation of insulin secretion from the pancreas, and many others that can influence its therapeutic potential.

In this sense, in the Annonaceae family, some genera are characterized by the economic interest of their fruits; such is the case of the genus Annona spp., which consists of many species, of which about 20 are cultivated for said interest [14]. Moreover, several species include compounds that have already been studied for their antidiabetic properties [15]. Among the most cultivated is *Annona cherimola* Miller (*A. cherimola*). It is a perennial tree of edible fruit whose leaves are present almost all year [16]. However, it is known that environmental conditions such as temperature and humidity can modify the growth of its leaves and modify the concentration of the bioactive compounds [17]. *A cherimola* constitutes part of the natural flora in Central America and South America, where it is known as "anona" or "cherimoya" and is widely cultivated and used as a traditional medicinal remedy by local populations to treat various illnesses, including gastrointestinal disorders, worms, and diarrhea [18]. Research has recently intensified mainly due to the discovery of the great potential of the natural products they contain [19]. Further, it is the only species within this genus to which special attention has been paid due to its medicinal and nutritional values, which have been exploited in Europe, where it has been preserved and consumed for the aroma and delicate flavor of its fruits. Hence, its acceptance from the commercial point of view as an exotic fruit is widely disseminated internationally, with a marked interest in its expansion [20]. Its marketing generally goes from the local scale to the international level, and as the cherimoya begins to be better known, it is the object of greater attention by researchers, growers, and consumers from many countries [21]. For this reason, it is necessary to stimulate scientific research related to the biological activity of some of its components, medicinal properties, and its various potentialities in human nutrition. In addition, this species is significant in the conservation and restoration of ecosystems.

Recent studies have provided information that the leaves of this species have antidepressant [22], pro-apoptotic [23], and antilipidemic activities [24]. Further, previous investigations showed that extract from the leaves of this species has an antidiabetic effect when it is administered orally in acute and subchronic treatment alone [25] or even in combination with the main antidiabetic drugs [26], with a wide frame of security with an LD_{50} over 3000 mg/kg without toxic effects in healthy organs [27].

It is known that the leaves of this species contain many kinds of compounds [28] that exert antihyperglycemic activities responsible for their medicinal potential [29], where flavonoids are highlighted due to their wide-ranging properties [30].

Although the antidiabetics [31] and other effects related to the antioxidant mechanisms [32] of the rutin constituent present in a greater quantity in the leaves of this species have already been studied [33], there are no studies that evaluate other components present in lower concentrations in the leaves of *Annona cherimola*.

Thus, the present study aims to assess the effect of the minor components obtained from the leaves of *Annona cherimola* in a diabetic model to show its antihyperglycemic potential that may contribute to validating its use in the treatment of diabetics.

2. Results

2.1. In Vivo Assays

2.1.1. Acute Evaluation of the Antidiabetic Effect of Ethanolic Extract from *Annona cherimola* and Its Polyphenols

Initially, the acute antihyperglycemic effect of the treatments was measured using a single dose; this was selected to determine the probable activity of the treatments in the short term (2 and 4 h) over the hyperglycemic values.

The ethanolic extract obtained from the leaves from *Annona cherimola* Miller (EEAch) was determined. It exhibited a significative reduction of hyperglycemia at 2 and 4 h after the administration of 300 mg/kg of EEAch; this effect was significative in comparison with the initial values and comparison with the alloxan-induced type 2 diabetic mice (AIT2D) control (Table 1).

Table 1. Blood glucose levels of normoglycemic mice (NM) and alloxan-induced type 2 diabetic mice (AIT2D) at 0, 2, and 4 h, on the acute antihyperglycemic test.

Treatment	Glycemia (mg/dL)		
	0 h	2 h	4 h
NM Control	154.3 ± 0.4	151.3 ± 1.2	146.6 ± 2.1
AIT2D Control	214.0 ± 5.7	218.5 ± 3.7	221.5 ± 3.9
AIT2D + EEAch	205.0 ± 4.0	143.7 ± 2.4 *,$^\Delta$	134.0 ± 5.1 *,$^{\Delta\Delta}$
AIT2D + AcRFr	204.0 ± 2.8	163.7 ± 3.6 *,$^\Delta$	174.7 ± 0.8 *,$^{\Delta\Delta}$
AIT2D + DCMFr	207.0 ± 5.1	181.0 ± 0.8 *,$^\Delta$	189.0 ± 0.4 *,$^{\Delta\Delta}$
AIT2D + Astragalin	203.3 ± 4.8	190.7 ± 1.3 $^\Delta$	200.0 ± 2.6 $^{\Delta\Delta}$
AIT2D + Chlorogenic acid	171.0 ± 12.5	193.0 ± 6.4 $^\Delta$	211.0 ± 3.4 $^{\Delta\Delta}$
AIT2D + Hyperin	203.0 ± 1.4	152.7 ± 5.5 *,$^\Delta$	184.0 ± 5.3 *,$^{\Delta\Delta}$
AIT2D + Isoquercitrin	206.3 ± 5.1	169.0 ± 3.2 *,$^\Delta$	197.7 ± 3.6 $^{\Delta\Delta}$
AIT2D + Myricetin	197.3 ± 2.5	161.0 ± 6.2 *,$^\Delta$	155.0 ± 3.1 *,$^{\Delta\Delta}$
AIT2D + Narcissin	204.7 ± 4.0	186.0 ± 4.1 $^\Delta$	167.3 ± 6.3 *,$^{\Delta\Delta}$
AIT2D + Nicotiflorin	206.7 ± 0.3	176.7 ± 2.1 *,$^\Delta$	179.7 ± 2.4 *,$^{\Delta\Delta}$
AIT2D + Rutin	214.3 ± 4.0	170.6 ± 8.3 *,$^\Delta$	162.3 ± 3.6 *,$^{\Delta\Delta}$
AIT2D + Acarbose	205.0 ± 1.6	190.0 ± 2.0 *,$^\Delta$	181.3 ± 3.0 *,$^{\Delta\Delta}$

EEAch, AcRFr, and DCMFr were administered at 300 mg/kg; astragalin, chlorogenic acid, hyperin, isoquercitrin, myricetin, narcissin, nicotiflorin rutin, and acarbose were administered at 50 mg/kg. Data are expressed as means ± SEM, $n = 6$; * $p < 0.05$ vs. initial values; Δ $p < 0.05$ vs. SIT2D control for 2 h; $\Delta\Delta$ $p < 0.05$ vs. SIT2D control for 4 h SEM: standard error of the mean; NM: normoglycemic mice; AIT2D: alloxan-induced type 2 diabetes mice; EEAch: ethanolic extract of *Annona cherimola* Miller; AcRFr: aqueous residual fraction; DCMFr: dichloromethane fraction.

After the fractionation of the extract, we obtained the dichloromethane fraction (DCMFr) and an aqueous residual fraction (AcRFr); both fractions were evaluated to determine their antihyperglycemic effect. When those products were administered, a significant reduction of hyperglycemia was observed at 2 and 4 h in both treatments (Table 1). Being more effective, the AcRFr reduces the hyperglycemic values near normoglycemic mice values.

The purification of AcRFr was carried out using preparative thin-layer chromatography, and this led to the isolation of eight compounds with polyphenolic characteristics, astragalin, chlorogenic acid, hyperin, isoquercitrin, myricetin, narcissin, nicotiflorin, and rutin (see Supplementary Materials). Following the scheme of work, all compounds were evaluated in the AIT2D model to determine which of them reduces hyperglycemia; the effect was compared with the oral antidiabetic drug (OAD) acarbose.

All compounds and acarbose were administered at the dose of 50 mg/kg. We observed that after administration, hyperin, myricetin, nicotiflorin, and rutin significantly reduced the hyperglycemic values at 2 and 4 h, and similar activity was observed in the group treated with acarbose. The effect over hyperglycemic values observed was significant in comparison with the initial values, and in comparison, with the AIT2D control at the respective times of measurement. In the case of isoquercitrin, it significantly reduces hyperglycemic values only at 2 h of the treatment and narcissin at 4 h; both effects were significant in comparison with AIT2D control. On the other hand, astragalin and chlorogenic acid did not generate a significant reduction in hyperglycemia (Table 1).

The results obtained allowed us to determine that myricetin and rutin were the compounds with the major antidiabetic effect; therefore, both compounds were selected to be evaluated in a subchronic assay as well as EEAc and AcRFr.

2.1.2. Subchronical Evaluation of the Antidiabetic Effect of Ethanolic Extract from *Annona cherimola*, AcRFr, Myricetin, and Rutin

The products with the best acute antihyperglycemic activity from *A. cherimola* were evaluated in a subchronic assay.

We observed that animals treated with EEAch showed a significant reduction of hyperglycemic values from week one, reaching normoglycemic values in week two; however, in weeks three and four, the glycemic values began to increase again. During the experiment, the hyperglycemia reduction was significant in comparison with the initial values and the AIT2D control (Figure 1A).

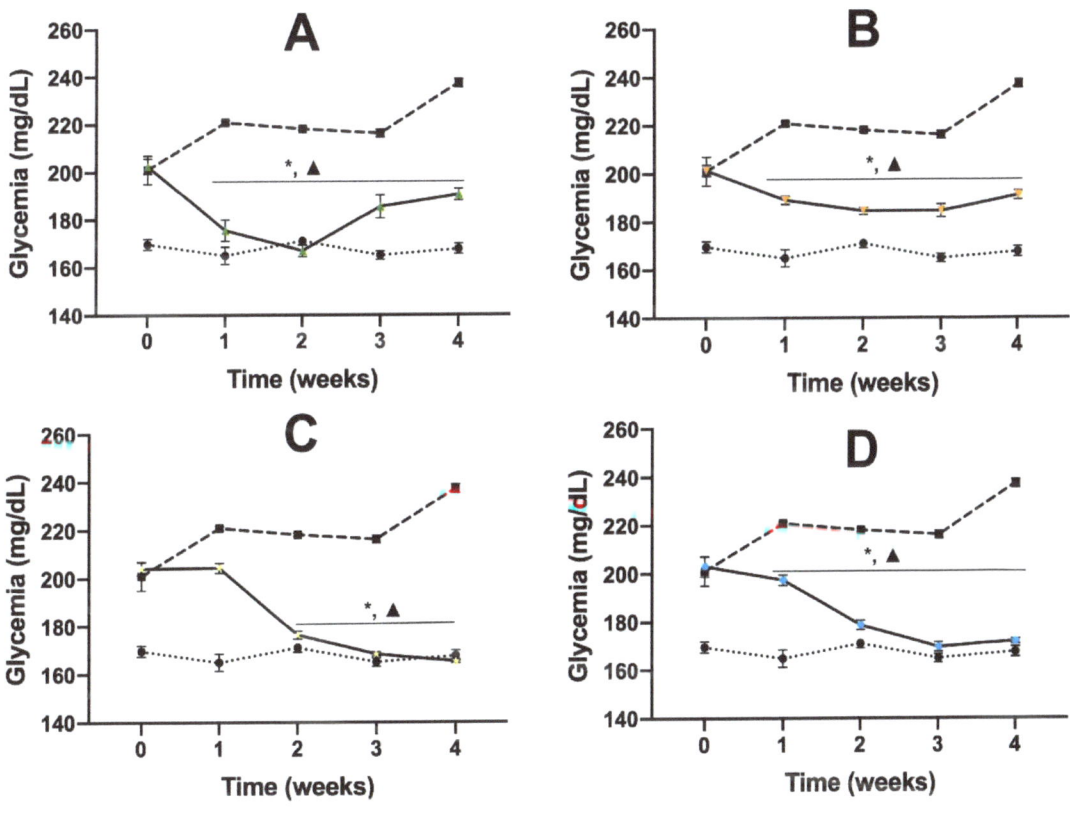

Figure 1. *Cont.*

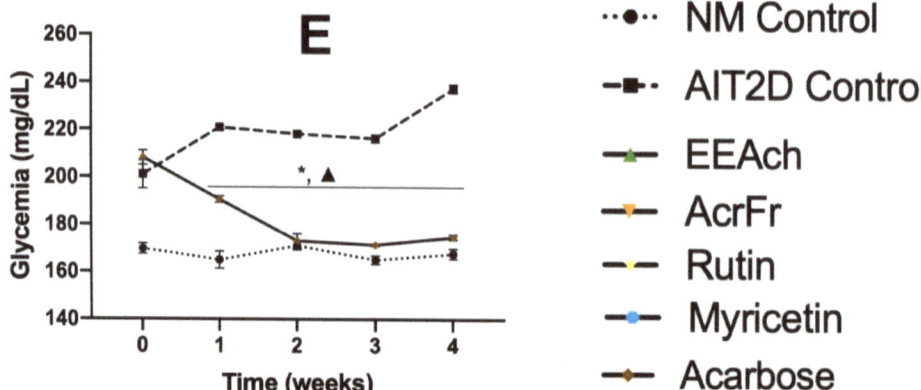

Figure 1. Effect over glycemic values of subchronic administration of the treatments in AIT2D mice. Groups treated with EEAch 300 mg/kg (**A**), AcRFr 300 mg/kg (**B**), rutin 50 mg/kg (**C**), myricetin 50 mg/kg (**D**), and acarbose 50 mg/kg (**E**). Results are expressed as the mean ± SEM, $n = 6$, * $p < 0.05$ vs. initial values; Δ $p < 0.05$ vs. AIT2D control at same week of treatment. NM: normoglycemic mice; AIT2D: alloxan-induced type 2 diabetes mice; EEAch: ethanolic extract of *Annona cherimola* Miller; AcRFr: aqueous residual fraction.

The group treated with AcRFr showed a significant reduction of hyperglycemia from week one, this reduction was constant during the experiment, and the antidiabetic effect was significant in comparison with the initial values and the AIT2D control (Figure 1B); however, in this case, the normoglycemic values was never reached.

In the case of rutin, this treatment shows a significant reduction of hyperglycemia from week two in comparison with the AIT2D control, and reaching normoglycemic values from week three, this effect was observed until the end of the assay (Figure 1C).

For the other flavonoid, the group treated with myricetin showed an effect similar to the group treated with rutin, i.e., a good reduction of hyperglycemic values from week one. This reduction was significant in comparison with the initial values as well as with the AIT2D control. Moreover, this group reached normoglycemic values from week two, and this activity was observed until the end of the assay (Figure 1D).

Finally, the group treated with acarbose showed a significant reduction from week one; this effect was similar to the observed in the groups treated with the flavonoids rutin and myricetin (Figure 1E).

The results showed us that rutin and myricetin were compounds with good antihyperglycemic activity in acute and subchronic assays; the next step of our study was to determine their potential inhibitory activity over a-glucosidase enzyme and SGLT-1 cotransporter, two important proteins involved in the carbohydrates metabolism. These determinations were made with in vivo oral glucose and sucrose tolerance test and in silico assays.

2.1.3. Oral Glucose and Sucrose Tolerance Test (OGTT and OSTT) of Ethanolic Extract from *Annona cherimola*, AcRFr, Myricetin, and Rutin

In the oral sucrose tolerance test (OSTT) assay, after the administration of EEAch, AcRFr, rutin, and myricetin, a significative reduction of the postprandial peak was observed. All the treatments were significant in comparison with the group treated with sucrose at 2 and 4 h (Figure 2A).

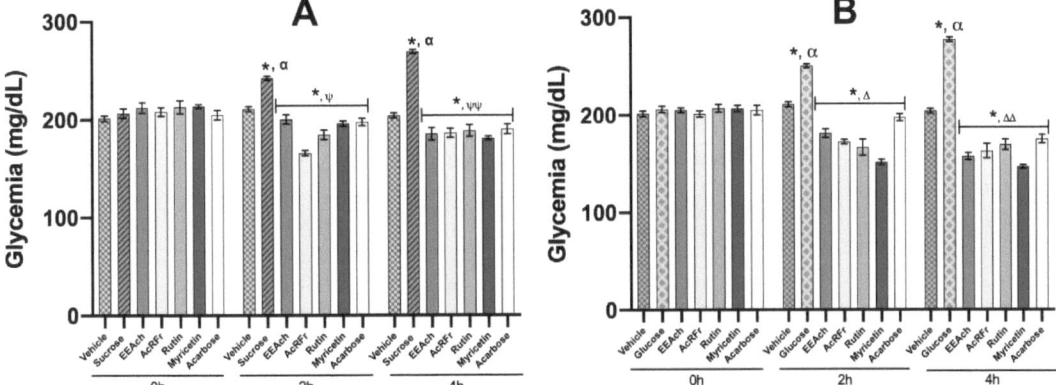

Figure 2. Effect of isolated products from *A. cherimola* on the oral sucrose (OSTT), and glucose tolerance test (OGTT). (**A**) OSTT assay, groups treated with vehicle, sucrose (3 g/kg), EEAch, AcRFr (300 mg/kg), rutin, myricetin, and acarbose (50 mg/kg). (**B**) OGTT assay, groups treated with vehicle, glucose (1.5 g/kg), EEAch, AcRFr (300 mg/kg), rutin, myricetin, and acarbose (50 mg/kg). Data are expressed as means ± SEM, $n = 6$; * $p < 0.05$ vs. initial values; ψ $p < 0.05$ vs. sucrose group 2 h; ψψ $p < 0.05$ vs. sucrose group 4 h; α $p < 0.05$ vs. vehicle 0 h; Δ $p < 0.05$ vs. glucose group 2 h; ΔΔ $p < 0.05$ vs. glucose group 2 h.

Further, we observed that the group treated with rutin showed lower glycemic levels in comparison with myricetin and acarbose at 2 h of the assay.

When the oral glucose tolerance test (OGTT) was carried out, the postprandial glucose peak was inhibited in all the treatments administered. The reduction observed was significant in comparison with the group treated with glucose at 2 and 4 h. Moreover, it is important to mention that in this assay, the group treated with myricetin showed lower glycemic levels than the other treatments, inclusive of the control acarbose group (Figure 2B).

Both results suggest that rutin may have more selectivity to prevent glucose uptake from complex carbohydrate hydrolysis and myricetin from simple carbohydrates.

2.2. In Silico Assays

2.2.1. Molecular Docking Studies of Rutin, Myricetin, and Acarbose on α-Glucosidase Enzyme

To determine the possible interaction of rutin and myricetin, a molecular docking study using as a target the α-glucosidase enzyme was carried out. This enzyme is involved in the hydrolysis of complex carbohydrates such as sucrose. As a control, we used acarbose, an inhibitor of the α-glucosidase enzyme and co-crystalized ligand of the protein 2QMJ.

The molecular docking analysis showed that rutin has the best affinity to the α-glucosidase enzyme with ΔG values of -6.03 kcal·mol^{-1}; it showed ten polar interactions with aminoacidic residues of the enzyme. In the case of myricetin, its affinity values were -3.32 kcal·mol^{-1}, with ten polar interactions. Both ligands also have four and three nonpolar interactions, respectively. For acarbose, it showed affinity values of -4.39 kcal·mol^{-1}, with sixteen polar and two nonpolar interactions (Table 2).

The analysis of the 3D model of binding suggests that the three ligands have the same binding pocket, and their position is similar (Figure 3). It is important to highlight that rutin showed the best affinity to the enzyme than the pharmacological control acarbose.

Table 2. Binding energy and interactions of ligands rutin, myricetin, and acarbose on α-glucosidase enzyme.

Ligand	ΔG (kcal·mol^{-1})	α-Glucosidase		
		H-BR	NPI	RMSD
Rutin	−6.03	Asp203, Asp327, Trp441, Met444, Ser448, Phe450, Arg526, Trp539 Asp542, His600	Tyr299, Trp406, Asp443, Phe575,	-
Myricetin	−3.32	Asp203, Thr204, Thr205, Trp406, Met444, Ser448, Asn449, Phe450, Arg526, Asp542	Tyr299, Lys480, Phe575	-
Acarbose	−4.39	Arg202, Thr204, Tyr299, Asp327, Ile328, Ile364, Trp441, Asp443, Phe450, Asp474, Lys480, Arg526, Trp539, Asp542, Phe575, His600	Trp406, Met444	1.93

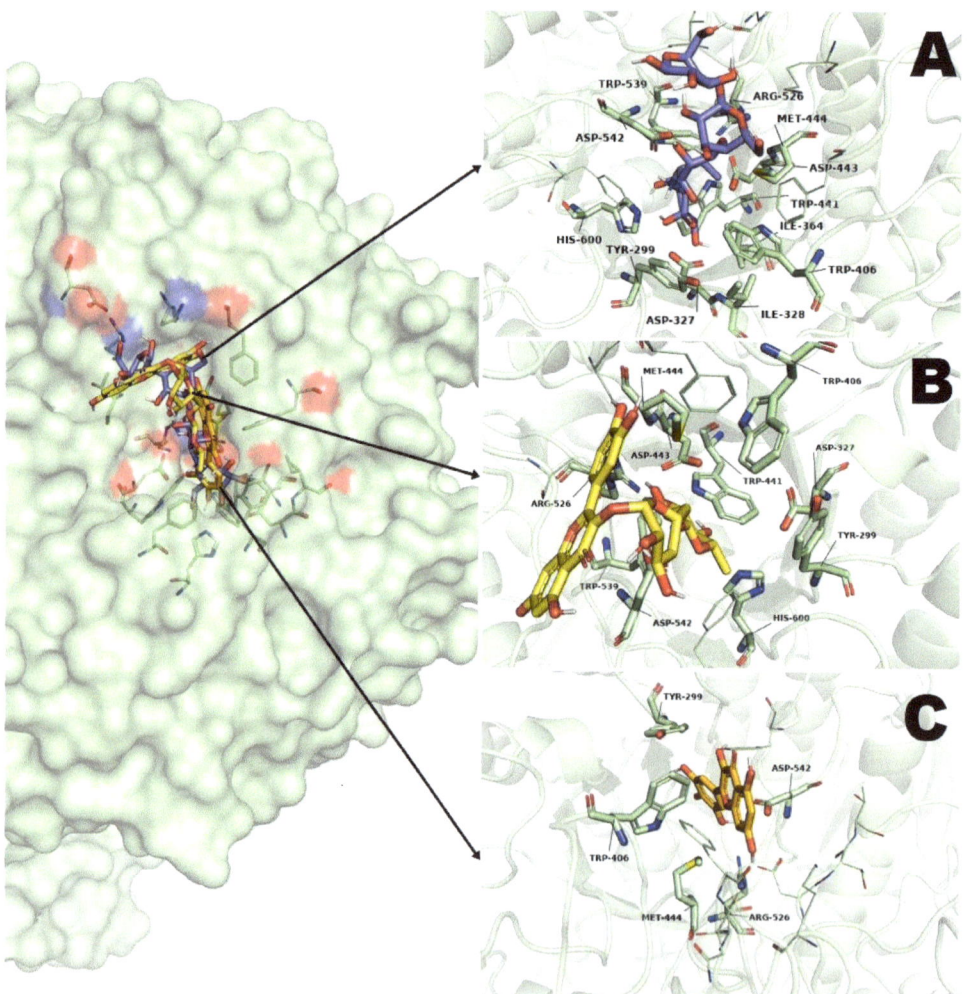

Figure 3. Results of molecular docking on α-glucosidase enzyme. (**A**) Interaction of acarbose and its binding site position; (**B**) Interaction of rutin and its binding site position; (**C**) Interaction of myricetin and its binding site position.

2.2.2. Molecular Docking Studies of Rutin, Myricetin and Canagliflozin on SGLT1 Cotransporter

The other molecular docking study was carried out using the SGLT1 cotransporter, a protein important involved in the monosaccharide's absorption on the enterocyte; as a control ligand, canagliflozin was used.

The analysis of results from molecular docking showed that rutin has binding free energy (ΔG) values of 22.82 kcal·mol^{-1}, with nineteen polar interactions and two nonpolar interactions with the amino acid residues from SGLT1 cotransporter. On the other hand, myricetin showed ΔG values of -7.89 kcal·mol^{-1}, with nine polar interactions and four nonpolar interactions. In the case of the pharmacological control canagliflozin, it showed the best ΔG values of -10.08 kcal·mol^{-1}, with sixteen polar and six nonpolar interactions (Table 3). The analysis of the 3D of the binding site suggests that the three ligands have the same binding position (Figure 4); however, the ΔG values shown for rutin suggest that this binding position is highly unlikely to take place.

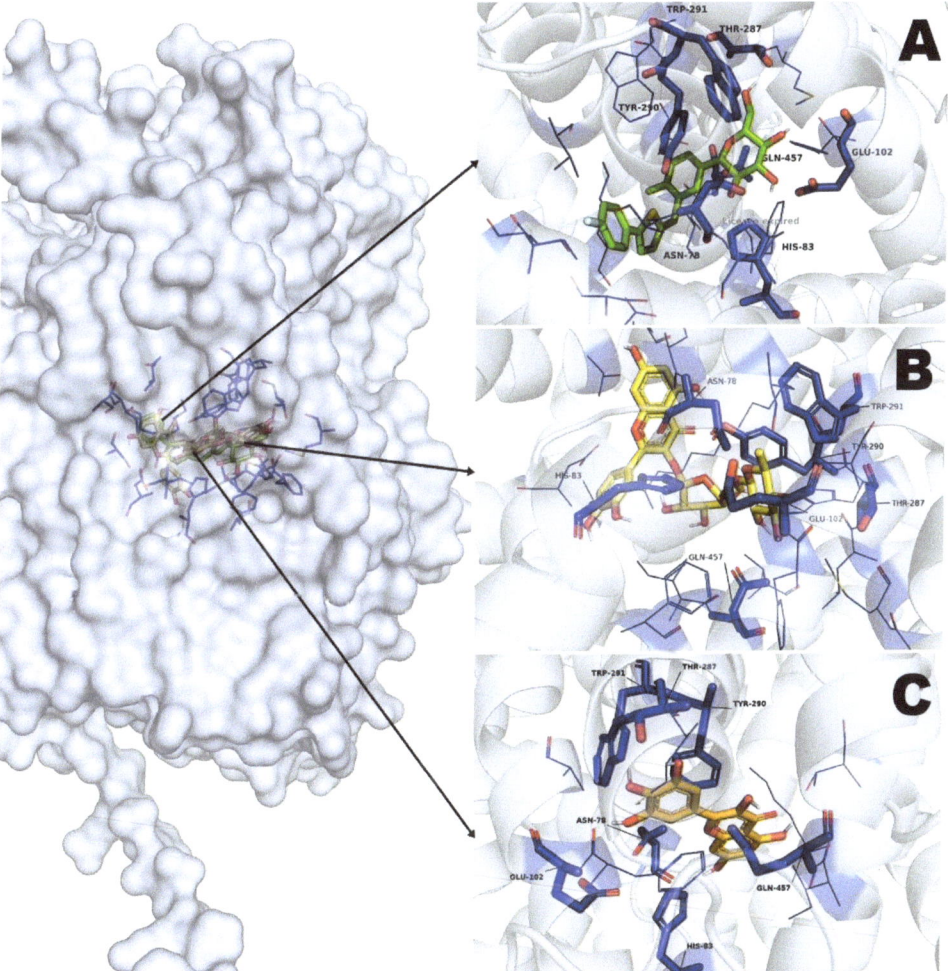

Figure 4. Results of molecular docking on SGLT1 cotransporter. (**A**) Interaction of canagliflozin and its binding site position; (**B**) Interaction of rutin and its binding site position; (**C**) Interaction of myricetin and its binding site position.

Table 3. Binding energy and interactions of ligands rutin, myricetin and acarbose on SGLT1 cotransporter.

Ligand	Sodium-Glucose Cotransporter (SGLT1)			
	ΔG (kcal·mol^{-1})	H-BR	NPI	RMSD
Rutin	22.82	Ser77, Asn78, His83, Phe101, Glu102, Ala105, Lys157, Gly282, Met283, Leu286, Thr287, Trp289, Tyr290, Lys321, Ser393, Ile397, Gln457, Thr460, Leu527	Asp161, Ile456	-
Myricetin	−7.89	Asn78, His83, Phe101, Glu102, Met283, Thr287, Tyr290, Gln457, Thr 460	Ala105, Lys157, Trp291, Ile456	-
Canagliflozin	−10.08	Thr56, Ser77, His83, Phe101, Glu102, Asp161, Met283, Thr287, Trp289, Trp291, Ser393, Ser396, Phe453, Gln457, Thr460	Asn78, Lys157, Tyr290, Val296, Ile397, Ile456	1.37

3. Discussion

Diabetes mellitus (DM) is a chronic progressive metabolic disorder of carbohydrates, lipids, and proteins. The prevalence of DM continues to increase worldwide, being a constant public health problem [1–3]. There are many treatments for DM, and all of them are classified according to their mechanism of action into seven principal groups: insulin sensitizers (thiazolidinediones and biguanides), secretagogues (meglitinides and sulfonylureas), dipeptidyl peptidase-4 (DPP-4) inhibitors, incretin mimetics, glucagon-like peptide-1 (GLP-1) inhibitors, α-glucosidase inhibitors and sodium-glucose cotransporter (SGLT) inhibitors [34,35]. All of them are focused on reducing and controlling hyperglycemia; however, in the long term, some of them can lose their pharmacological activity. Moreover, in all cases, they are accompanied by undesirable side effects for the patient. Insulin sensitizer may cause adverse gastrointestinal effects such as nausea, vomiting, and abdominal discomfort. Secretagogues mostly generate hypoglycemia, DPP-4 inhibitors principally generate gastrointestinal discomfort, incretin mimetics generate hypoglycemia and nausea, GLP-1 inhibitors cause intestinal discomfort, vomiting, and in some cases diarrhea, with respect to a-glucosidase inhibitors, the principal side effect is flatulence generation and abdominal distension, and finally, the SGLT inhibitors can cause urinary tract infections, genital infections and a possible risk of bladder cancer [35,36]. Due to the wide variety of side effects that all treatments of DM can generate, it is necessary to continue searching for new alternatives [4–6].

The present study aimed to determine the potential antidiabetic activity of an ethanolic extract obtained from the leaves of *Annona cherimola* Miller (*A. cherimola*), one species of the *Annonaceae* family, isolate the minor components from the extract and determine their acute and subchronic activity, as well as to suggest the possible antidiabetic mechanism of action. This study was carried out using activity-guided fractionation as a strategy.

First, the acute activity of the ethanolic extract from *Annona cherimola* Miller (EEAch) was carried out using female mice with alloxan-induced diabetes type 2 (AIT2D); the results showed that EEAch reduces the hyperglycemic values at 300 mg/kg dose, this was according to other studies that have been made to *A. cherimola*, where several authors have been determined their potential antidiabetic activity in different animal models [28–31]. To continue the study, the EEAch was fractionated. As a result, the aqueous residual fraction (AcRFr) and dichloromethane fraction (DCMFr) were obtained.

The aqueous fractions and the dichloromethane fraction were evaluated in the same model, observing that they have an antihyperglycemic effect; however, this effect does not reach the levels of glycemia values of the healthy control group. From both fractions, as observed in Table 1, the fraction that shows a better antihyperglycemic effect is AcRFr, confirming that this fraction contains the compounds responsible for the activity observed with the extract [29]. The next step of the investigation was to isolate the compounds, identify them, and evaluate their activity on the AIT2D model. In other studies, there have been isolated the flavonoid rutin, and this was responsible in part for the antihyperglycemic activity of *A. cherimola*; however, in the EEAch and AcRFr, there are more compounds that need to be studied to search for more alternatives for the treatment of DM.

The purification of AcRFr led us to the isolation of eight compounds with polyphenolic characteristics. They were identified as seven flavonoids (narcissin, hyperin, nicotiflorin, astragalin, isoquercitrin, rutin, and myricetin) and chlorogenic acid. All the compounds evaluated in the AIT2D model, hyperin, myricetin, nicotiflorin, rutin, isoquercitrin, and narcissin showed a reduction of the hyperglycemic values. Only astragalin and chlorogenic acid did not present antihyperglycemic activity. The activity of the compounds was compared with acarbose, an oral antidiabetic drug (OAD), being more effective in some of the compounds evaluated compared to acarbose (Table 1). The antihyperglycemic activity reported in our study is according to the described by other authors, which indicates that polyphenols are good candidates for the treatment of DM and its complications. The activity of polyphenols as antidiabetic agents varies according to their composition and their substituents [24,37–39].

Myricetin and rutin were selected as the compounds with the best antihyperglycemic activity due to showing the best reduction of hyperglycemic values; therefore, the study was continued with these compounds.

Once demonstrated the acute antidiabetic activity of the compounds was, only those with the best antihyperglycemic activity (EEAch, AcRFr, myricetin, and rutin) were evaluated in a subchronic assay using the AIT2D model. After the subchronic evaluation of the products obtained from *A. cherimola*, we observed that EEAch and AcRFr help to reduce hyperglycemic values after 2 weeks of treatment and avoid the exponential increase in hyperglycemic values characteristic of the AIT2D model that normally evolves in DM1 and the hyperglycemic values constantly increase as we can see in Figure 1. This activity is according to that observed in previous studies with *A. cherimola* [30]; this activity is also too observed in other species of the family Annonaceae [40].

The groups treated with myricetin and rutin showed a better regulation of hyperglycemic values due to both treatments reaching normoglycemic values from the second week until the end of the treatment. Those activities were similar to those observed in the group treated with acarbose. Our results suggest that myricetin and rutin have a similar activity of acarbose; in this sense, we continue the investigation, and it was proposed to evaluate the possible mechanism of action of both compounds. We propose firstly the evaluation of an α-glucosidase inhibitor due to their having reported activity for rutin [29]; however, myricetin did not have been reported with this activity. Additionally, we propose both compounds be evaluated as an SGLT1 cotransporter. These mechanisms of action were selected due to one alternative to reduce hyperglycemic values that did not generate hypoglycemia is the reduction of postprandial peaks of glucose. In this sense, α-glucosidase enzyme and SGLT1 cotransporters were two proteins involved in the metabolism of complex carbohydrates and absorption of simple carbohydrates, respectively [41,42].

In order to determine the potential α-glucosidase and SGLT1 inhibition, two in vivo experiments (OSTT and OGTT) were carried out according to previous investigations [40]. In OSTT, we observed that all treatments reduce the postprandial peak after sucrose load (Figure 2). Further, we observed that the group treated with AcRFr reduced their glycemic values below their initial values and the vehicle control. We hypothesize that in the AcRFr, there are many compounds, and some of them can have activity over other mechanisms of action that, added to the α-glucosidase inhibition, have a synergic activity and generate the hypoglycemia observed. In the case of rutin, we observed that the activity of this compound is better than the pharmacological control acarbose; this is according to the described in the literature, which indicates that rutin is a flavonoid that avoids the postprandial peak after a sucrose load in rat and mice models [22,25].

When the OGTT test was carried out, we observed a similar activity to the OSTT, i.e., all treatments significantly reduced the glucose postprandial peak. Moreover, we observed that in this case, all the compounds obtained from *A. cherimola* showed to development of SIT2D was determined by measuring postprandial blood glucose levels using a conventional glucometer (ACC CHECK® Performa Blood Glucose Systems, Roche®, DC, Basel, Switzerland).

Additionally, to confirm the AIT2D model, the β-cell function was evaluated with the administration of 5 mg/kg glibenclamide orally and measuring the decrease in glucose values 2 and 4 h after administration; according to the results, there can be confirmed the existence of functional β-cell [40]; therefore, the generated model was classified as an experimental type 2 diabetes mellitus model.

4.4.3. Grouping

For the evaluations of the antidiabetic effect of the ethanolic extract, BALB/c mice were randomly divided into groups of 6 each as follows: ethanolic extract of *A. cherimola* (EEAch) at the dose of 300 mg/kg, aqueous fraction (AcRFr) at 300 mg/kg, and dichloromethane fraction (DCMFr). In the case of the compounds isolated from the EEAch, the dose used was 50 mg/kg in all cases. Moreover, the oral antidiabetic drug (OAD) metformin acarbose (Aca) at 50 mg/kg bw was used as the positive control. Further, normoglycemic and AIT2D control groups were carried out. In all cases, the treatments were dissolved in 2% Tween 80 in water as vehicle and were given orally through a gavage; the volume was calculated according to international guidelines [48] as 2 mL/100 g body weight.

4.4.4. Acute Evaluation of the Antidiabetic Effect of Ethanolic Extract from *Annona cherimola*, Fractions, and Isolated Compounds

Animals with blood glucose levels between 190–220 mg/dL were used for this study. The treatments described above were administered orally; once the treatments were administered, the blood samples were collected from the tail vein at the beginning (0 h), 2 and 4 h after administration using a conventional glucometer described previously.

4.4.5. Subchronic Evaluation of the Antidiabetic Effect of Ethanolic Extract from *Annona cherimola*, Fractions, and Isolated Compounds

Experimental-induced diabetes type 2 animals in the same conditions previously described were used for the subchronic evaluation. In this case, the animals were administered with the treatments as described above once daily for 4 weeks. Blood glucose levels were measured weekly, as previously described.

4.4.6. Oral Glucose and Sucrose Tolerance Test (OGTT and OSTT) of Ethanolic Extract from *Annona cherimola*, Fractions, and Isolated Compounds

The oral sucrose tolerance test (OSTT) was conducted according to published protocols [36]. Diabetic fasted female mice were randomly divided into eight groups of 6 animals each as follows: control group treated only with water as vehicle, EEAc (300 mg/kg), AcRFr (300 mg/kg), DCMFr (300 mg/kg), myricetin (50 mg/kg), rutin (50 mg/kg), and acarbose (50 mg/kg) as pharmacological control. In order to perform the test, the time 0 was set before treatments; then, treatments were given orally, and 30 min after the administration, a sucrose load (3 g/kg) was administered to the mice. Measures of the blood glucose level from the tail vein were performed at 2 and 4 h after administration of the carbohydrate by applying the glucose oxidase method using a standard glucometer (Accu-Chek® Performa Glucometer, Boehringer Mannheim, Germany) [49]. The oral glucose tolerance test (OGTT) was performed under the same conditions as the OSTT assay, but in this case, a glucose load (1.5 g/kg) was given to the groups, and the blood glucose measurements were recorded following the same method for the OGTT.

4.5. In Silico Studies

The chemical structure of ligands rutin (CID: 5280805), myricetin (CID: 5281672), canagliflozin (CID: 24812758), and acarbose (CID: 41774) were retrieved from the chemical library PubChem (https://pubchem.ncbi.nlm.nih.gov/) (accessed on 12 December 2022), these were optimized and submitted to energetic and geometrical minimization using

Avogadro software [50]. The α-glucosidase enzyme (crystal structure of the N-terminal of Human Maltase–Glucoamylase, RCSB, PDB ID: 2QMJ) and SGLT-1 cotransporter (crystal structure of human sodium/glucose cotransporter, Uniprot ID: P13866) were used as a target of the study. These were retrieved from the Protein Data Bank (http://www.rcsb.org/) (accessed on 12 December 2022) and the Uniprot database (https://www.uniprot.org/) (accessed on 12 December 2022). Total molecules of water and ions not needed for catalytic activity were stripped to preserve the entire protein. All polar hydrogen atoms were added and ionized in a basic environment (pH = 7.4), and Gasteiger charges were assigned; the computed output topologies from the previous steps were used as input files to docking simulations.

The molecular docking experiments were carried out using Autodock 4.2 software [51]; the search parameters were as follows: a grid-base procedure was employed to generate the affinity maps delimiting a grid box of $126 \times 126 \times 126$ Å^3 in each space coordinate, with a grid points spacing of 0.375 Å, the Lamarckian genetic algorithm was employed as scoring function with a randomized initial population of 100 individuals and a maximum number of energy evaluations of 1×10^7 cycles, the analysis of the interactions in the enzyme/inhibitor complex was visualized with PyMOL software (The PyMOL Molecular Graphics System, Ver 2.0, Schrödinger, LLC, DeLano Scientific, San Carlos, CA, USA).

The validation of the molecular docking was carried out by re-docking the co-crystallized ligand in the proteins (α-glucosidase and SGLT-1). The lowest energy pose of the co-crystallized ligand was superimposed, and it was observed whether it maintained the same bind position. The RMSD was calculated, and a reliable range within 2 Å is reported.

4.6. Statistical Analysis

All the results are expressed as mean values standard error of the mean (SEM). All statistical analyses were performed using GraphPad Prism version 8.2.1 (GraphPad Software Inc., San Diego, CA, USA). The statistical evaluation was conducted through an analysis of variance (ANOVA) followed by a Tukey test for multiple comparisons considering the p-value ≤ 0.05 was a statistically significant difference.

5. Conclusions

The acute and subchronic in vivo evaluations showed that in the current AIT2D model, EEAch, AcRFr, DCMFr, rutin, and myricetin reduced the hyperglycemic values. The oral glucose and sucrose tolerance test and the molecular docking suggest that the antidiabetic activity of the products obtained from *A. cherimola* is mediated in part by α-glucosidase enzyme inhibition and SGLT1 cotransporter inhibition.

This research supports the phytochemical and pharmacological bases of *A. cherimola* and its use as a source for the development of new potential antidiabetic agents for T2D control based on flavonoid molecules.

Supplementary Materials: The following supporting information can be downloaded at: https://www.mdpi.com/article/10.3390/ph16050724/s1.

Author Contributions: Conceptualization, M.V. and F.C.; Formal analysis, J.M.-S., C.V. and E.B.; Funding acquisition, F.C.; Investigation, M.V. and J.M.-S.; Project administration, F.C.; Resources, F.C.; Supervision, F.C.; Writing—original draft, M.V., J.M.-S., C.V. and E.B. Writing—review and editing, M.V. and F.C. All authors have read and agreed to the published version of the manuscript.

Funding: This research was supported by grants from Instituto Mexicano del Seguro Social (IMSS): FIS/IMSS/PROT/PRIO/19/110 and FIS/IMSS/PROT/G17-2/1722. Awarded to F.C.

Institutional Review Board Statement: The study was conducted according to the guidelines of the Declaration of Helsinki and the Official Mexican Regulations on animal care and experimental management NOM-062-ZOO-1999. This study was approved by the Local Ethics Committee of CMN SXXI in the Instituto Mexicano del Seguro Social under protocol codes R-2020-3601-038 and R-2019-3601-004.

Informed Consent Statement: Not applicable.

Data Availability Statement: Not applicable.

Acknowledgments: We would like to thank QFB Erika Hernández Salvador for your assistance. Further, we would like to thank IMSS for the contract grant sponsor FIS/IMSS/PROT/PRIO/19/110 and FIS/IMSS/PROT/G17-2/1722.

Conflicts of Interest: The authors declare no conflict of interest.

References

1. American Diabetes Association. Classification and diagnosis of diabetes: Standards of Medical Care in Diabetes 2020. *Diabetes Care* **2021**, *43*, S14–S31.
2. DF Diabetes Atlas 10th Edition. 2021. Available online: https://diabetesatlas.org/idfawp/resource-files/2021/07/IDF_Atlas_10th_Edition_2021.pdf (accessed on 6 May 2022).
3. World Health Organization. Diabetes. Available online: https://www.who.int/news-room/fact-sheets/detail/diabetes (accessed on 22 August 2022).
4. DeFronzo, R. From the Triumvirate to the Ominous Octet: A New Paradigm for the Treatment of Type 2 Diabetes Mellitus. *Diabetes* **2009**, *58*, 773–795. [CrossRef]
5. Strain, W.D.; Paldánius, P.M. Diabetes, Cardiovascular Disease and the Microcirculation. *Cardiovasc. Diabetology* **2018**, *17*, 57. [CrossRef] [PubMed]
6. American Diabetes Association. Pharmacologic Approaches to Glycemic Treatment: Standards of Medical Care in Diabetes—2021. *Diabetes Care* **2021**, *44*, S111–S124. [CrossRef] [PubMed]
7. Tan, S.Y.; Wong, J.L.M.; Sim, Y.J.; Wong, S.S.; Elhassan, S.A.M.; Tan, S.H.; Lim, G.P.L.; Rong Tay, N.W.; Annan, N.C.; Bhattamisra, S.K.; et al. Type 1 and 2 Diabetes Mellitus: A Review on Current Treatment Approach and Gene Therapy as Potential Intervention. *Diabetes Metab. Syndr.* **2019**, *13*, 364–372. [CrossRef] [PubMed]
8. Rajasekaran, P.; Ande, C.; Vankar, Y.D. Synthesis of zero sugar (5,6 and 6,6)-oxa-oxa as glucosidase inhibitors from 2-formylgalactal using iodocyclization as a key step. *ARKIVOC* **2022**, *6*, 5–23. [CrossRef]
9. Tseng, P.S.; Ande, C.; Moremen, K.W.; Crich, D. Influence of the conformation of the side chain on the activity of glucosidase inhibitors. *Angew. Chem. Int. Ed.* **2023**, *135*, e202217809. [CrossRef]
10. Giovannini, P.; Howes, M.; Edwards, S. Medicinal plants used in the traditional management of diabetes and its sequelae in Central America: A review. *J. Ethnopharmacol.* **2016**, *184*, 58–71. [CrossRef] [PubMed]
11. El-Tantawy, W.; Temraz, A. Management of diabetes using herbal extracts: Review. *Arch. Physiol. Biochem.* **2018**, *124*, 383–389. [CrossRef] [PubMed]
12. Chawla, R.; Thakur, P.; Chowdhry, A.; Jaiswal, S.; Sharma, A.; Goel, R.; Sharma, J.; Priyadarshi, S.S.; Kumar, V.; Sharma, R.K.; et al. Evidence-Based Herbal Drug Standardization Approach in Coping with Challenges of Holistic Management of Diabetes: ADreadful Lifestyle Disorder of 21st Century. *J. Diabetes Metab. Disord.* **2013**, *12*, 35. [CrossRef] [PubMed]
13. Choudhury, H.; Pandey, M.; Hua, C. An update on natural compounds in the remedy of diabetes mellitus: A systematic review. *J. Tradit. Complement. Med.* **2017**, *8*, 361–376. [CrossRef]
14. González Vega, M.E. Cherimoya (*Annona cherimola* Miller), fruit-bearing tropical and sub-tropical of promissory values. *Cultiv. Trop.* **2013**, *34*, 52–63.
15. Quilez, A.M.; Fernández-Arche, M.A.; García-Giménez, M.M.; De la Puerta, R. Potential therapeutic applications of the genus Annona Local and traditional uses and pharmacology. *J. Ethnopharmacol.* **2018**, *225*, 244–270. [CrossRef]
16. CABI. *Annona cherimola (Cherimoya); Invasive Species Compendium*; CAB International: Wallingford, UK, 2014; Available online: https://www.cabi.org/isc/datasheet/5806 (accessed on 28 April 2022).
17. Amador, M.D.C.V.; Rodríguez, F.M.; Rodríguez, Z.M.; Guerra, M.J.M.; Barreiro, M.L. Tamizaje Fitoquímico, Actividad Antiinflamatoria y Toxicidad Aguda de Extractos de Hojas de *Annona Squamosa* L. *Rev. Cuba. Plantas Med.* **2006**, *11*, 1–12.
18. Larranaga, N.; Albertazzi, F.; Fontecha, G. A Mesoamerican origin of cherimoya (*Annona cherimola* Mill.): Implications for the conservation of plant genetic resources. *Mol. Ecol.* **2017**, *26*, 4116–4130. [CrossRef]
19. Young, A. Tropical forests and their crops: N. J. H. Smith, J.T. Williams, D.L. Plucknett and J. P. Talbot, Comstock Publishing Associates, Ithaca and London. *Agric. Syst.* **1994**, *45*, 235–237. [CrossRef]
20. Gentile, C.; Mannino, G.; Palazzolo, E.; Gianguzzi, G.; Perrone, A.; Serio, G.; Farina, V. Pomological, Sensorial, Nutritional and Nutraceutical Profile of Seven Cultivars of Cherimoya (*Annona cherimola* Mill). *Foods* **2020**, *10*, 35. [CrossRef]
21. Grossberger, D. The California cherimoya industry. Proceedings of the First International Symposium on Cherimoya. *Acta Hortic.* **1999**, *497*, 131–142.
22. Martínez-Vázquez, M.; Estrada-Reyes, R.; Escalona, A.A.; Velázquez, I.L.; Martínez-Mota, L.; Moreno, J.; Heinze, G. Antidepressant-like Effects of an Alkaloid Extract of the Aerial Parts of *Annona cherimola* in Mice. *J. Ethnopharmacol.* **2012**, *139*, 164–170. [CrossRef]

23. Ammoury, C.; Younes, M.; El Khoury, M.; Hodroj, M.H.; Haykal, T.; Nasr, P.; Sily, M.; Taleb, R.I.; Sarkis, R.; Khalife, R.; et al. The Pro-Apoptotic Effect of a Terpene-Rich *Annona cherimola* Leaf Extract on Leukemic Cell Lines. *BMC Complement. Altern. Med.* **2019**, *19*, 365. [CrossRef]
24. Martínez-Solís, J.; Calzada, F.; Barbosa, E.; Valdés, M. Antihyperglycemic and Antilipidemic Properties of a Tea Infusion of the Leaves from *Annona cherimola* Miller on Streptozocin-Induced Type 2 Diabetic Mice. *Molecules* **2021**, *9*, 2408. [CrossRef] [PubMed]
25. Calzada, F.; Solares-Pascasio, J.I.; Ordoñez-Razo, R.M.; Velazquez, C.; Barbosa, E.; García-Hernández, N.; Mendez-Luna, D.; Correa-Basurto, J. Antihyperglycemic Activity of the Leaves from *Annona Cherimola* Miller and Rutin on Alloxan-Induced Diabetic Rats. *Pharmacogn. Res.* **2017**, *9*, 1–6. [CrossRef] [PubMed]
26. Valdes, M.; Calzada, F.; Martínez-Solís, J.; Martínez-Rodríguez, J. Antihyperglycemic Effects of *Annona cherimola* Miller and the Flavonoid Rutin in Combination with Oral Antidiabetic Drugs on Streptozocin-Induced Diabetic Mice. *Pharmaceuticals* **2023**, *16*, 112. [CrossRef] [PubMed]
27. Martínez-Solís, J.; Calzada, F.; Barbosa, E.; Gutiérrez-Meza, J.M. Antidiabetic and Toxicological Effects of the Tea Infusion of Summer Collection from *Annona cherimola* Miller Leaves. *Plants* **2022**, *11*, 3224. [CrossRef]
28. Díaz-de-Cerio, E.; Aguilera-Saez, L.M.; Gómez-Caravaca, A.M.; Verardo, V.; Fernández-Gutiérrez, A.; Fernández, I.; Arráez-Román, D. Characterization of Bioactive Compounds of *Annona cherimola* L. Leaves Using a Combined Approach Based on HPLC-ESI-TOF-MS and NMR. *Anal. Bioanal. Chem.* **2018**, *410*, 3607–3619. [CrossRef]
29. Albuquerque, T.G.; Santos, F.; Sanches-Silva, A.; Oliveira, M.; Bento, A.; Costa, H. Nutritional and Phytochemical Composition of *Annona cherimola* Mill. Fruits and by-Products: Potential Health Benefits. *Food Chem.* **2014**, *193*, 187–195. [CrossRef]
30. Mannino, G.; Gentile, C.; Porcu, A.; Agliassa, C.; Caradonna, F.; Bertea, C.M. Chemical Profile and Biological Activity of Cherimoya (*Annona cherimola* Mill.) and Atemoya (*Annona Atemoya*) Leaves. *Molecules* **2020**, *25*, 2612. [CrossRef]
31. Ghorbani, A. Mechanisms of Antidiabetic Effects of Flavonoid Rutin. *Biomed. Pharmacother.* **2017**, *96*, 305–312. [CrossRef]
32. Yang, J.; Guo, J.; Yuan, J. In Vitro Antioxidant Properties of Rutin. *LWT-Food Sci. Technol.* **2008**, *41*, 1060–1066. [CrossRef]
33. Kamalakkannan, N.; Prince, P.S.M. Antihyperglycaemic and Antioxidant Effect of Rutin, a Polyphenolic Flavonoid, in Streptozotocin-Induced Diabetic Wistar Rats. *Basic Clin. Pharmacol. Toxicol.* **2006**, *98*, 97–103. [CrossRef]
34. Llave, F. Actualización en el manejo de los antidiabéticos orales en atención primaria. *Med. Fam.* **2008**, *8*, 98–111.
35. Gonzales-Duhart, D.; Tamay-Cach, F.; Álvarez-Almazán, S.; Mendieta-Wejebe, J. Current advances in the biochemical and physiological aspects of the treatment of type 2 Diabetes Mellitus with thiazolidinediones. *PPAR Res.* **2016**, *2016*, 7614270.
36. Alam, U.; Usghar, O.; Azmi, S.; Malik, R. General aspects of diabetes mellitus. *Handb. Clin. Neurol.* **2014**, *126*, 211–222.
37. Blanco-Salas, J.; Vazquez, F.; Hortigó-Vinagre, M.; Ruiz-Tellez, T. Bioactive Pytochemicals from Mercurialis spp. Used in Traditional Spanish Medicine. *Plants* **2019**, *8*, 193. [PubMed]
38. Bai, L.; Li, X.; He, L.; Zheng, H.; Li, J.; Zhong, L.; Tong, R.; Jiang, Z.; Shi, J.; Li, J. Antidiabetic Potential of Flavonoids from Traditional Chinese Medicine: A Review. *Am. J. Chin. Med.* **2019**, *47*, 933–957. [CrossRef] [PubMed]
39. Shamsudin, N.; Ahmed, Q.; Mahmood, S.; Shah, S.; Sarian, M.; Khattak, M.; Khatib, A.; Sabere, A.; Yusoff, Y.; Latip, J. Flavonoids as Antidiabetic and Anti-Inflammatory Agents: A Review on Structural Activity Relationship-Based Studies and Meta-Analysis. *Int. J. Mol. Sci.* **2022**, *23*, 12605. [CrossRef] [PubMed]
40. Valdés, M.; Calzada, F.; Mendieta-Wejebe, J.; Merlín-Lucas, V.; Veláquez, C.; Barbosa, E. Antihyperglycemic Effects of *Annona diversifolia* Safford and Its Acyclic Terpenoids: α-Glucosidase and Selective SGLT-1 Inhibitiors. *Molecules* **2020**, *25*, 3361. [CrossRef]
41. Jhong, C.H.; Riyaphan, J.; Lin, S.H.; Chia, Y.C.; Weng, C.F. Screening alpha-glucosidase and alpha-amylase inhibitors from natural compounds by molecular docking in silico. *BioFactors* **2015**, *41*, 242–251. [CrossRef] [PubMed]
42. Röder, P.V.; Geillinger, K.E.; Zietek, T.S.; Thorens, B.; Koepsell, H.; Daniel, H. The role of SGLT1 and GLUT2 in intestinal glucose transport and sensing. *PLoS ONE* **2014**, *9*, 20–22. [CrossRef] [PubMed]
43. Lehmann, A.; Hornby, P. Intestinal SGLT1 in metabolic health and disease. *Am. J. Physiol. Gastrointest. Liver Physiol.* **2016**, *310*, G887–G898. [CrossRef]
44. Sim, L.; Willemsma, C.; Mohan, S.; Naim, H.Y.; Mario Pinto, B.; Rose, D.R. Structural Basis for Substrate Selectivity in Human Maltase-Glucoamylase and Sucrase-Isomaltase N-terminal Domains. *J. Biol. Chem.* **2010**, *285*, 17763. [CrossRef]
45. Kashton, H.; Kwang-Hyun, B. Recent Updates on Phytoconstituent Alpha-Glucosidase Inhibitors: An Approach towards the Treatment of Type Two Diabetes. *Plants* **2022**, *11*, 2722. [CrossRef] [PubMed]
46. Wright, E.; Loo, D.; Hirayama, B. Biology of human Sodium Glucose Transporters. *Physiol. Rev.* **2011**, *91*, 733–794. [CrossRef]
47. Diario Oficial de la Federación. NOM-062-ZOO-1999, 2001. *Norma Oficial Mexicana. Especificaciones Técnicas Para La Producción, Cuidado y Uso de Los Animales de Laboratorio*; Diario Oficial de La Federación: México City, México, 1999; p. 58. Available online: https://www.gob.mx/cms/uploads/attachment/file/203498/NOM-062-ZOO-1999_220801.pdf (accessed on 14 October 2022).
48. OECD Test Guidelines for Chemicals—OECD. Available online: http://www.oecd.org/chemicalsafety/testing/oecdguidelinesforthetestingofchemicals.htm (accessed on 25 April 2023).
49. Valdes, M.; Calzada, F.; Mendieta-Wejebe, J. Structure-activity relationship study of acyclic terpenes in blood glucose levels: Potential α-glucosidase and sodium-glucose cotransporter (SGLT-1) inhibitors. *Molecules* **2019**, *24*, 4020. [CrossRef] [PubMed]

50. Hanwell, M.; Curtis, D.; Lonie, D.; Vandermeersch, T.; Zurek, E.; Hutchison, G. Avogadro: An advanced semantic chemical editor, visualization, and analysis platform. *J. Cheminform.* **2012**, *4*, 17. [CrossRef] [PubMed]
51. Morris, G.; Lindstrom, W.; Sanner, M.; Belew, R.; Goodshell, D.; Olson, A. Autodock4 and AutodockTools4: Automated docking with selective receptor flexibility. *J. Comput. Chem.* **2009**, *30*, 2785–2791. [CrossRef]

Disclaimer/Publisher's Note: The statements, opinions and data contained in all publications are solely those of the individual author(s) and contributor(s) and not of MDPI and/or the editor(s). MDPI and/or the editor(s) disclaim responsibility for any injury to people or property resulting from any ideas, methods, instructions or products referred to in the content.

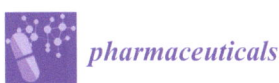

Article

Hesperidin Mitigates Cyclophosphamide-Induced Testicular Dysfunction via Altering the Hypothalamic Pituitary Gonadal Axis and Testicular Steroidogenesis, Inflammation, and Apoptosis in Male Rats

Tarek Khamis [1,*], Abdelmonem Awad Hegazy [2,3], Samaa Salah Abd El-Fatah [3], Eman Ramadan Abdelfattah [3], Marwa Mohamed Mahmoud Abdelfattah [3], Liana Mihaela Fericean [4,*] and Ahmed Hamed Arisha [5,6,*]

1. Department of Pharmacology and Laboratory of Biotechnology, Faculty of Veterinary Medicine, Zagazig University, Zagazig 44519, Egypt
2. Anatomy and Embryology, Faculty of Dentistry, Zarqa University, Zarqa 13110, Jordan
3. Human Anatomy & Embryology Department, Faculty of Medicine, Zagazig University, Zagazig 44519, Egypt
4. Biology Department, Faculty of Agriculture, University of Life Sciences "King Michael I of Romania" from Timisoara, Aradului St. 119, 300645 Timisoara, Romania
5. Department of Animal Physiology and Biochemistry, Faculty of Veterinary Medicine, Badr University in Cairo, Badr City 11829, Egypt
6. Department of Physiology, Laboratory of Biotechnology, Faculty of Veterinary Medicine, Zagazig University, Zagazig 44519, Egypt
* Correspondence: t.khamis@vet.zu.edu.eg (T.K.); mihaelafericean@usab-tm.ro (L.M.F.); vetahmedhamed@zu.edu.eg (A.H.A.); Tel.: +20-55-228-3683 (T.K. & A.H.A.)

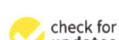

Citation: Khamis, T.; Hegazy, A.A.; El-Fatah, S.S.A.; Abdelfattah, E.R.; Abdelfattah, M.M.M.; Fericean, L.M.; Arisha, A.H. Hesperidin Mitigates Cyclophosphamide-Induced Testicular Dysfunction via Altering the Hypothalamic Pituitary Gonadal Axis and Testicular Steroidogenesis, Inflammation, and Apoptosis in Male Rats. *Pharmaceuticals* **2023**, *16*, 301. https://doi.org/10.3390/ph16020301

Academic Editors: Fernando Calzada and Miguel Valdes

Received: 10 December 2022
Revised: 7 February 2023
Accepted: 13 February 2023
Published: 15 February 2023

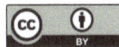

Copyright: © 2023 by the authors. Licensee MDPI, Basel, Switzerland. This article is an open access article distributed under the terms and conditions of the Creative Commons Attribution (CC BY) license (https:// creativecommons.org/licenses/by/ 4.0/).

Abstract: Cyclophosphamide (CP) is a cytotoxic, cell cycle, non-specific, and antiproliferative drug. This study aimed to address the toxic effects of CP on male fertility and the possible ameliorative role of hesperidin (HSP). Thirty-two adult albino rats were randomly divided into four groups, namely, the negative control, HSP, CP-treated, and CP+HSP-treated groups. The CP-treated rats showed a significant reduction in the levels of serum LH, FSH, testosterone, prolactin, testicular glutathione peroxidase (GPx), and total antioxidant capacity (TAC) with an elevation in levels of malondialdehyde (MDA), and p53, and iNOS immune expression, compared to the control group. A significant downregulation in hypothalamic KISS-1, KISS-1r, and GnRH, hypophyseal GnRHr, and testicular mRNA expression of steroidogenesis enzymes, PGC-1α, PPAR-1, IL10, and GLP-1, as well as a significant upregulation in testicular mRNA of P53 and IL1β mRNA expression, were detected in the CP-treated group in comparison to that in the control group. The administration of HSP in CP-treated rats significantly improved the levels of serum LH, FSH, testosterone, prolactin, testicular GPx, and TAC, with a reduction in levels of MDA, and p53, and iNOS immune expression compared to the CP-treated group. A significant upregulation in hypophyseal GnRHr, and testicular mRNA expression of CYP19A1 enzymes, PPAR-1, IL10, and GLP-1, as well as a significant downregulation in testicular mRNA of P53 and IL1β mRNA expression, were detected in the CP+HSP-treated group in comparison to that in the CP-treated group. In conclusion, HSP could be a potential auxiliary agent for protection from the development of male infertility.

Keywords: cyclophosphamide; hesperidin; apoptosis; P53; iNOS; oxidative stress

1. Introduction

The incidence of cancer has increased significantly throughout the world in recent years [1]. Formerly, surgery used to be the sole option for treating patients with solid tumors, which had a high fatality rate. Chemotherapy has improved such patient survival rates over the past 40 years [2]. Various chemotherapeutic agents, including cyclophosphamide (CP), are widely used as a part of their treatment regimen [3]. Unfortunately, it is non-selective for diseased cells [4,5]. CP has two active metabolites, namely, phosphoramide mustard and acrolein. While phosphoramide mustard has been associated with the antineoplastic and immunosuppressive actions of CP, acrolein is responsible for the toxic side effects of CP that include apoptosis and necrosis in normal tissue [6]. CP administration has been linked to significant side effects, such as hemorrhagic cystitis, gonadotoxicity, nephrotoxicity, and cardiotoxicity, limiting its therapeutic use. Moreover, female patients who are treated with CP are susceptible to early menopause. The risk of irreversible infertility increases significantly in both male and female patients when exposed to a cumulative medical dose [7,8]. CP has been reported to impact male fertility both centrally and peripherally via downregulating the hypothalamic–pituitary–gonadal (HPG) axis through affecting the hypothalamic Kiss1 mRNA expression and gonadotropin secretion, testicular steroidogenesis, testosterone synthesis, and eventually spermatogenesis [9,10]. Furthermore, Cp has been linked to direct testicular oxidative stress and DNA damage leading to testicular degeneration [11,12].

Flavonoids, found in many medicinal plants, fruit, and vegetables, can be useful in treating a variety of diseases. Flavonoids possess various pharmacological properties, including vasodilation, anti-allergic, immunostimulant, and antiviral effects [13,14]. They are reported to be effective as an antioxidant, anticarcinogen, antiproliferative, and in combating multidrug resistance, as well as in preventing chemotherapy-associated injury [15]. Hesperidin (HSP) is a bioflavonoid that is found mainly in citrus fruit such as oranges and lemons, as well as plant-derived liquids such as tea and olive oil. It has a wide range of pharmacological effects, including antioxidant, anti-inflammatory, anticarcinogenic, antiviral, antibacterial, antifungal, antiulcer, analgesic, and anticancer properties [16]. The main objective of the current work was to examine the potential therapeutic effect of HSP in preventing the progression of male infertility in rats treated with CP and its effects on the various molecular processes involved in male reproduction.

2. Results

2.1. Effect on the Final Body, Testicular Weights and Serum Hormone Levels

The final body and testicular weights of the CP-treated group were significantly lower ($p < 0.05$) compared to the control group in Figure 1A,B. The CP+HSP-treated group showed a significant increase in final body and testicular weights compared to the CP-treated group in Figure 1A,B.

The serum levels of testosterone, FSH, LH, and prolactin showed a significant decrease in the CP-treated group in comparison to the control group ($p < 0.05$) in Figure 1C–F. The serum levels of testosterone, FSH, LH, and prolactin in the CP+HSP-treated group showed a significant increase compared to the CP-treated group, shown in Figure 1C–F.

2.2. Effect on Testicular Lipid Peroxidation and Oxidative Stress Markers

CP-induced oxidative stress was indicated, with a significant decrease in GPx and TAC levels in the CP-treated group in comparison to that in the control group ($p < 0.05$), shown in Figure 2B,C. A significant increase in the MDA level, the lipid peroxidation marker, in the CP-treated group in comparison to that in the control group ($p < 0.05$) is also shown in Figure 2A. The CP+HSP-treated rats showed a significant decrease in testicular MDA levels, as well as a significant increase in testicular GPx and TAC levels, in comparison to those in the CP-treated group, shown in Figure 2A–C.

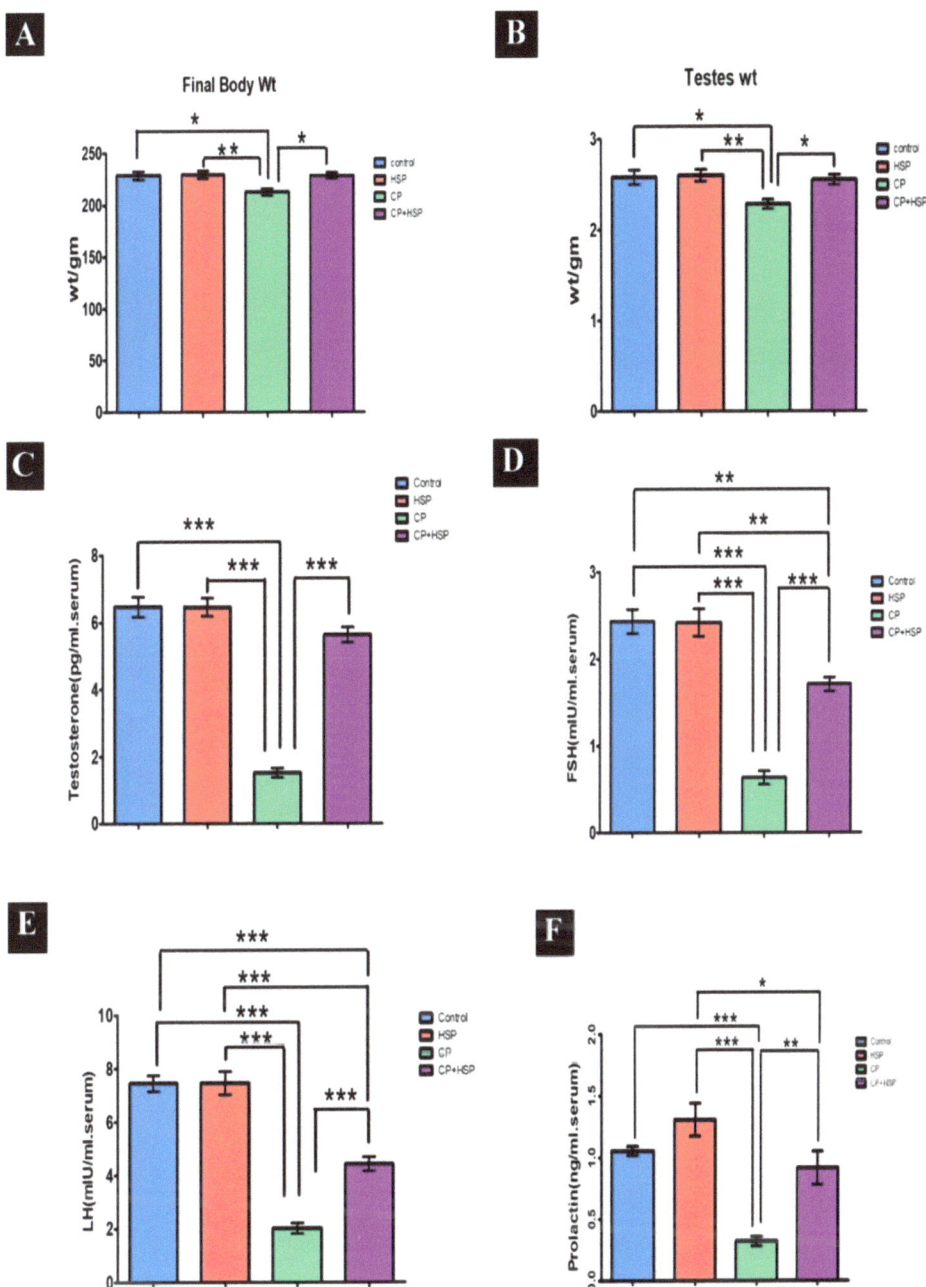

Figure 1. Effect on the final body, testicular weights and serum hormones (**A–F**). (**A**) Body weight (g), and (**B**) weight (g), (**C**) serum testosterone level (pg/mL), (**D**) serum FSH (mIU/mL) level, (**E**) serum LH (mIU/mL) level, and (**F**). serum prolactin (ng/mL) level. Data are expressed as means ± SEM. N = 8. *, **, *** indicate significant difference ($p < 0.05$).

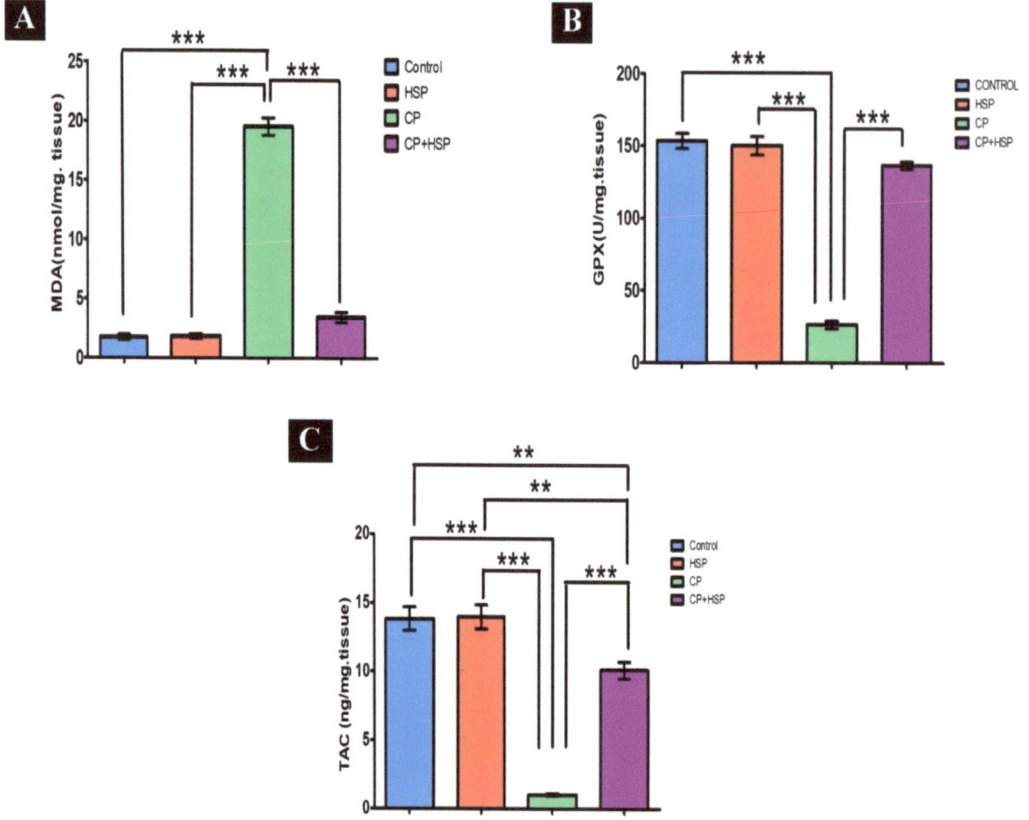

Figure 2. Effect of hesperidin administration in cyclophosphamide-induced testicular impairment in male rats on testicular lipid peroxidation and oxidative stress markers (**A–C**). (**A**) Testicular MDA level (nmol/mg. tissue), (**B**) testicular GPx level (U/mg. tissue), and (**C**) testicular TAC level (ng/mg. tissue). Data are expressed as means ± SEM. N = 8. **, *** indicate significant difference ($p < 0.05$).

2.3. Effect on Testicular Histopathology and Morphology

The control and the HSP groups showed normal morphology. The majority of seminiferous tubules were rounded in shape with a regular contour and few interstitial spaces containing clusters of interstitial cells. The lumina of most tubules revealed aggregated sperm bundles in Figure 3A,B. A complete series of spermatogenic cells were seen (spermatogonia, primary spermatocytes, secondary spermatocytes and spermatids). The seminiferous tubules were covered by a single layer of myoid cells with flattened nuclei. The interstitial spaces were narrow and contained normal Leydig cells and blood vessels, as shown in Figure 3E,F.

Sections from CP-treated groups revealed degenerative testicular changes, including loss of their normal architecture, compared with the control group. Distorted seminiferous tubules with exfoliation of germ cells within their lumina and irregular outlines and germinal epithelium with some atrophic part. The spermatogenic cells appeared with darkly stained pyknotic nuclei and multinucleated giant cells were also seen. The interstitial tissues were wide and edematous. Numerous vacuolations were also seen, as shown in Figure 3C,G.

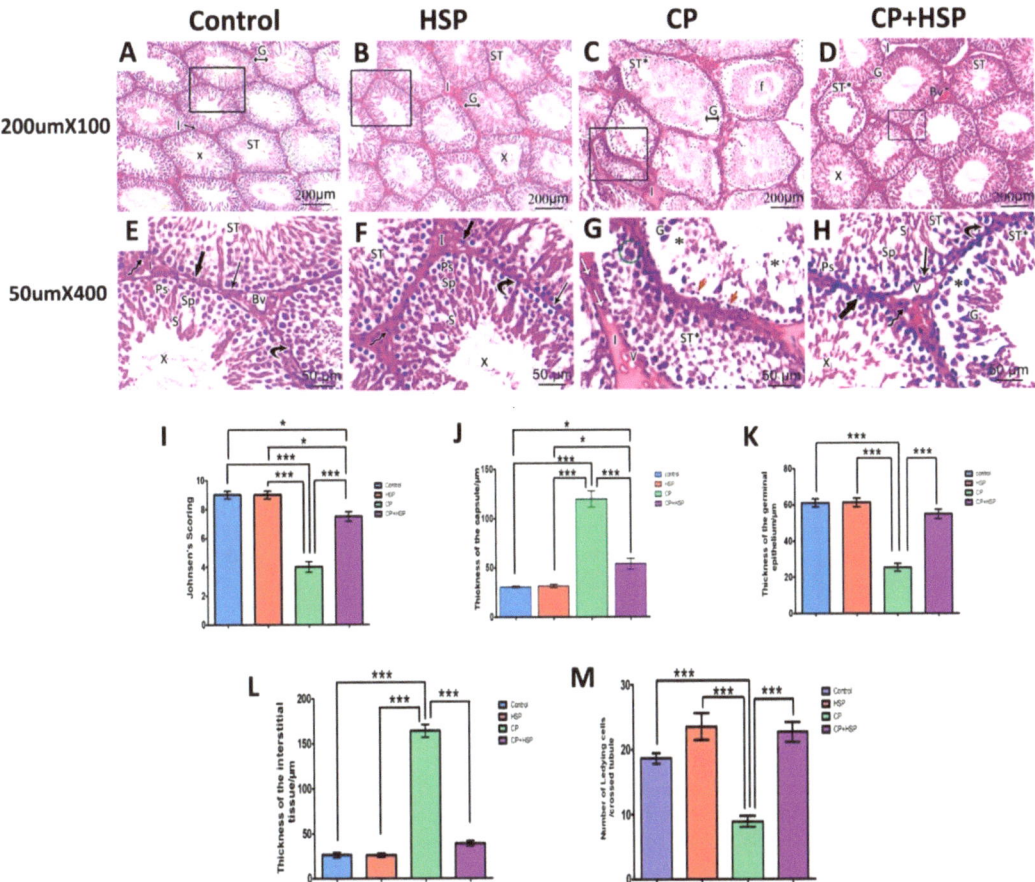

Figure 3. Effect of hesperidin administration in cyclophosphamide-induced testicular impairment in male rats on testicular histopathological and morphometric analysis (**A–M**). (**A**) Seminiferous tubules (ST) lined with stratified germinal epithelium (G). Aggregation of sperm is seen in their lumina (X). Narrow interstitial spaces (I), H&E X100. (**B**) Seminiferous tubules are closely packed (ST) and lined by stratified germinal epithelium (G). Clumps of sperm are seen in their lumina (X). A narrow interstitium is seen in between the tubules and contains clusters of cells (I), H&E X100. (**C**) Distorted seminiterous tubule (ST*) with irregular outlines and atrophied layers of germinal epithelium (G) with exfoliation of some germ cells towards the lumen (f). The interstitial tissues are wide and edematous (I), H&E X100. (**D**) Well-organized seminiferous tubules (ST) with a normal regular outline of germinal epithelium (G) and aggregation of sperm in their lumina (X). Other tubules appear affected with detached germinal epithelium and empty lumen (ST*). Relatively narrow interstitial spaces (I) between tubules and congested blood vessels (Bv*) are seen, H&E X 100.

(**E**) The higher magnification of the figure (**A**) shows seminiferous tubules lined with; spermatogonia (thick arrow), primary spermatocytes (Ps), secondary spermatocytes (Sp), spermatids (S), and sperms (X) are seen. Sertoli cells (curved arrow) are resting on the basement membrane. The seminiferous tubule is ensheathed by a single layer of flattened myoid cells (long thin arrow). The interstitial space (I) shows blood vessels (Bv) and Leydig cells (zigzag arrow), H&E X400. (**F**) The higher magnification of the figure (**B**) shows seminiferous tubule (ST) with different spermatogenic cells that include spermatogonia (thick arrow), primary spermatocytes (Ps), secondary spermatocytes (Sp), spermatids (S) and sperms (X). Sertoli cells (curved arrow) are seen on a regular basement membrane. The tubules are ensheathed by a single layer of flat myoid cells (long thin arrow). Clusters of Leydig cells (zigzag arrow) are seen in the narrow interstitial spaces (I), H&E X400. (**G**) The higher magnification of the figure (**C**) shows degenerated seminiferous tubule (ST*) with disorganization of germinal epithelium (G) and the presence of atrophic parts (*). Darkly stained nuclei (red short arrow) and multinucleated giant cells (green circle) are also observed. The interstitial space (I) showing inflammatory cells infiltration (white arrow) and vacuolated acidophilic hyaline material (V), H&E X400. (**H**) The higher magnification of the figure (**D**) shows one seminiferous tubule (ST*) lined by disorganized germinal epithelium (G) with atrophic parts in between (*). The other tubules appear nearly normal (ST) and retain their stratified germinal epithelium; spermatogonia (thick arrow), primary spermatocytes (Ps), secondary spermatocytes (Sp), spermatids (S) and sperms (X). Sertoli cells (curved arrow) are seen between spermatogenic cells. The tubule is ensheathed by a single layer of flattened myoid cells (long thin arrow). The interstitium contains clusters of Leydig cells (zigzag arrow) and some vacuolations are noticed (V). (**I**) Johnson's testicular score. (**J**) The thickness of the capsule. (**K**) The thickness of the germinal epithelium. (**L**) The thickness of the interstitial space. (**M**) Number of Leydig cells. Scale bar = 50 µm, X400. Data are expressed as means ± SEM. *, *** indicate significant difference ($p < 0.05$).

Sections from CP+HSP-treated groups showed a marked improvement in the histological structure of testicular tissue in comparison to the CP-treated group. The majority of the seminiferous tubules almost regained their normal architecture, had nearly regular outlines, and were lined by stratified germinal epithelium. A few seminiferous tubules were lined by disorganized germinal epithelium separated from the underlying basement membrane. The lumina of most of them showed aggregations of sperms, while others were empty. Normal blood vessels and clusters of Leydig cells were also noticed in the relatively narrow interstitium with some vacuolations still observed, as shown in Figure 3D,H.

Evaluation of Johnsen's scores in histopathological sections indicated that there was a significant decrease in spermatogenesis quality in the CP-treated group compared to that in the control group ($p < 0.001$). When compared with the CP-treated group, the CP+HSP-treated group showed a significant rise, but was still significantly different to the control group in Figure 3I. Evaluation of the mean thickness of the capsule showed a significant increase in the CP-treated group in comparison to that of the control group ($p < 0.001$). The CP+HSP-treated group showed a significant decline when compared with the CP-treated group, but was still significantly different from that in the control group, as shown in Figure 3J. The CP-treated group's mean thickness of the germinal epithelium was significantly decreased when compared to that of the control group ($p < 0.001$). The CP+HSP-treated group showed a significant increase in the thickness of germinal epithelium when compared with the CP-treated group, as shown in Figure 3K. The mean thickness of the interstitial space in the CP-treated group showed a significant increase in comparison to the control group ($p < 0.001$). When compared to the CP-treated group, the CP+HSP-treated group showed a significant decline in Figure 3L. The number of Leydig cells was significantly decreased in the CP-treated group compared to that in the control group ($p < 0.001$). However, the CP+HSP-treated group showed a significant increase in comparison to the CP-treated group, as shown in Figure 3M.

2.4. Effect on Testicular Immunohistochemistry of iNOS and P53

Examination of the iNOS immunohistochemical stained section of the control and HSP-treated group revealed mild expression of iNOS immune reactivity in the cytoplasm of the germ cells of seminiferous tubules, shown in Figure 4A,B,E,F. The CP-treated group expressed a significant increase in iNOS immune reactivity in the cytoplasm of the germ cells and the interstitial cells, shown in Figure 4C,G, whereas administration of HSP led to a marked decrease in iNOS immunoreactivity in the cytoplasm of the germ cells of seminiferous tubules and the interstitial cells in Figure 4D,H. The mean area % of iNOS expression in the testes sections (X400) of the four experimental groups, was considerably higher in the CP-treated group in comparison to the control and CP+HSP-treated group, shown in Figure 4M.

In the seminiferous tubules of the control group and HSP-treated group, the P53 immunopositive reaction was primarily found in the nucleus of apoptotic cells, and is hardly noticeable in Figure 4I,J. Nevertheless, the seminiferous tubules of the CP-treated group had a large number of P53 immunopositive cells, shown in Figure 4K; however, the seminiferous tubules of the CP+HSP-treated group contained fewer P53 immunopositive cells, shown in Figure 4L. Regarding the average area % of P53 expression and the number of P53 immunopositive cells per tubule in the testes sections (X400) of the four experimental groups, the CP-treated group showed a significant increase compared to the control and CP+HSP-treated groups, shown in Figure 4N,O. The CP+HSP-treated group showed a significant decrease in comparison to the CP-treated group, shown in Figure 4N,O.

2.5. Effect on mRNA Expression of Hypothalamic KISS-1, KISS-1r, GnRH, Hypophyseal GnRHr and Testicular Steroidogenic Enzymes

A significant downregulation in hypothalamic KISS-1, KISS-1r, and GnRH and hypophyseal GnRHr mRNA expression in the CP-treated group in comparison to that in the control group were noticed. Treatment with HSP significantly upregulated hypothalamic KISS-1 and GnRH and hypophyseal GnRHr, but not KISS-1r, in comparison to that in the CP-treated group, as shown in Figure 5A–D. In comparison to the control group, a significant downregulation in the testicular mRNA expression of StAR, CYP11A1, CYP17A1, HSD17B3, and CYP19A1 in the CP-treated group was noticed. In comparison to the CP-treated group, the CP+HSP-treated group showed considerable upregulation in the testicular StAR, CYP11A1, CYP17A1, HSD17B3, and CYP19A1, as shown in Figure 5E–I.

2.6. Effect on Testicular mRNA Expression of GLP-1, PGC-1, and PPAR-α

A significant decrease in testicular GLP-1, PGC-1, and PPAR-a was shown in the CP-treated group compared to the control group in Figure 6A–C. HSP administration showed a significant increase in testicular GLP-1, PGC-1, and PPAR-α when compared to that in the CP-treated group, shown in Figure 6A–C.

2.7. Effect on Testicular Apoptotic and Inflammatory Marker

A significant upregulation in testicular P53 and IL1B mRNA expression and downregulation in testicular IL10 mRNA expression were detected in the CP-treated group when compared to that of the control group, as shown in Figure 7A–C. The CP+HSP-treated group showed significant downregulation of testicular P53 and IL1B and upregulation in testicular IL10 mRNA expression when compared to CP-treated group, shown in Figure 7A–C.

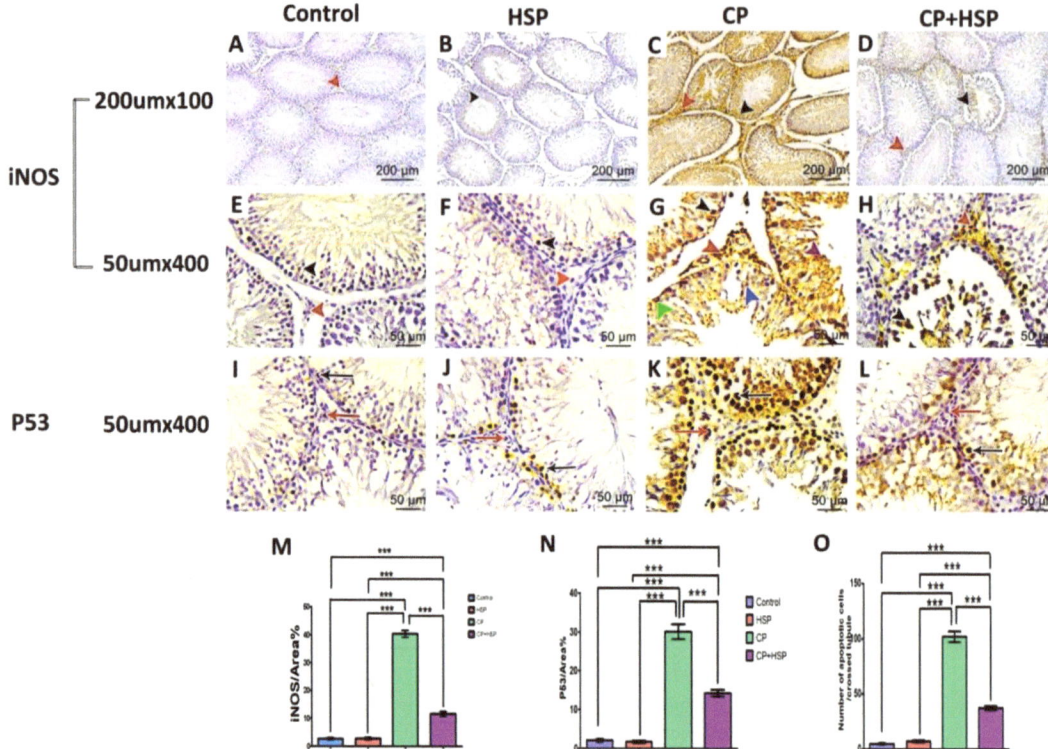

Figure 4. Effect of hesperidin administration in cyclophosphamide-induced testicular impairment in male rats on testicular immunohistochemical staining of iNOs and P53, as indicated by a positive immune reaction (arrowheads and arrows) in the cytoplasm and nuclei of the Leydig cells and germ cells of different studied groups (**A–O**). (**A**) Testicular immunohistochemical stained sections of iNOs in control-treated groups. Scale bar = 200 μm, X100. (**B**) Testicular immunohistochemical stained sections of iNOs in HSP-treated group. Scale bar = 200 μm, X100. (**C**) Testicular immunohistochemical stained sections of iNOs in CP-treated group. Scale bar = 200 μm, X100. (**D**) Testicular immunohistochemical stained sections of iNOs in CP+HSP-treated group. Scale bar = 200 μm, X100. (**E**) Testicular immunohistochemical stained sections of iNOs in control-treated groups. Scale bar = 50 μm, X400. (**F**) Testicular immunohistochemical stained sections of iNOs in HSP-treated group. Scale bar = 50 μm, X400. (**G**) Testicular immunohistochemical stained sections of iNOs in CP-treated group. Scale bar = 50 μm, X400. (**H**) Testicular immunohistochemical stained sections of iNOs in CP+HSP-treated group. Scale bar = 50 μm, X400. (**I**) Testicular immunohistochemical stained sections of P53 in control-treated groups. Scale bar = 50 μm, X400. (**J**) Testicular immunohistochemical stained sections of P53 in HSP-treated group. Scale bar = 50 μm, X400. (**K**) Testicular immunohistochemical stained sections of P53 in CP-treated group. Scale bar = 50 μm, X400. (**L**) Testicular immunohistochemical stained sections of P53 in CP+HSP-treated group. Scale bar = 50 μm, X400. (**M**) Immunostaining intensity of testicular iNOs (% area). (**N**) Immunostaining intensity of testicular P53 (% area). (**O**) Number of apoptotic cells per crossed tubule. Data are expressed as means ± SEM. *** indicate significant difference ($p < 0.05$).

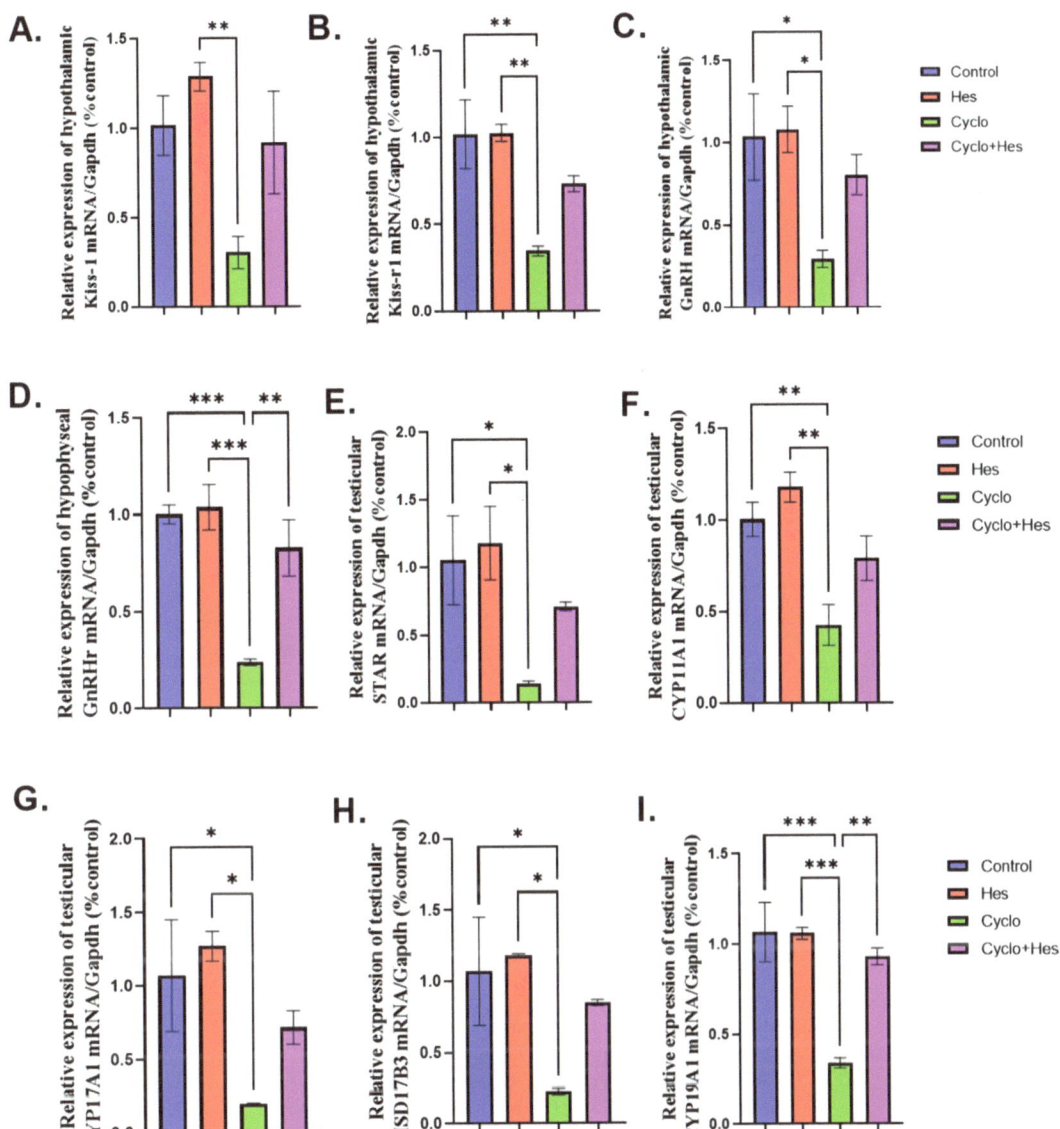

Figure 5. Effect of hesperidin administration in cyclophosphamide-induced testicular impairment in male rats on mRNA expression of hypothalamic KISS-1, KISS-1r, GnRH, hypophyseal GnRHr and testicular steroidogenic enzymes (**A–I**). (**A**) Hypothalamic KISS-1/Gapdh (% control), (**B**) mRNA expression of hypothalamic KISS-1r/Gapdh (% control), (**C**) mRNA expression of hypothalamic GnRH/Gapdh (% control), (**D**) mRNA expression of hypophyseal GnRHr/Gapdh (% control), (**E**) Testicular Star/Gapdh (% control), (**F**) Testicular Cyp11a1/Gapdh (% control), (**G**) Testicular Cyp17A1/Gapdh (% control), (**H**) Testicular HSD17B3/Gapdh (% control), and (**I**) Testicular Cyp19A1/Gapdh (% control). Data are expressed as means ± SEM. *, **, *** indicate significant difference ($p < 0.05$).

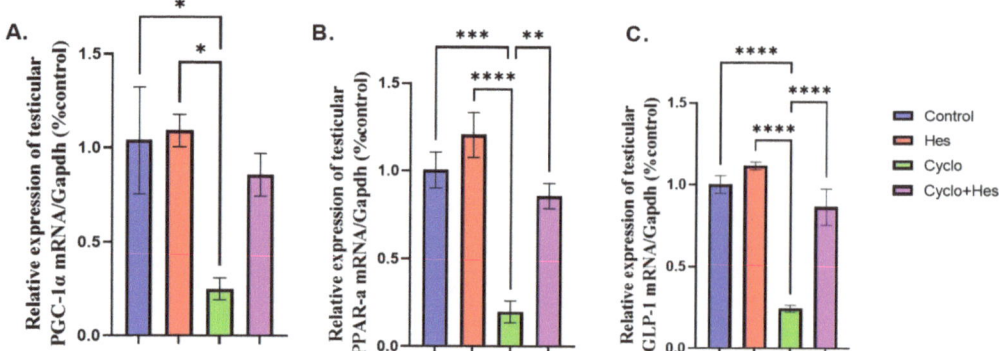

Figure 6. Effect of hesperidin administration in cyclophosphamide-induced testicular impairment in male rats on mRNA expression of testicular GLP-1, PGC-1, and PPAR-a (**A–C**). (**A**) Testicular PGC-1/Gapdh (% control), (**B**) mRNA expression of testicular PPAR-a/Gapdh (% control), and (**C**) mRNA expression of testicular GLP-1/Gapdh (% control). Data are expressed as means ± SEM. *, **, ***, **** indicate significant difference ($p < 0.05$).

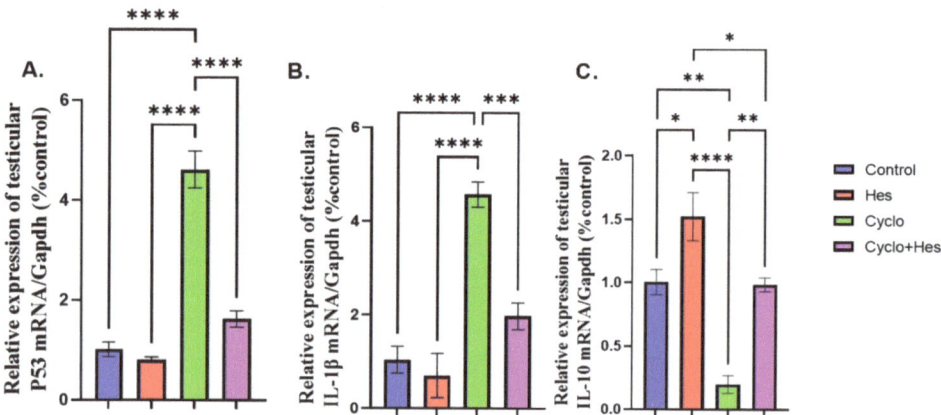

Figure 7. Effect of hesperidin administration in cyclophosphamide-induced testicular impairment in male rats on mRNA expression of testicular P53, IL1B, and IL10 (**A–C**). (**A**) Testicular P53/Gapdh (% control), (**B**) mRNA expression of testicular IL1B/Gapdh (% control), and (**C**) mRNA expression of testicular IL10/Gapdh (% control). Data are expressed as means ± SEM. *, **, ***, **** indicate significant difference ($p < 0.05$).

3. Discussion

Cancer is a leading cause of death worldwide [17]. As a result, researchers have been looking for different therapeutic strategies to improve the quality of life for patients. CP is a regularly used form of chemotherapy particularly in multiple myeloma, sarcoma, lymphoma, neuroblastoma, leukemia, and prostate and breast cancer [18]. CP has been shown to affect rapidly proliferating tissues such as gonads by interfering with their cell growth and differentiation [19]. CP treatment combined with several protective supplements, including polyphenols, vitamins, and minerals, has been suggested [20] to overcome such damaging impacts. HSP, owing to its antioxidant/anti-inflammatory effects, could be beneficial [21,22].

In the present work, the final body weight of rats receiving CP treatment was significantly decreased when compared with the control group, as previously reported [23]. A single intraperitoneal injection of a lesser dose of 120 mg/kg/b.wt [24] or 50 mg/kg/day for three days [25] also was reported to decrease body weight in rats. This decline could be caused by metabolic alterations causing appetite loss and decreased food intake. Yet, no weight change was noticed after administering CP in a single intraperitoneal dose of 200 mg/kg/b.wt. in rats [26]. HSP administration at a dose of 200 mg/kg/b.wt has been linked to improving the body weight in the aluminum phosphatide-treated group [27,28]. In the present study, the CP-treated group's testicular weight significantly decreased when compared with the control group [29]. Administration of CP in a dose of 15 mg/kg once a week for 35 days has been linked to reduced testicular size in mice [30]. Other reports administering single CP at a dose of 100 mg/kg showed no difference in the weight of testis between groups [31,32]. HSP in a dose of 25–50 mg/kg for 60 days, revealed that HSP co-administration normalizes testicular weight [33]. Collectively, this could suggest a potential effect for the administration route, dose, treatment duration, and sensitivity of the animals in body and testicular weight changes.

The hypothalamic–pituitary–gonadal (HPG) axis controlling gonadal function in males starts by hypothalamic secretion of GnRH to stimulate the pituitary generation of FSH and LH. Additionally, FSH and LH play a role in regulating Leydig cell function to produce testosterone in males [8]. CP markedly reduced the serum levels of testosterone, FSH, LH, and prolactin [11], even at a single dose of 100 mg/kg [34]. The results of this study indicated that CP affected spermatogenesis by interfering with cellular processes as well as the pituitary–testicular axis. HSP significantly enhanced the serum testosterone, FSH, LH, and prolactin levels following bisphenol A administration [35,36]. Also, the administration of other flavonoids, including quercetin [11] or morin [37,38], or rutin [38], improved serum levels of testosterone, FSH, LH, and prolactin. This could be attributed to the protective roles of flavonoids in terms of anti-inflammatory and antioxidant ability.

CP disrupts the antioxidant defense mechanisms by producing large amounts of ROS in conjunction with its harmful metabolite, acrolein, which is known to increase oxidative stress, causing a marked reduction in GPx and TAC levels and a marked elevation in MDA levels [39,40]. Oxidative stress is a major contributor to male infertility [41] via modifications in microvascular blood flow leading to elevated rates of germ cell death. HSP co-administration reduced the level of the lipid peroxidation marker, MDA, and also strengthened the body's natural antioxidant defense system by boosting the activity of antioxidant enzymes such as SOD and GPx [27,42–44]. Oxidative stress, lipid peroxidation, and inflammation usually manifest histological and functional abnormalities in testicular tissue [45,46]. CP intraperitoneal administration at a dose of 5 mg/kg daily for four weeks, showed intraepithelial vacuoles as an indication of seminiferous tubules atrophy, as well as spacing and separation of germ cells, which may be caused by sloughing and exfoliation of the germ cells due to the primary impact on the cell-to-cell junction in between Sertoli cells and germ cells [47,48].

Other reports of single CP administration at a dose of 200 mg/kg showed marked testicular damage, including interstitial bleeding, and separation of spermatogenic cells with the presence of vacuoles, and explained how CP could cause oxidative stress, lipid peroxidation, and apoptosis [49]. CP intraperitoneal administration at a dose of 60 mg/kg per week for eight weeks revealed that the seminiferous tubules exhibited morphological changes, including interstitial edema, vacuolization, multinucleated giant cell development, desquamation, degeneration, and disorganization. In addition, reactive oxygen species and oxidative stress have been linked to the pathogenesis of CP toxicity [50].

The CP-treated group revealed a significant increase in iNOS, only formed during inflammation, ischemia, and apoptosis [51], immune reactivity in the cytoplasm of the cells of the seminiferous tubules [52]. Exposure to cisplatin, aluminum chloride, methotrexate, and silica nanoparticles reported an increase in testicular iNOS expression [53–56]. Anticancer drugs, including cyclophosphamide, methotrexate, tamoxifen, doxorubicin, and

5-fluorouracil administration, have been associated with the induction of oxidative stress and inflammation [57]. Such results, confirmed by another flavonoid (quercetin), [54] found that coadministration of quercetin to the aluminum chloride-treated group decreased the iNOS expression in testis tissue. HSP caused a marked decrease in the CP-induced expression of iNOS in the liver [58] and renal tissue [59]. Coadministration of another antioxidant as melatonin decreased the expression of iNOS in testicular tissue in the cisplatin-treated group [60].

Increased testicular apoptosis, as indicated by increased P53 expression, results in spermatogenic arrest and a reduction in spermatogonia, spermatocytes, and spermatid numbers [61]. The CP-treated group revealed a marked increase in P53 immune reactivity in the nucleus of the cells of the seminiferous tubules and revealed an increased number of apoptotic cells in the CP-treated group [62]. Exposure to potassium dichromate, D-gal/$NaNO_2$, bleomycin, etoposide, and cisplatin resulted in an increase in testicular P53 expression [63–65]. Treatment with hesperidin might protect mice's testis against apoptosis [66]. HSP administration at a dose of 50 mg/kg daily via gavage for 14 days, reported mitigated testicular alterations brought on by cisplatin [67]. Additionally, HSP treatment reduced the testicular seminiferous tubules deterioration process and lowered ischemia/reperfusion-induced reproductive damage [68]. HSP caused a marked decrease in the expression of P53 in the corneal tissue [69], liver [22], and colon [70]. Regarding other flavonoids, co-administration of quercetin to the cisplatin-treated group decreased the expression of P53 in testicular tissue [71].

The mean testicular Johnsen's score in the CP-treated group decreased significantly in comparison with the control group [52]. The thickness of germinal epithelium had significantly decreased and the lumina were large and empty [72]. They linked these findings to the inhibition of B-spermatogonia mitosis, which denotes an extension of the G1 phase of the cell cycle growth. Additionally, it has been demonstrated that this epithelial thinning results in a deficiency in sperm production. A significant decline in epithelial height and increase in the interstitial space in the cisplatin-treated group [73] could be attributed to oxidative stress that was responsible for all cisplatin-induced damage in the testis. The thickness of the capsule of the testis was significantly increased in the iprodione-treated group [35]. The number of Leydig cells decreased significantly in the CP-treated group [74,75]. In the present study, there was a significant improvement in testicular Johnsen's score in the CP+HSP-treated group when compared to the CP-treated group. This result was consistent with previous reports indicating that diabetic rats treated with HSP showed considerable improvement in the mean testicular biopsy score [76].

In the present study, the number of Leydig cells in the CP+HSP-treated group increased significantly when compared to the CP-treated group [77]. HSP treatment with cisplatin causes considerable improvement in the thickness of germinal epithelium [67]. Quercetin co-treatment showed a significant reduction in the interstitial space in the arsenic-treated group [78]. Melatonin co-treatment showed a significant reduction in the thickness of tunica albuginea in the taxol-treated group [79].

In this study, there was significant downregulation of hypothalamic KISS, KISSr, GnRH, and hypophyseal GnRHr in the CP-treated group when compared with the control group. Oxidative stress induced by extensive exercise has been reported to downregulate the expression of KISS, KISSr, GnRH, and GnRHr [80]. A significant upregulation in gene expression of hypothalamic KISS, GnRH, and hypophyseal GnRHr in the CP+HSP-treated group if compared with the CP-treated group was noticed. This could be attributed to the flavonoid's ability to prevent tissue damage, prevent the inactivation of steroidogenesis, and increase gonadotropin release [81,82]. CP treatment significantly decreases steroidogenic genes that include StAR, CYP11A1, CYP17A1, HSD17B, and CYP1719A1 compared with other groups [11,83]. Cisplatin has been reported to induce similar impacts [84,85]. HSP administration enhances testicular functions through the upregulation of steroidogenesis-related genes [86]. Additionally, isorhamnetin, a bioflavonoid treatment, significantly improved testosterone production through the upregulation of steroidogenic genes and antioxidant ability [87]. On the other hand, studies have also suggested that flavonoids may interact with estrogen receptors (ERs) to modulate the activity of the endocrine system [88,89]. This interaction has been linked to a variety of health outcomes, including testicular dysfunction in rats [88]. The interaction between flavonoids and ERs is complex and depends on the type of flavonoid, duration of administration and its concentration. Such interaction should be in focus in future research.

GLP-1 is essential for maintaining male fertility, since it controls spermatogenesis and steroidogenesis directly. It is released by Leydig cells and works on Sertoli, germinal epithelial, and Leydig cells (all of which have GLP-1 receptors). This procedure increases the metabolism of Sertoli cells and raises sperm cell quality [90]. PPAR-α and PGC-1α, stimulate fatty acid oxidation and impact the testicular energy balance [91]. Testicular torsion, similar to CP administration, caused significant downregulation of testicular GLP-1, PPAR-α, and PGC-1α and affect the metabolism of testicular cells and worsens oxidative stress by raising reactive oxygen species and reactive nitrogen species, which promote apoptosis and inflammation inside testis [92]. A significant upregulation of testicular GLP-1, PPAR-α, and PGC-1α in the CP+HSP-treated group was noticed, indicating a positive effect on testicular metabolism. CP-treated rats showed a significant upregulation of testicular apoptotic P53 [83] and pro-inflammatory IL1β and downregulation of anti-inflammatory IL10. Cisplatin caused a significant elevation in pro-inflammatory IL1β and significant downregulation of the anti-inflammatory IL10 gene respectively [84,93]. HSP's antioxidant properties cleared the ROS, preventing the pro-inflammatory genes from activating, and protecting testicular tissue from inflammation [94]. CP and HSP-combined treatment downregulated the testicular apoptotic P53 gene and pro-inflammatory IL1β and significant upregulated the anti-inflammatory IL10 gene when compared with CP-treated group. Co-treatment with bilobetin, a natural bioflavonoid, significantly reduced testicular P53 expression and significantly increased testicular IL10 expression in the cisplatin-treated group [95].

4. Materials and Methods

4.1. Chemicals

Cyclophosphamide in the form of powder acquired from Baxter oncology GmbH in Germany. CP was injected at a dose of 150 mg/kg/B.wt. Hesperidin (>80% purity powder CAS NO 520-26-3) was produced by Sigma-Aldrich Company St. Louis, MO, USA, and acquired from Sigma-Egypt. Hesperidin was orally administrated by gavage at a dose of 200 mg/kg/B.wt.

4.2. Experimental Animals

Thirty-two adult healthy male Sprague Dawley rats (12–14 weeks) weighing 210 ± 10 g were obtained from Zagazig scientific and medical research center (ZSMRC). The animals were then kept at a constant 23 ± 2 °C and operated on a 12-h light/12-h dark cycle. Throughout the study, the animals were kept on a regular diet and ad libitum water supply. All rats received humane care and the experimental methods were approved by the Institutional Animal Care and Use Committee of Zagazig University (No. ZU-IACUC/3/F/172/2019).

4.3. Experimental Design and Sample Collection

The rats were randomly assigned into four main groups (n = 8), namely, the control group that received normal saline for eight days, the HSP-treated group that received HSP 200 mg/kg/d orally for eight days [27,96], the CP-treated group that received CP 150 mg/kg single intraperitoneal injection on the 1st day of the experiment [87], and CP+HSP-treated group that received CP 150 mg/kg single intraperitoneal injection on the 1st day of the experiment and HSP 200 mg/kg/d orally for eight days. Rats were euthanized 48 h after the last HSP dose. The body weights were determined and venous blood samples were taken from their retro-orbital plexus using a capillary glass tube, blood was left to clot at room temperature, then centrifuged at 3000 rpm for 10 min to separate the serum. The samples were then kept at $-20\,°C$ to be used subsequently for hormonal assay estimation. Then, the rats were anesthetized by intraperitoneal injection of thiopental (75 mg/kg BW) and subjected to cervical dislocation, the abdomen was then opened to collect both testes outside the body, weighted and then divided into three parts; the first part was collected on 10% neutral buffered formalin for histopathological and immunohistochemical examination, the second part (30 mg) was removed directly on liquid nitrogen and then kept at $-80\,°C$ to be used for total RNA extraction and the third part (1 g) was homogenized to be used for different biochemical tests. After being dissected, the hypothalamus and pituitary gland were stored in liquid nitrogen and kept there at $-80\,°C$ until total RNA extraction as previously described [97].

4.4. Hormonal and Biochemical Analysis

The levels of serum of FSH, LH, total testosterone, and prolactin were determined by using a commercially available rat enzyme-linked immunosorbent assay (ELISA) (Catalog No. CSB-E12654r) for LH as well as (Catalog No. CSB-E06869r) for FSH and (Catalog No. MBS282195) for testosterone and (Catalog No. CSB-E06881r) for prolactin [98,99]. The levels of malondialdehyde (MDA), glutathione peroxidase enzyme activity (GPx), and total antioxidant capacity (TAC) were assessed using (Catalog No. (ELA-E0597r) for MDA, (Catalog No. ELA-E0295r) for GPx, (Catalog No. STA-360) for TAC.

4.5. Real-Time Quantitative RT-PCR (qRT-PCR) Analysis

Briefly, total RNA was extracted using Trizol (Invitrogen; Thermo Fisher Scientific, Waltham, MA, USA), and for evaluating the RNA quality, the A260/A280 ratio was analyzed using the NanoDrop VR ND-1000 Spectrophotometer (NanoDrop Technologies; Wilmington, DE, USA). For cDNA synthesis, a High-Capacity cDNA Reverse Transcription Kit cDNA Kit (Applied Biosystems™, USA) was used, followed by the preparation of the primers according to their manufacturer instructions, Sangon Biotech (Beijing, China), as provided in Table 1.

Table 1. Forward and reverse primers sequence of targeted genes.

Gene	Forward Primer Sequence (5' to 3')	Reverse Primer Sequence (5' to 3')	Product Size	Accession No.
GLP1	CACCTCCTCTCAGCTCAGTC	CGTTCTCCTCCGTGTCTTGA	128	NM_012707.2
Pparα	GTCCTCTGGTTGTCCCCTTG	GTCAGTTCACAGGGAAGGCA	176	NM_013196.2
PGC1α	TTCAGGAGCTGGATGGCTTG	GGGCAGCACACTCTATGTCA	70	NM_031347.1
Gapdh	GCATCTTCTTGTGCAGTGCC	GGTAACCAGGCGTCCGATAC	91	NM_017008.4
Kiss-1	TGCTGCTTCTCCTCTGTGTGG	ATTAACGAGTTCCTGGGGTCC	110	NM_181692.1
Kiss-1r	CTTTCCTTCTGTGCTGCGTA	CCTGCTGGATGTAGTTGACG	102	NM_023992.1
GnRH1	AGGAGCTCTGGAACGTCTGAT	AGCGTCAATGTCACACTCGG	100	NM_012767.2
GnRHr	TCAGGACCCACGCAAACTAC	CTGGCTCTGACACCCTGTTT	182	NM_031038.3
StAr	CCCAAATGTCAAGGAAATCA	AGGCATCTCCCCAAAGTG	187	NM_031558.3
CYP11A1	AAGTATCCGTGATGTGGG	TCATACAGTGTCGCCTTTTCT	127	NM_017286.3
CYP17A1	TGGCTTTCCTGGTGCACAATC	TGAAAGTTGGTGTTCGGCTGAAG	90	NM_012753.2
HSD17B3	AGTGTGTGAGGTTCTCCCGGTACCT	TACAACATTGAGTCCATGTCTGGCCAG	161	NM_054007.1
CYP19A1	GCTGAGAGACGTGGAGACCTG	CTCTGTCACCAACAACAGTGTGG	178	NM_017085.2
IL10	GTAGAAGTGATGCCCCAGGC	AGAAATCGATGACAGCGTCG	116	NM_012854.2
IL1β	CACCTCTCAAGCAGAGCACAGA	ACGGGTTCCATGGTGAAGTC	81	NM_031512.2
P53	GTTCGTGTTTGTGCCTGTCC	TGCTCTCTTTGCACTCCCTG	108	NM_030989.3

Real-time RT-PCR was performed in Mx3005P real-time PCR system (Agilent Stratagene, USA) using TOPrealTM qPCR 2X PreMIX (SYBR Green with low ROX) (Cat. # P725 or P750) (Enzynomics, Korea) following the manufacturer's instructions. The PCR cycling conditions included initial denaturation at 95 °C for 12 min followed by 40 cycles of denaturation at 95 °C for 20 s, annealing at 60 °C for 30 s, and extension at 72 °C for 30 s. A melting curve analysis was performed following PCR amplification. The expression level of the target genes was normalized using the mRNA expression of a known housekeeping gene, Gapdh. Results are expressed as fold-changes compared to the control group following the $2^{-\Delta\Delta Ct}$ method [100].

4.6. Histopathological and Immunohistochemical Examination

All the testicular specimens from all groups were installed in Bouin solution for 4 to 5 h till converted to a hard consistency then kept for paraffin block preparation. For the light microscopic analysis, tissue sections of 5 μm thickness were stained with H and E stain to examine the structural light microscopic alterations [101]. For immunohistochemical staining, a rabbit monoclonal antibody of IgG type was designed for specific localization of inducible nitric oxide synthase (iNOS) marker for oxidative stress and P53 (apoptosis marker) in paraffin sections. The kits were delivered from DAKO life trade Egypt (Catalog No. A0312 for iNOS and Catalog No. A5761 for P53). Following the manufacturer's recommendations, sections were inspected and photographed by light microscope LEICA DM500 in the Anatomy Department, Faculty of Medicine, Zagazig University

The Johnsen scoring system was used to assess the histological alterations in testicular tissue. Each tubule received a Johnsen's score between 1 (extremely poor) and 10 (excellent) following Johnsen's criteria [102]. Image J analysis software (Fiji image j; 1.51 n, NIH, USA) was used for measuring the thickness of the capsule, the thickness of the germinal epithelium, the thickness of the interstitial space, and the count of Leydig cells in sections stained with H&E per 100 high powers fields for the thickness of capsule and 400 high powers fields for the thickness of the germinal epithelium, the thickness of the interstitial space and count of Leydig cells [103]. After immunostaining, the number of apoptotic cells (in P53 stained sections) was counted and analysis of the mean area % of P53 (in P53 stained sections) or iNOS (in iNOS stained sections) was performed in nearly 150 seminiferous tubules from 8 animals/group, and the findings were statistically analyzed [104].

4.7. Statistical Analysis

Continuous variables were represented by the mean ± standard error mean (SEM). All data were normally distributed and were analyzed by one-way analysis of variance (ANOVA) followed by Tukey's honest significant difference test in homogenous data for multiple group comparison. p values less than 0.05 ($p < 0.05$) was statistically significant using the statistical software package SPSS for Windows (Version 20; SPSS Inc., Chicago, IL, USA).

5. Conclusions

Our study concludes that hesperidin's antioxidant, anti-inflammatory, and anti-apoptotic activities could modulate testicular disturbances induced by cyclophosphamide. The findings of our study raise the prospect of hesperidin, a bioflavonoid, as a therapeutic intervention for delaying testicular dysfunction. Such findings could be an important entry point for preserving fertility while using antineoplastic drugs such as cyclophosphamide against a wide spectrum of malignancies. Although the therapeutic applications of bioflavonoids, including hesperidin, should be promising, any future clinical application should be preceded by rigorous clinical studies.

Author Contributions: Conceptualization, A.A.H., E.R.A., S.S.A.E.-F., T.K. and M.M.M.A.; methodology, A.A.H., E.R.A., S.S.A.E.-F., T.K., L.M.F. and A.H.A.; software, T.K., L.M.F. and A.H.A.; validation, A.A.H., E.R.A., S.S.A.E.-F., T.K., L.M.F., A.H.A. and M.M.M.A.; formal analysis, S.S.A.E.-F., T.K., L.M.F., A.H.A. and M.M.M.A.; investigation, A.A.H., E.R.A., S.S.A.E.-F., T.K., L.M.F., A.H.A. and M.M.M.A.; resources, S.S.A.E.-F., T.K., L.M.F. and A.H.A.; data curation, S.S.A.E.-F., T.K. and A.H.A.; writing—original draft preparation, S.S.A.E.-F., T.K. and A.H.A.; writing—review and editing, A.A.H., E.R.A., S.S.A.E.-F., T.K., L.M.F., A.H.A. and M.M.M.A.; visualization, supervision, project administration, A.A.H., E.R.A., T.K., L.M.F., A.H.A. and M.M.M.A.; funding acquisition, S.S.A.E.-F., M.M.M.A., T.K., L.M.F. and A.H.A. All authors have read and agreed to the published version of the manuscript.

Funding: This research received no external funding, and the APC was funded by the project 6PFE of the University of Life Sciences "King Mihai I" from Timisoara and Research Institute for Biosecurity and Bioengineering from Timisoara, Romania.

Institutional Review Board Statement: All rats received humane care and the experimental methods were approved by the Institutional Animal Care and Use Committee of Zagazig University (No. ZU-IACUC/3/F/172/2019).

Informed Consent Statement: Not applicable.

Data Availability Statement: The data presented in this study are available upon reasonable request from the corresponding author. The data are not publicly available as it contains information that could compromise the privacy of an ongoing research.

Conflicts of Interest: The authors declare no conflict of interest.

References

1. Yilmaz, E.; Coskun, E.I.; Sahin, N.; Ciplak, B.; Ekici, K. MPV, NLR, and platelet count: New hematologic markers in diagnosis of malignant ovarian tumor. *Eur. J. Gynaecol. Oncol.* **2017**, *38*, 346–349. [PubMed]
2. Klareskog, L.; van der Heijde, D.; de Jager, J.P.; Gough, A.; Kalden, J.; Malaise, M.; Mola, E.M.; Pavelka, K.; Sany, J.; Settas, L.; et al. Therapeutic effect of the combination of etanercept and methotrexate compared with each treatment alone in patients with rheumatoid arthritis: Double-blind randomised controlled trial. *Lancet* **2004**, *363*, 675–681. [CrossRef] [PubMed]
3. Veal, G.J.; Cole, M.; Chinnaswamy, G.; Sludden, J.; Jamieson, D.; Errington, J.; Malik, G.; Hill, C.R.; Chamberlain, T.; Boddy, A.V. Cyclophosphamide pharmacokinetics and pharmacogenetics in children with B-cell non-Hodgkin's lymphoma. *Eur. J. Cancer* **2016**, *55*, 56–64. [CrossRef] [PubMed]
4. Boisseaux, P.; Noury, P.; Thomas, H.; Garric, J. Immune responses in the aquatic gastropod Lymnaea stagnalis under short-term exposure to pharmaceuticals of concern for immune systems: Diclofenac, cyclophosphamide and cyclosporine A. *Ecotoxicol. Environ. Saf.* **2017**, *139*, 358–366. [CrossRef] [PubMed]
5. Grzesiuk, M.; Mielecki, D.; Pilżys, T.; Garbicz, D.; Marcinkowski, M.; Grzesiuk, E. How cyclophosphamide at environmentally relevant concentration influences Daphnia magna life history and its proteome. *PLoS ONE* **2018**, *13*, e0195366. [CrossRef]
6. Temel, Y.; Çağlayan, C.; Ahmed, B.M.; Kandemir, F.M.; Çiftci, M. The effects of chrysin and naringin on cyclophosphamide-induced erythrocyte damage in rats: Biochemical evaluation of some enzyme activities in vivo and in vitro. *Naunyn Schmiedebergs Arch Pharm.* **2021**, *394*, 645–654. [CrossRef]
7. Spears, N.; Lopes, F.; Stefansdottir, A.; Rossi, V.; De Felici, M.; Anderson, R.A.; Klinger, F.G. Ovarian damage from chemotherapy and current approaches to its protection. *Hum. Reprod. Update* **2019**, *25*, 673–693. [CrossRef]
8. Akomolafe, S.F.; Aluko, B.T. Protective effect of curcumin on fertility in cyclophosphamide exposed rats: Involvement of multiple pathways. *J. Food Biochem.* **2020**, *44*, e13095. [CrossRef]
9. Khamis, T.; Abdelalim, A.F.; Saeed, A.A.; Edress, N.M.; Nafea, A.; Ebian, H.F.; Algendy, R.; Hendawy, D.M.; Arisha, A.H.; Abdallah, S.H. Breast milk MSCs upregulated β-cells PDX1, Ngn3, and PCNA expression via remodeling ER stress/inflammatory/apoptotic signaling pathways in type 1 diabetic rats. *Eur. J. Pharmacol.* **2021**, *905*, 174188. [CrossRef]
10. Khamis, T.; Abdelalim, A.F.; Abdallah, S.H.; Saeed, A.A.; Edress, N.M.; Arisha, A.H. Early intervention with breast milk mesenchymal stem cells attenuates the development of diabetic-induced testicular dysfunction via hypothalamic Kisspeptin/Kiss1r-GnRH/GnIH system in male rats. *Biochim. Et Biophys. Acta-Mol. Basis Dis.* **2020**, *1866*, 165877. [CrossRef]
11. Ebokaiwe, A.P.; Obasi, D.O.; Njoku, R.C.; Osawe, S. Cyclophosphamide-induced testicular oxidative-inflammatory injury is accompanied by altered immunosuppressive indoleamine 2, 3-dioxygenase in Wister rats: Influence of dietary quercetin. *Andrologia* **2022**, *54*, e14341. [CrossRef]
12. Van den Boogaard, W.M.C.; Komninos, D.S.J.; Vermeij, W.P. Chemotherapy Side-Effects: Not All DNA Damage Is Equal. *Cancers* **2022**, *14*, 627. [CrossRef]
13. Naz, S.; Imran, M.; Rauf, A.; Orhan, I.E.; Shariati, M.A.; Iahtisham Ul, H.; IqraYasmin; Shahbaz, M.; Qaisrani, T.B.; Shah, Z.A.; et al. Chrysin: Pharmacological and therapeutic properties. *Life Sci.* **2019**, *235*, 116797. [CrossRef]
14. Gulcin, İ. Antioxidants and antioxidant methods: An updated overview. *Arch. Toxicol.* **2020**, *94*, 651–715. [CrossRef]

15. Kopustinskiene, D.M.; Jakstas, V.; Savickas, A.; Bernatoniene, J. Flavonoids as Anticancer Agents. *Nutrients* **2020**, *12*, 457. [CrossRef]
16. Shoorei, H.; Banimohammad, M.; Kebria, M.M.; Afshar, M.; Taheri, M.M.; Shokoohi, M.; Farashah, M.S.; Eftekharzadeh, M.; Akhiani, O.; Gaspar, R.; et al. Hesperidin improves the follicular development in 3D culture of isolated preantral ovarian follicles of mice. *Exp. Biol. Med.* **2019**, *244*, 352–361. [CrossRef]
17. Lehmann, V.; Chemaitilly, W.; Lu, L.; Green, D.M.; Kutteh, W.H.; Brinkman, T.M.; Srivastava, D.K.; Robison, L.L.; Hudson, M.M.; Klosky, J.L. Gonadal Functioning and Perceptions of Infertility Risk Among Adult Survivors of Childhood Cancer: A Report From the St Jude Lifetime Cohort Study. *J. Clin. Oncol. Off. J. Am. Soc. Clin. Oncol.* **2019**, *37*, 893–902. [CrossRef]
18. Fusco, R.; Salinaro, A.T.; Siracusa, R.; D'Amico, R.; Impellizzeri, D.; Scuto, M.; Ontario, M.L.; Crea, R.; Cordaro, M.; Cuzzocrea, S.; et al. Hidrox($^®$) Counteracts Cyclophosphamide-Induced Male Infertility through NRF2 Pathways in a Mouse Model. *Antioxidants* **2021**, *10*, 778. [CrossRef]
19. Ghobadi, E.; Moloudizargari, M.; Asghari, M.H.; Abdollahi, M. The mechanisms of cyclophosphamide-induced testicular toxicity and the protective agents. *Expert Opin. Drug Metab. Toxicol.* **2017**, *13*, 525–536. [CrossRef]
20. Yasueda, A.; Urushima, H.; Ito, T. Efficacy and Interaction of Antioxidant Supplements as Adjuvant Therapy in Cancer Treatment: A Systematic Review. *Integr. Cancer Ther.* **2016**, *15*, 17–39. [CrossRef]
21. Zouchoune, B. How the ascorbic acid and hesperidin do improve the biological activities of the cinnamon: Theoretical investigation. *Struct. Chem.* **2020**, *31*, 2333–2340. [CrossRef] [PubMed]
22. Afzal, S.M.; Vafa, A.; Rashid, S.; Barnwal, P.; Shahid, A.; Shree, A.; Islam, J.; Ali, N.; Sultana, S. Protective effect of hesperidin against N,N'-dimethylhydrazine induced oxidative stress, inflammation, and apoptotic response in the colon of Wistar rats. *Environ. Toxicol.* **2020**, *36*, 642–653. [CrossRef] [PubMed]
23. Khorwal, G.; Chauhan, R.; Nagar, M.; Khorwal, G. Effect of cyclophosphamide on liver in albino rats: A comparative dose dependent histomorphological study. *Int. J. Biomed. Adv. Res.* **2017**, *8*, 102–107. [CrossRef]
24. Yao, Y.; Xu, Y.; Wang, Y. Protective roles and mechanisms of rosmarinic acid in cyclophosphamide-induced premature ovarian failure. *J. Biochem. Mol. Toxicol.* **2020**, *34*, e22591. [CrossRef]
25. Omole, J.G.; Ayoka, O.A.; Alabi, Q.K.; Adefisayo, M.A.; Asafa, M.A.; Olubunmi, B.O.; Fadeyi, B.A. Protective Effect of Kolaviron on Cyclophosphamide-Induced Cardiac Toxicity in Rats. *J. Evid.-Based Integr. Med.* **2018**, *23*, 2156587218757649. [CrossRef]
26. Razak, R.; Ismail, F.; Isa, M.L.M.; Wahab, A.Y.A.; Muhammad, H.; Ramli, R.; Ismail, R. Ameliorative Effects of Aquilaria malaccensis Leaves Aqueous Extract on Reproductive Toxicity Induced by Cyclophosphamide in Male Rats. *Malays. J. Med. Sci.: MJMS* **2019**, *26*, 44–57. [CrossRef]
27. Afolabi, O.K.; Wusu, A.D.; Ugbaja, R.; Fatoki, J.O. Aluminium phosphide-induced testicular toxicity through oxidative stress in Wistar rats: Ameliorative role of hesperidin. *Toxicol. Res. Appl.* **2018**, *2*, 2397847318812794. [CrossRef]
28. Hamdy, S.M.; Sayed, O.N.; Abdel Latif, A.K.M.; Abd-Elazeez, A.M.; Amin, A.M. Protective Effect Of Hesperidin And Tiger Nut Against DMBA Carcinogenicity In Female Rats. *Biochem. Lett.* **2016**, *12*, 150–167. [CrossRef]
29. Rezaei, S.; Hosseinimehr, S.J.; Zargari, M.; Karimpour Malekshah, A.; Mirzaei, M.; Talebpour Amiri, F. Protective effects of sinapic acid against cyclophosphamide-induced testicular toxicity via inhibiting oxidative stress, caspase-3 and NF-kB activity in BALB/c mice. *Andrologia* **2021**, *53*, e14196. [CrossRef]
30. Mehraban, Z.; Ghaffari Novin, M.; Golmohammadi, M.G.; Sagha, M.; Ziai, S.A.; Abdollahifar, M.A.; Nazarian, H. Protective Effect of Gallic Acid on Testicular Tissue, Sperm Parameters, and DNA Fragmentation against Toxicity Induced by Cyclophosphamide in Adult NMRI Mice. *Urol. J.* **2020**, *17*, 78–85. [CrossRef]
31. Mohammadi, F.; Nikzad, H.; Taghizadeh, M.; Taherian, A.; Azami-Tameh, A.; Hosseini, S.M.; Moravveji, A. Protective effect of Zingiber officinale extract on rat testis after cyclophosphamide treatment. *Andrologia* **2014**, *46*, 680–686. [CrossRef] [PubMed]
32. Xie, R.; Chen, L.; Wu, H.; Chen, T.; Wang, F.; Chen, X.; Sun, H.; Li, X. GnRH Antagonist Improves Pubertal Cyclophosphamide-Induced Long-Term Testicular Injury in Adult Rats. *Int. J. Endocrinol.* **2018**, *2018*, 4272575. [CrossRef] [PubMed]
33. Helmy, H.S.; Senousy, M.A.; El-Sahar, A.E.; Sayed, R.H.; Saad, M.A.; Elbaz, E.M. Aberrations of miR-126-3p, miR-181a and sirtuin1 network mediate Di-(2-ethylhexyl) phthalate-induced testicular damage in rats: The protective role of hesperidin. *Toxicology* **2020**, *433–434*, 152406. [CrossRef] [PubMed]
34. Shabaan, S.; Madi, N.; Elgharib, M.; Nasif, E. Study the Effect of Silymarin on Cyclophosphamide Induced Testicular Damage in Adult Albino Rats. *Bull. Egypt. Soc. Physiol. Sci.* **2021**, *41*, 553–564. [CrossRef]
35. Hassan, M.A.; El Bohy, K.M.; El Sharkawy, N.I.; Imam, T.S.; El-Metwally, A.E.; Hamed Arisha, A.; Mohammed, H.A.; Abd-Elhakim, Y.M. Iprodione and chlorpyrifos induce testicular damage, oxidative stress, apoptosis and suppression of steroidogenic- and spermatogenic-related genes in immature male albino rats. *Andrologia* **2021**, *53*, e13978. [CrossRef]
36. Kasem, S.E.; Abdelnaby, A.A.; Mohammed, P.A.; Hemdan, S.B.; Abd El-Fattah, R.M.Z.; Elsayed, R.M. Protective Effect of Hesperidin on Kidneys and Testes of Adult Male Rats Exposed to Bisphenol A. *Egypt. J. Hosp. Med.* **2022**, *88*, 3005–3013. [CrossRef]
37. Arisha, A.H.; Ahmed, M.M.; Kamel, M.A.; Attia, Y.A.; Hussein, M.M.A. Morin ameliorates the testicular apoptosis, oxidative stress, and impact on blood–testis barrier induced by photo-extracellularly synthesized silver nanoparticles. *Environ. Sci. Pollut. Res.* **2019**, *26*, 28749–28762. [CrossRef]

38. Hussein, M.M.A.; Gad, E.; Ahmed, M.M.; Arisha, A.H.; Mahdy, H.F.; Swelum, A.A.A.; Tukur, H.A.; Saadeldin, I.M. Amelioration of titanium dioxide nanoparticle reprotoxicity by the antioxidants morin and rutin. *Environ. Sci. Pollut. Res.* **2019**, *26*, 29074–29084. [CrossRef]
39. Salimnejad, R.; Soleimani Rad, J.; Nejad, D. Protective Effect of Ghrelin on Oxidative Stress and Tissue Damages of Mice Testes Followed By Chemotherapy With Cyclophosphamide. *Crescent J. Med. Biol. Sci.* **2018**, *5*, 138–143.
40. Ekeleme-Egedigwe, C.A.; Famurewa, A.C.; David, E.E.; Eleazu, C.O.; Egedigwe, U.O. Antioxidant potential of garlic oil supplementation prevents cyclophosphamide-induced oxidative testicular damage and endocrine depletion in rats. *J. Nutr. Intermed. Metab.* **2019**, *18*, 100109. [CrossRef]
41. Alkhalaf, M.I.; Alansari, W.S.; Alshubaily, F.A.; Alnajeebi, A.M.; Eskandrani, A.A.; Tashkandi, M.A.; Babteen, N.A. Chemoprotective effects of inositol hexaphosphate against cyclophosphamide-induced testicular damage in rats. *Sci. Rep.* **2020**, *10*, 12599. [CrossRef]
42. Shokoohi, M.; Khaki, A.; Shoorei, H.; Khaki, A.A.; Moghimian, M.; Abtahi-Eivary, S.H. Hesperidin attenuated apoptotic-related genes in testicle of a male rat model of varicocoele. *Andrology* **2020**, *8*, 249–258. [CrossRef]
43. Saber, T.M.; Arisha, A.H.; Abo-Elmaaty, A.M.A.; Abdelgawad, F.E.; Metwally, M.M.M.; Saber, T.; Mansour, M.F. Thymol alleviates imidacloprid-induced testicular toxicity by modulating oxidative stress and expression of steroidogenesis and apoptosis-related genes in adult male rats. *Ecotoxicol. Environ. Saf.* **2021**, *221*, 112435. [CrossRef]
44. Saber, T.M.; Mansour, M.F.; Abdelaziz, A.S.; Mohamed, R.M.S.; Fouad, R.A.; Arisha, A.H. Argan oil ameliorates sodium fluoride-induced renal damage via inhibiting oxidative damage, inflammation, and intermediate filament protein expression in male rats. *Environ. Sci. Pollut. Res. Int.* **2020**, *27*, 30426–30436. [CrossRef]
45. Iqubal, A.; Syed, M.A.; Najmi, A.K.; Ali, J.; Haque, S.E. Ameliorative effect of nerolidol on cyclophosphamide-induced gonadal toxicity in Swiss Albino mice: Biochemical-, histological- and immunohistochemical-based evidences. *Andrologia* **2020**, *52*, e13535. [CrossRef]
46. Hamzeh, M.; Hosseinimehr, S.J.; Karimpour, A.; Mohammadi, H.R.; Khalatbary, A.R.; Talebpour Amiri, F. Cerium Oxide Nanoparticles Protect Cyclophosphamide-induced Testicular Toxicity in Mice. *Int. J. Prev. Med.* **2019**, *10*, 5. [CrossRef]
47. Anan, H.H.; Zidan, R.A.; Abd El-Baset, S.A.; Ali, M.M. Ameliorative effect of zinc oxide nanoparticles on cyclophosphamide induced testicular injury in adult rat. *Tissue Cell* **2018**, *54*, 80–93. [CrossRef]
48. Afkhami-Ardakani, M.; Hasanzadeh, S.; Shahrooz, R.; Delirezh, N.; Malekinejad, H. Antioxidant effects of Spirulina platensis (Arthrospira platensis) on cyclophosphamide-induced testicular injury in rats. *Vet. Res. Forum: Int. Q. J.* **2018**, *9*, 35–41.
49. Cengiz, M.; Sahinturk, V.; Yildiz, S.C.; Şahin, İ.K.; Bilici, N.; Yaman, S.O.; Altuner, Y.; Appak-Baskoy, S.; Ayhanci, A. Cyclophosphamide induced oxidative stress, lipid per oxidation, apoptosis and histopathological changes in rats: Protective role of boron. *J. Trace Elem. Med. Biol. Organ Soc. Miner. Trace Elem. (GMS)* **2020**, *62*, 126574. [CrossRef]
50. Torabi, F.; Malekzadeh Shafaroudi, M.; Rezaei, N. Combined protective effect of zinc oxide nanoparticles and melatonin on cyclophosphamide-induced toxicity in testicular histology and sperm parameters in adult Wistar rats. *Int. J. Reprod. Biomed.* **2017**, *15*, 403–412. [CrossRef]
51. Nakazawa, H.; Chang, K.; Shinozaki, S.; Yasukawa, T.; Ishimaru, K.; Yasuhara, S.; Yu, Y.M.; Martyn, J.A.; Tompkins, R.G.; Shimokado, K.; et al. iNOS as a Driver of Inflammation and Apoptosis in Mouse Skeletal Muscle after Burn Injury: Possible Involvement of Sirt1 S-Nitrosylation-Mediated Acetylation of p65 NF-κB and p53. *PLoS ONE* **2017**, *12*, e0170391. [CrossRef] [PubMed]
52. Salama, R.M.; Abd Elwahab, A.H.; Abd-Elgalil, M.M.; Elmongy, N.F.; Schaalan, M.F. LCZ696 (sacubitril/valsartan) protects against cyclophosphamide-induced testicular toxicity in rats: Role of neprilysin inhibition and lncRNA TUG1 in ameliorating apoptosis. *Toxicology* **2020**, *437*, 152439. [CrossRef] [PubMed]
53. Hamza, A.A.; Elwy, H.M.; Badawi, A.M. Fenugreek seed extract attenuates cisplatin-induced testicular damage in Wistar rats. *Andrologia* **2016**, *48*, 211–221. [CrossRef] [PubMed]
54. Olanrewaju, J.A.; Akinpade, T.G.; Olatunji, S.Y.; Owolabi, J.O.; Enya, J.I.; Adelodun, S.T.; Fabiyi, S.O.; Desalu, A.B. Observable Protective Activities of Quercetin on Aluminum Chloride-Induced Testicular Toxicity in Adult Male Wistar Rat. *J. Hum. Reprod. Sci.* **2021**, *14*, 113–120. [CrossRef] [PubMed]
55. Sayed, A.M.; Hassanein, E.H.M.; Ali, F.E.M.; Omar, Z.M.M.; Rashwan, E.K.; Mohammedsaleh, Z.M.; Abd El-Ghafar, O.A.M. Regulation of Keap-1/Nrf2/AKT and iNOS/NF-κB/TLR4 signals by apocynin abrogated methotrexate-induced testicular toxicity: Mechanistic insights and computational pharmacological analysis. *Life Sci.* **2021**, *284*, 119911. [CrossRef]
56. Azouz, R.A.; Korany, R.M.S.; Noshy, P.A. Silica Nanoparticle-Induced Reproductive Toxicity in Male Albino Rats via Testicular Apoptosis and Oxidative Stress. *Biol. Trace Elem. Res.* **2022**. [CrossRef]
57. Famurewa, A.C.; Ekeleme-Egedigwe, C.A.; Onwe, C.S.; Egedigwe, U.O.; Okoro, C.O.; Egedigwe, U.J.; Asogwa, N.T. Ginger juice prevents cisplatin-induced oxidative stress, endocrine imbalance and NO/iNOS/NF-κB signalling via modulating testicular redox-inflammatory mechanism in rats. *Andrologia* **2020**, *52*, e13786. [CrossRef]
58. Fouad, A.; Albuali, W.; Jresat, I. Protective Effect of Hesperidin against Cyclophosphamide Hepatotoxicity in Rats. *Int. J. Bioeng. Life Sci.* **2014**, *8*, 730–733.
59. Siddiqi, A.; Hasan, S.K.; Nafees, S.; Rashid, S.; Saidullah, B.; Sultana, S. Chemopreventive efficacy of hesperidin against chemically induced nephrotoxicity and renal carcinogenesis via amelioration of oxidative stress and modulation of multiple molecular pathways. *Exp. Mol. Pathol.* **2015**, *99*, 641–653. [CrossRef]

60. Filobbos, S.; Amin, N.; Yacoub, M.; Abd El_Hakim, K.R. Possible Protective Effect of Melatonin on Cisplatin-Induced Testicular Toxicity in Adult Albino Rats. A Histological and Immunohistochemical Study. *Egypt. J. Histol.* **2020**, *43*, 891–901. [CrossRef]
61. Zickri, M.B.; Moustafa, M.H.; Fasseh, A.E.; Kamar, S.S. Antioxidant and antiapoptotic paracrine effects of mesenchymal stem cells on spermatogenic arrest in oligospermia rat model. *Ann. Anat. Anat. Anz. Off. Organ Anat. Ges.* **2021**, *237*, 151750. [CrossRef]
62. Wang, Y.; Bai, L.; Zhang, J.; Li, H.; Yang, W.; Li, M. Lepidium draba L. leaves extract ameliorated cyclophosphamide-induced testicular toxicity by modulation of ROS-dependent Keap1/Nrf2/HO1, Bax/Bcl2/p53/caspase-3, and inflammatory signaling pathways. *J. Food Biochem.* **2021**, *45*, e13987. [CrossRef]
63. Bashandy, S.A.E.; Ebaid, H.; Al-Tamimi, J.; Ahmed-Farid, O.A.; Omara, E.A.; Alhazza, I.M. Melatonin Alleviated Potassium Dichromate-Induced Oxidative Stress and Reprotoxicity in Male Rats. *BioMed. Res. Int.* **2021**, *2021*, 3565360. [CrossRef]
64. Li, L.; Chen, B.; An, T.; Zhang, H.; Xia, B.; Li, R.; Zhu, R.; Tian, Y.; Wang, L.; Zhao, D.; et al. BaZiBuShen alleviates altered testicular morphology and spermatogenesis and modulates Sirt6/P53 and Sirt6/NF-κB pathways in aging mice induced by D-galactose and NaNO(2). *J. Ethnopharmacol.* **2021**, *271*, 113810. [CrossRef]
65. Moradi, M.; Goodarzi, N.; Faramarzi, A.; Cheraghi, H.; Hashemian, A.H.; Jalili, C. Melatonin protects rats testes against bleomycin, etoposide, and cisplatin-induced toxicity via mitigating nitro-oxidative stress and apoptosis. *Biomed. Pharmacother. = Biomed. Pharmacother.* **2021**, *138*, 111481. [CrossRef]
66. Li, S.; Che, S.; Chen, S.; Ruan, Z.; Zhang, L. Hesperidin partly ameliorates the decabromodiphenyl ether-induced reproductive toxicity in pubertal mice. *Environ. Sci. Pollut. Res. Int.* **2022**, *29*, 90391–90403. [CrossRef]
67. Kaya, K.; Ciftci, O.; Cetin, A.; Doğan, H.; Başak, N. Hesperidin protects testicular and spermatological damages induced by cisplatin in rats. *Andrologia* **2015**, *47*, 793–800. [CrossRef]
68. Celik, E.; Oguzturk, H.; Sahin, N.; Turtay, M.G.; Oguz, F.; Ciftci, O. Protective effects of hesperidin in experimental testicular ischemia/reperfusion injury in rats. *Arch. Med. Sci.* **2016**, *12*, 928–934. [CrossRef]
69. Elwan, W.M.; Kassab, A.A. The Potential Protective Role of Hesperidin Against Capecitabine-Induced Corneal Toxicity in Adult Male Albino Rat. Light and Electron Microscopic Study. *Egypt. J. Histol.* **2017**, *40*, 201–215. [CrossRef]
70. Turk, E.; Kandemir, F.M.; Yildirim, S.; Caglayan, C.; Kucukler, S.; Kuzu, M. Protective Effect of Hesperidin on Sodium Arsenite-Induced Nephrotoxicity and Hepatotoxicity in Rats. *Biol. Trace Elem. Res.* **2019**, *189*, 95–108. [CrossRef]
71. El-Diasty, H.H.; El-Sayyad, H.; Refaat, S.; El-Ghaweet, H.A. Efficacy of Quercetin-Sensitized Cisplatin against N-Nitroso-NMethylurea Induced Testicular Carcinogenesis in Wistar Rats. *Asian Pac. J. Cancer Prev.* **2021**, *22*, 75–84. [CrossRef] [PubMed]
72. Adana, M.Y.; Imam, A.; Bello, A.A.; Sunmonu, O.E.; Alege, E.P.; Onigbolabi, O.G.; Ajao, M.S. Oral thymoquinone modulates cyclophosphamide-induced testicular toxicity in adolescent Wistar rats. *Andrologia* **2022**, *54*, e14368. [CrossRef] [PubMed]
73. Ijaz, M.; Tahir, A.; Samad, A.; Ashraf, A.; Ameen, M.; Imran, M.; Yousaf, S.; Sarwar, N. Casticin Alleviates Testicular and Spermatological Damage Induced by Cisplatin in Rats. *Pak. Vet. J.* **2020**, *40*, 234–238. [CrossRef]
74. Delgarm, N.; Morovati-Sharifabad, M.; Salehi, E.; Afkhami-Ardakani, M.; Heydarnejad, M.S. Exploring the main effects of phoenix dactylifera on destructive changes caused by cyclophosphamide in male reproductive system in mice. *Vet. Res. Forum Int. Q. J.* **2022**, *13*, 249–255. [CrossRef]
75. Bakhtiary, Z.; Shahrooz, R.; Ahmadi, A.; Soltanalinejad, F. Ethyl Pyruvate Ameliorates The Damage Induced by Cyclophosphamide on Adult Mice Testes. *Int. J. Fertil. Steril.* **2016**, *10*, 79–86. [CrossRef]
76. Samie, A.; Sedaghat, R.; Baluchnejadmojarad, T.; Roghani, M. Hesperetin, a citrus flavonoid, attenuates testicular damage in diabetic rats via inhibition of oxidative stress, inflammation, and apoptosis. *Life Sci.* **2018**, *210*, 132–139. [CrossRef]
77. Alanbaki, A.; Al-Mayali, H.; Al-Mayali, H. Ameliorative effect of Quercetin and Hesperidin on Antioxidant and Histological Changes in the Testis of Etoposide-Induced Adult Male Rats. *Res. J. Pharm. Technol.* **2018**, *11*, 564. [CrossRef]
78. Jahan, S.; Iftikhar, N.; Ullah, H.; Rukh, G.; Hussain, I. Alleviative effect of quercetin on rat testis against arsenic: A histological and biochemical study. *Syst. Biol. Reprod. Med.* **2015**, *61*, 89–95. [CrossRef]
79. Abdelwafa, H.R.; Ramadan, R.A.; El-Kott, A.F.; Abdelhamid, F.M. The protective effect of melatonin supplementation against taxol-induced testicular cytotoxicity in adult rats. *Braz. J. Med. Biol. Res. Rev. Bras. Pesqui. Med. Biol.* **2022**, *55*, e11614. [CrossRef]
80. Arisha, A.H.; Moustafa, A. Potential inhibitory effect of swimming exercise on the Kisspeptin–GnRH signaling pathway in male rats. *Theriogenology* **2019**, *133*, 87–96. [CrossRef]
81. Osawe, S.O.; Farombi, E.O. Quercetin and rutin ameliorates sulphasalazine-induced spermiotoxicity, alterations in reproductive hormones and steroidogenic enzyme imbalance in rats. *Andrologia* **2018**, *50*, e12981. [CrossRef]
82. Sharma, P.; Aslam Khan, I.; Singh, R. Curcumin and Quercetin Ameliorated Cypermethrin and Deltamethrin-Induced Reproductive System Impairment in Male Wistar Rats by Upregulating The Activity of Pituitary-Gonadal Hormones and Steroidogenic Enzymes. *Int. J. Fertil. Steril.* **2018**, *12*, 72–80. [CrossRef]
83. Nayak, G.; Rao, A.; Mullick, P.; Mutalik, S.; Kalthur, S.G.; Adiga, S.K.; Kalthur, G. Ethanolic extract of Moringa oleifera leaves alleviate cyclophosphamide-induced testicular toxicity by improving endocrine function and modulating cell specific gene expression in mouse testis. *J. Ethnopharmacol.* **2020**, *259*, 112922. [CrossRef]
84. Nna, V.U.; Ujah, G.A.; Suleiman, J.B.; Mohamed, M.; Nwokocha, C.; Akpan, T.J.; Ekuma, H.C.; Fubara, V.V.; Kekung-Asu, C.B.; Osim, E.E. Tert-butylhydroquinone preserve testicular steroidogenesis and spermatogenesis in cisplatin-intoxicated rats by targeting oxidative stress, inflammation and apoptosis. *Toxicology* **2020**, *441*, 152528. [CrossRef]

85. Adelakun, S.A.; Akintunde, O.W.; Jeje, S.O.; Alao, O.A. Ameliorating and protective potential of 1-isothiocyanato-4-methyl sulfonyl butane on cisplatin induced oligozoospermia and testicular dysfunction via redox-inflammatory pathway: Histomorphometric and immunohistochemical evaluation using proliferating cell nuclear antigen. *Phytomedicine Plus* **2022**, *2*, 100268. [CrossRef]
86. Noshy, P.A.; Khalaf, A.A.A.; Ibrahim, M.A.; Mekkawy, A.M.; Abdelrahman, R.E.; Farghali, A.; Tammam, A.A.; Zaki, A.R. Alterations in reproductive parameters and steroid biosynthesis induced by nickel oxide nanoparticles in male rats: The ameliorative effect of hesperidin. *Toxicology* **2022**, *473*, 153208. [CrossRef]
87. Can, S.; Çetik Yıldız, S.; Keskin, C.; Şahintürk, V.; Cengiz, M.; Appak Başköy, S.; Ayhanci, A.; Akıncı, G. Investigation into the protective effects of Hypericum Triquetrifolium Turra seed against cyclophosphamide-induced testicular injury in Sprague Dawley rats. *Drug Chem. Toxicol.* **2022**, *45*, 1679–1686. [CrossRef]
88. Ye, H.; Ng, H.W.; Sakkiah, S.; Ge, W.; Perkins, R.; Tong, W.; Hong, H. Pathway Analysis Revealed Potential Diverse Health Impacts of Flavonoids that Bind Estrogen Receptors. *Int. J. Environ. Res. Public Health* **2016**, *13*, 373. [CrossRef]
89. Huang, Z.; Fang, F.; Wang, J.; Wong, C.-W. Structural activity relationship of flavonoids with estrogen-related receptor gamma. *FEBS Lett.* **2010**, *584*, 22–26. [CrossRef]
90. Cannarella, R.; Calogero, A.E.; Condorelli, R.A.; Greco, E.A.; Aversa, A.; La Vignera, S. Is there a role for glucagon-like peptide-1 receptor agonists in the treatment of male infertility? *Andrology* **2021**, *9*, 1499–1503. [CrossRef]
91. Starovlah, I.M.; Radovic Pletikosic, S.M.; Kostic, T.S.; Andric, S.A. Reduced spermatozoa functionality during stress is the consequence of adrenergic-mediated disturbance of mitochondrial dynamics markers. *Sci. Rep.* **2020**, *10*, 16813. [CrossRef] [PubMed]
92. Abdullah, D.M.; Alsemeh, A.E.; Khamis, T. Semaglutide early intervention attenuated testicular dysfunction by targeting the GLP-1-PPAR-α-Kisspeptin-Steroidogenesis signaling pathway in a testicular ischemia-reperfusion rat model. *Peptides* **2022**, *149*, 170711. [CrossRef] [PubMed]
93. Almeer, R.S.; Abdel Moneim, A.E. Evaluation of the Protective Effect of Olive Leaf Extract on Cisplatin-Induced Testicular Damage in Rats. *Oxid Med. Cell Longev.* **2018**, *2018*, 8487248. [CrossRef] [PubMed]
94. Gur, C.; Kandemir, O.; Kandemir, F.M. Investigation of the effects of hesperidin administration on abamectin-induced testicular toxicity in rats through oxidative stress, endoplasmic reticulum stress, inflammation, apoptosis, autophagy, and JAK2/STAT3 pathways. *Environ. Toxicol.* **2022**, *37*, 401–412. [CrossRef]
95. Negm, W.A.; El-Kadem, A.H.; Hussein, I.A.; Alqahtani, M.J. The Mechanistic Perspective of Bilobetin Protective Effects against Cisplatin-Induced Testicular Toxicity: Role of Nrf-2/Keap-1 Signaling, Inflammation, and Apoptosis. *Biomedicines* **2022**, *10*, 1134. [CrossRef]
96. Selvaraj, P.; Pugalendi, K.V. Efficacy of hesperidin on plasma, heart and liver tissue lipids in rats subjected to isoproterenol-induced cardiotoxicity. *Exp. Toxicol. Pathol. Off. J. Ges. Fur Toxikol. Pathol.* **2012**, *64*, 449–452. [CrossRef]
97. Al-Shahat, A.; Hulail, M.A.E.; Soliman, N.M.M.; Khamis, T.; Fericean, L.M.; Arisha, A.H.; Moawad, R.S. Melatonin Mitigates Cisplatin-Induced Ovarian Dysfunction via Altering Steroidogenesis, Inflammation, Apoptosis, Oxidative Stress, and PTEN/PI3K/Akt/mTOR/AMPK Signaling Pathway in Female Rats. *Pharmaceutics* **2022**, *14*, 2769. [CrossRef]
98. Zirkin, B.R.; Chen, H. Regulation of Leydig cell steroidogenic function during aging. *Biol. Reprod.* **2000**, *63*, 977–981. [CrossRef]
99. Moustafa, A. Effect of Light-Dark Cycle Misalignment on the Hypothalamic-Pituitary-Gonadal Axis, Testicular Oxidative Stress, and Expression of Clock Genes in Adult Male Rats. *Int. J. Endocrinol.* **2020**, *2020*, 1426846. [CrossRef]
100. Livak, K.J.; Schmittgen, T.D. Analysis of Relative Gene Expression Data Using Real-Time Quantitative PCR and the $2^{-\Delta\Delta CT}$ Method. *Methods* **2001**, *25*, 402–408. [CrossRef]
101. Bancroft, J.D.; Layton, C. 12—Connective and other mesenchymal tissues with their stains. In *Bancroft's Theory and Practice of Histological Techniques*, 8th ed.; Suvarna, S.K., Layton, C., Bancroft, J.D., Eds.; Elsevier: Amsterdam, The Netherlands, 2019; pp. 153–175.
102. Johnston, D.S.; Russell, L.D.; Friel, P.J.; Griswold, M.D. Murine germ cells do not require functional androgen receptors to complete spermatogenesis following spermatogonial stem cell transplantation. *Endocrinology* **2001**, *142*, 2405–2408. [CrossRef]
103. Sharpe, R.M. Sperm counts and fertility in men: A rocky road ahead. Science & Society Series on Sex and Science. *EMBO Rep.* **2012**, *13*, 398–403. [CrossRef]
104. Jensen, E.C. Quantitative analysis of histological staining and fluorescence using ImageJ. *Anat. Rec.* **2013**, *296*, 378–381. [CrossRef] [PubMed]

Disclaimer/Publisher's Note: The statements, opinions and data contained in all publications are solely those of the individual author(s) and contributor(s) and not of MDPI and/or the editor(s). MDPI and/or the editor(s) disclaim responsibility for any injury to people or property resulting from any ideas, methods, instructions or products referred to in the content.

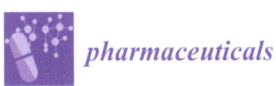

Article

Phytofabrication and Characterisation of Zinc Oxide Nanoparticles Using Pure Curcumin

Batoul Alallam [1], Abd Almonem Doolaanea [2], Mulham Alfatama [3] and Vuanghao Lim [1,*]

[1] Advanced Medical and Dental Institute, Universiti Sains Malaysia, Bertam, Kepala Batas 13200, Penang, Malaysia
[2] Department of Pharmaceutical Technology, Faculty of Pharmacy, Kolej Universiti Antarabangsa Maiwp, Taman Batu Muda, Batu Caves, Kuala Lumpur 68100, Selangor, Malaysia
[3] Faculty of Pharmacy, Universiti Sultan Zainal Abidin, Besut Campus, Besut 22200, Terengganu, Malaysia
* Correspondence: vlim@usm.my; Tel.: +60-4-562-2427

Abstract: Zinc oxide and curcumin, on their own and in combination, have the potential as alternatives to conventional anticancer drugs. In this work, zinc oxide nanoparticles (ZnO NPs) were prepared by an eco-friendly method using pure curcumin, and their physicochemical properties were characterised. ATR-FTIR spectra confirmed the role of curcumin in synthesising zinc oxide curcumin nanoparticles (Green-ZnO-NPs). These nanoparticles exhibited a hexagonal wurtzite structure with a size and zeta potential of 27.61 ± 5.18 nm and −16.90 ± 0.26 mV, respectively. Green-ZnO-NPs showed good activity towards studied bacterial strains, including *Escherichia coli*, *Staphylococcus aureus* and methicillin-resistant *Staphylococcus aureus*. The minimum inhibitory concentration of Green-ZnO-NPs was consistently larger than that of chemically synthesised ZnO NPs (Std-ZnO-NPs) or mere curcumin, advocating an additive effect between the zinc oxide and curcumin. Green-ZnO-NPs demonstrated an efficient inhibitory effect towards MCF-7 cells with IC$_{50}$ (20.53 ± 5.12 µg/mL) that was significantly lower compared to that of Std-ZnO-NPs (27.08 ± 0.91 µg/mL) after 48 h of treatment. When Green-ZnO-NPs were tested against *Artemia* larvae, a minimised cytotoxic effect was observed, with LC$_{50}$ being almost three times lower compared to that of Std-ZnO-NPs (11.96 ± 1.89 µg/mL and 34.60 ± 9.45 µg/mL, respectively). This demonstrates that Green-ZnO-NPs can be a potent, additively enhanced combination delivery/therapeutic agent with the potential for anticancer therapy.

Keywords: zinc oxide nanoparticles; antimicrobial; curcumin; green synthesis; drug discovery from natural products

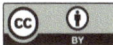

Citation: Alallam, B.; Doolaanea, A.A.; Alfatama, M.; Lim, V. Phytofabrication and Characterisation of Zinc Oxide Nanoparticles Using Pure Curcumin. *Pharmaceuticals* 2023, *16*, 269. https://doi.org/10.3390/ph16020269

Academic Editors: Fernando Calzada and Miguel Valdes

Received: 22 December 2022
Revised: 10 January 2023
Accepted: 29 January 2023
Published: 10 February 2023

Copyright: © 2023 by the authors. Licensee MDPI, Basel, Switzerland. This article is an open access article distributed under the terms and conditions of the Creative Commons Attribution (CC BY) license (https://creativecommons.org/licenses/by/4.0/).

1. Introduction

The rapid emergence and growth of nanobiotechnology has created a varied range of new applications for the biomedical and pharmaceutical industries [1–4]. Currently, metal oxide nanoparticles are becoming more popular owing to their useful physicochemical and biological characteristics [5]. Specifically, zinc oxide nanoparticles (ZnO NPs) are commonly used due to their broad range of applications in many fields. ZnO NPs possess potential biological applications, including antioxidant, antimicrobial and anticancer [6,7]. Their preparation process is simple, and they are considered biocompatible and safe materials [8]. Therefore, they are ideal for biomedical applications such as nanomedicine carriers, nanodiagnostics, biomolecular detection and luminescence materials [9]. Several physical and chemical synthesis methods have been used to synthesise ZnO NPs, including sol–gel [10], microwave-assisted [11], and thermal decomposition [12] methods; however, these techniques could produce toxic materials. The green production approach of ZnO NPs, which predominantly uses phytocompounds, is currently gaining popularity since it is a safer, low-cost, and environmentally friendly process.

In recent decades, functional foods and nutraceuticals have been widely investigated for the prevention and treatment of various diseases. Natural products play an essential role in the pharmaceutical sector as medications and supplements due to their multimechanistic biological activity, safety, and long-term availability. Plants are the most abundant source of bioactive natural compounds as well as a variety of macro- and micronutrients [13,14].

Curcuma longa (turmeric), a member of the ginger family (*Zingiberaceae*), is a short-stemmed perennial plant that grows naturally all over the Indian subcontinent and South East Asia [15]. It has been used for thousands of years as a remedy in traditional Indian and folk medicine for the cure of a large variety of illnesses, such as inflammation, infectious diseases, and gastric, hepatic, and blood disorders [16]. Curcumin (diferuloylmethane) is the main polyphenol isolated from the rhizomes of *Curcuma longa* [13]. It has a wide range of pharmacological effects, such as antioxidant, antibacterial, anticarcinogenic, and antiproliferative activities [17,18]. Curcumin can regulate the expression and the activity of various biological processes, which may explain its potential use in cancer chemotherapy [14,19]. It has the ability for the green synthesis of metal nanoparticles due to the presence of polyphenol acting as a reducing agent [20]. However, the application of curcumin has been limited in the production of ZnO NPs due to low water solubility and sensitivity to heat, light, and alkaline. Various methods have been reported for the green synthesis of ZnO NPs from curcumin using hydroxides or chemical mediators [21–25]. However, several disadvantages including time consumption [25], the toxicity of the chemicals used as a mediator [23,25,26], and the large size of ZnO NPs [21] are the major limitations of these methods.

Therefore, this study reported the synthesis of zinc oxide nanoparticles (Green-ZnO-NPs) which can be considered green, eco-friendly and safe for producing nanoparticles as an anticancer agent. Zinc acetate was used as the zinc precursor, while pure curcumin was used as the reducing agent. The prepared nanoparticles were characterised for their physicochemical properties, as well as their antioxidant activity. The antibacterial activity of Green-ZnO-NPs, as well as their anticancer activity against MCF-7 cells, were evaluated and compared to chemically synthesised zinc oxide nanoparticles (Std-ZnO-NPs) and mere curcumin. The impact of Green-ZnO-NPs on the ecotoxicity against brine shrimp larvae was also examined.

2. Results and Discussion

2.1. Synthesis of Green-ZnO-NPs

Green-ZnO-NPs were prepared by a green method using curcumin as a reductant and stabiliser. The change in the reaction mixture's colour and the resulting orangish-white precipitate were used as indicators of the formation of the nanoparticles [27], as illustrated in Figure 1. Curcumin (diferuloylmethane) is a polyphenolic compound derived from the spices turmeric, consisting of bis-α, β-unsaturated β-diketone which exists in equilibrium with its enol tautomer [28]. Results of the NMR studies have confirmed that curcumin exists in solution in the form of the keto–enol tautomer [29]. The majority of the reductants have phenolic group or a β-diketone group in their structure [30]. Hence, the highest reducing ability of curcumin can be obtained when the phenolic hydroxyl group is sterically hindered by the introduction of two methyl groups at the ortho position of the benzene ring [31]. Therefore, the presence of two structural elements, namely, the β-diketone structure and the hydroxyl group at the ortho position in the aromatic ring, are the governing factors for the reducing potential of curcumin [31].

The possible mechanism for the formation of ZnO NPs is by the reaction of zinc acetate (precursor) with the polyphenols (from curcumin) to form an intermediate compound (zinc hydroxide). This compound is then transformed into zinc oxide mediated by the heat produced in the drying step, according to the following reactions:

$Zn(CH_3CO_2)_2$ (aq) + 2R–OH (aq) → $Zn(OH)_2$ (s) + 2R–CH_3CO_2 (aq)

$Zn(OH)_2$ (s) + heat → ZnO (s) + H_2O (v)

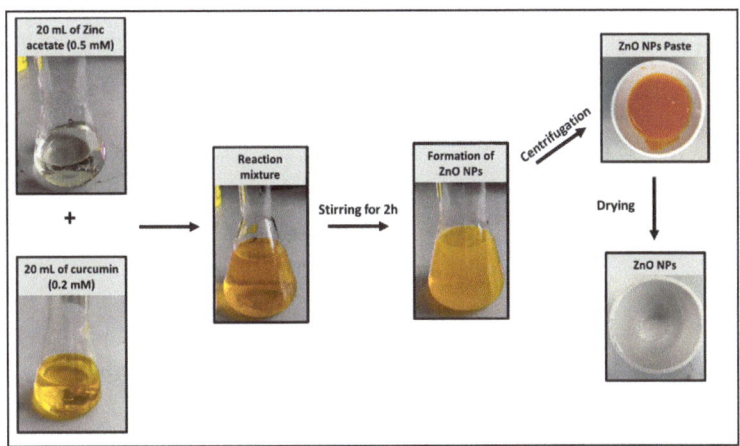

Figure 1. Synthesis scheme of Green-ZnO-NPs.

2.2. Characterisation of Green-ZnO-NPs

2.2.1. Ultraviolet–Visible (UV–Vis)

The optical properties of Green-ZnO-NPs, Std-ZnO-NPs and curcumin were recorded from 300 to 700 nm using a UV–Vis spectrophotometer (Figure 2). Green-ZnO-NPs and Std-ZnO-NPs displayed an absorption peak at 366 nm and 376 nm, respectively. The peak at 366 nm has confirmed the successful synthesis of the nanoparticles with the aid of curcumin. It is claimed that ZnO NPs had a characteristic absorption peak at a range of 330–460 nm [32]. This peak is related to the intrinsic band-gap absorption of zinc oxide driven by UV-induced electron transitions (O2p → Zn3d) [33]. Curcumin exhibited a wide band with a maximum absorbance peak at 425 nm, which could be correlated to the low energy π–π* excitation of the curcumin [34]. The synthesis of ZnO NPs using curcumin may be elucidated by the capability to bioaccumulate metal ions, besides the ability to stabilise the process [35].

2.2.2. Attenuated Total Reflectance-Fourier-Transform Infrared (ATR-FTIR) Analysis

FTIR analysis was conducted to examine the role of curcumin molecules in reducing and stabilising Green-ZnO-NPs. Std-ZnO-NPs showed the characteristic Zn–O bond at 475 cm^{-1} (Figure 3) [36], while no peaks were observed at 1600 cm^{-1}, which represents the surface bending vibration of H-OH. The peak that appeared at 3500 cm^{-1} represents the stretching vibration of O-H, confirming the absence of hydroxyl groups on ZnO NPs surfaces, indicating that ZnO was formed rather than $Zn(OH)_2$. Other peaks with a low intensity at 1250, 1340, and 1750 cm^{-1} could be correlated to the adsorbed carbonate moieties [37,38].

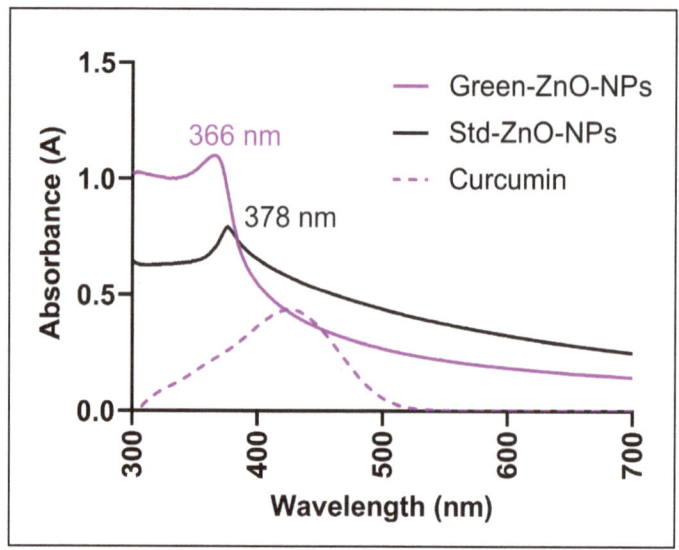

Figure 2. UV-Vis absorption spectra of the aqueous suspension of Green-ZnO-NPs (100 µg/mL), the aqueous suspension of Std-ZnO-NPs (100 µg/mL), and the ethanolic solution of curcumin (10 µg/mL).

The band at 475 cm^{-1} in the Std-ZnO-NPs spectrum was shifted to 479 cm^{-1} and was less pronounced in the spectrum of Green-ZnO-NPs, proving the alternation of the Zn–O bond as it could interact with curcumin, and it is attributed to the vibration of hexagonal ZnO. The frequency region of curcumin phenolic vibrations was reported at 3595 cm^{-1}; however, it was shifted to 3492 cm^{-1}, which could be due to the intra- and intermolecular H-bonding in curcumin [39]. This band was not present in the spectrum of the Green-ZnO-NPs, demonstrating the absence of interaction between phenolic hydroxyls and ZnO.

The β-diketone group is one of the most prominent functional groups in curcumin molecules, with a high affinity for chelating metal ions [40,41]. Curcumin spectra showed a peak in the carbonyl region (1800–1650 cm^{-1}), revealing that curcumin mainly exists in keto form. In the spectrum of Green-ZnO-NPs, the peak at 1739 cm^{-1} is associated with the asymmetric vibration of carbonyl in the keto form, while the symmetric mode was not observed. On the other hand, the band of enolic vibration (OH) appeared weak at 2979 cm^{-1}, demonstrating the presence of both keto/enol forms in curcumin molecules. Accordingly, the β-diketone moiety most probably interacts (weakly or strongly) with zinc atoms at the bulk ZnO surface. The broadness and intensity of the enol peak are dependent on intramolecular hydrogen bond strength. As hydrogen bond strength rises, the intensity of the enol band decreases and its broadness increases [42]. The hydroxy and methoxy groups on the curcumin phenyl rings (electron-donor) are anticipated to cause a stronger hydrogen bonding. As a result, any reduction of the electronegativity of these groups via conjugating or bonding with other moieties could decrease the hydrogen bonding strength; consequently, this would allow the enol band to appear more clearly. Thus, the absence of a clearly defined enolic vibration band (OH) suggests that there was a weak complexation between zinc and curcumin at the methoxy group of phenolic rings. In the spectrum of curcumin, the peak at 1630 cm^{-1} has mixed C=O and C=C vibrations. In Green-ZnO-NPs, this band shifted to 1602 cm^{-1}, which indicates strong coordination of the carbonyl moiety [43]. In the spectrum of curcumin, the band at 1510 cm^{-1} represents highly mixed CC=O, C=O and CC=C vibrations [39], while the peaks in the region of 1430–1460 cm^{-1} are attributed to the methyl vibration. Most peaks in the range of 1450–1300 cm^{-1} are mixed.

Curcumin chelates with zinc via the carbonyl moity and a weak interaction between the curcumin phenyl ring (methoxy groups) and zinc moieties occurs.

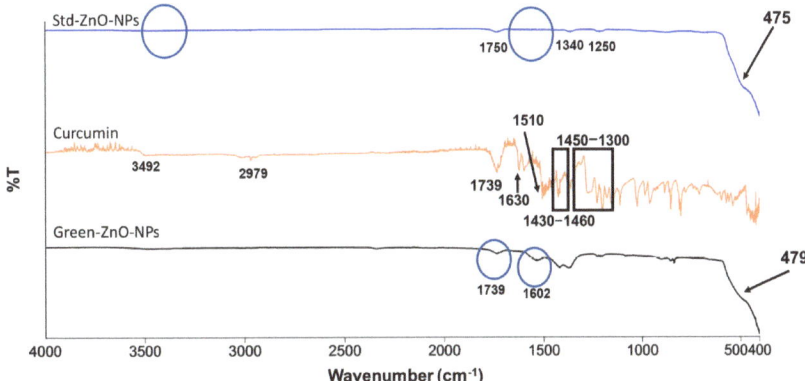

Figure 3. FTIR spectra of Std-ZnO-NPs (**up**), curcumin (**middle**), and Green-ZnO-NPs (**down**). The circles in Std-ZnO-NPs show that there were no peaks at 3500 cm^{-1} and 1600 cm^{-1}, confirming the absence of hydroxyl groups on ZnO NPs surfaces.

2.2.3. X-ray Powder Diffraction (XRD)

The crystallinity of Green-ZnO-NPs, Std-ZnO-NPs and curcumin was investigated by XRD. The experimental pattern of Green-ZnO-NPs (Figure 4) was consistent with the typical hexagonal zincite ZnO structure diffraction. All ZnO diffraction peaks were found in Green-ZnO-NPs at 31.85°, 34,50°, 36.20°, 47.50°, 56.45°, 62.71°, 67.73°, and 68.87°, corresponding to 110, 002, 101, 102, 110, 103, 200 and 112 lattice planes, respectively. These reported peaks comply with those obtained from the hexagonal phase of Std-ZnO-NPs with a wurtzite structure. All of the diffraction peaks are well correlated with the hexagonal phase of ZnO described in JCPDS card No. 36-1451 (space group *P63mc*). The diffraction peaks were sharp, highly intense and narrow, indicating the high crystallinity of Green-ZnO-NPs. No typical peaks of impurities or other phases of the zinc oxide were found, indicating the purity of the compound. The XRD pattern of curcumin exhibits peaks at the 2-theta range 20–30°, but these were not observed in Green-ZnO-NPs except for a peak at 30°.

2.2.4. Surface Morphology Analysis

Figure 5A,B show the typical hexagonal shape for Std-ZnO-NPs with an average size of 49.39 ± 22.54 nm. The morphology of Green-ZnO-NPs was predominantly grain-shaped or half-grain-shaped, while some were spherical (Figure 5C) with an average size of 68.12 ± 26.13 nm (Figure 5D). Using zinc acetate as a precursor, the ZnO nanoparticles developed slowly, forming small spherical structures that accumulate like bullets. The shape, size and size distribution of Green-ZnO-NPs and Std-ZnO-NPs were determined by using transmission electron microscopy (TEM) (Figure 6). Std-ZnO-NPs appeared mostly hexagonal in shape (Figure 6A), and the particle size was 20.72 ± 9.33 nm (Figure 6B). Green-ZnO-NPs mainly showed a grain shape with an average particle size of 27.61 ± 5.18 nm (Figure 6C,D). TEM indicates that both ZnO NPs showed aggregates.

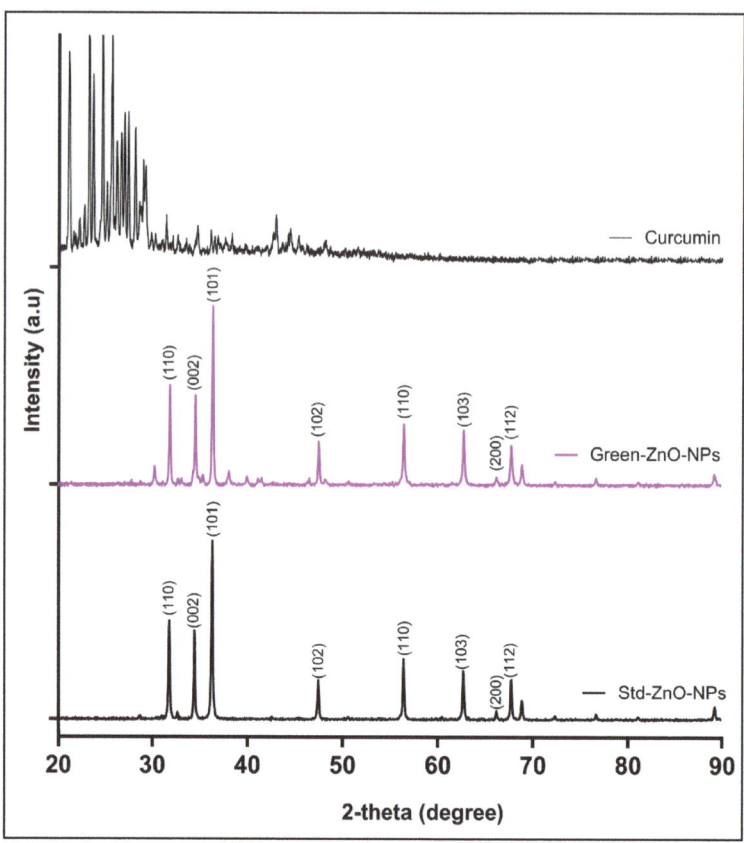

Figure 4. X-ray powder diffraction patterns of curcumin (**up**), Green-ZnO-NPs (**middle**) and Std-ZnO-NPs (**down**).

The difference in particle sizes obtained by scanning electron microscopy (SEM) and TEM can be explained by the sample supplied for these analyses. For the SEM samples analysis, the powder of nanoparticles is placed onto an SEM stub, and it is later coated by platinum or conductors for nonconductive samples, while for the TEM samples analysis, the nanoparticles are dispersed in a solvent and then homogenised using a sonicator before the sample is placed onto a grid and the solution is allowed to air-dry to obtain a thinly sliced sample. Hence, TEM image analysis showed a smaller size of particles as the sample was homogenised, whereas the SEM images usually displayed agglomerated particles with larger sizes.

Several reports have been conducted to synthesise curcumin-conjugated zinc oxide nanoparticles with different methods and the particles were formed in various shapes and sizes. For instance, researchers have synthesised ZnO NPs complexed with curcumin to improve the potency and reduce the cytotoxicity, and the formed nanoparticles were spherical in shape [44]. Curcumin-doped ZnO nanospheres were effectively synthesised using zinc nitrate hexahydrate, with a size of 100–200 nm [45]. The size and shape of zinc oxide nanoparticles in these studies were dependent on many factors, such as the concentration and ratio of the reactants and pH.

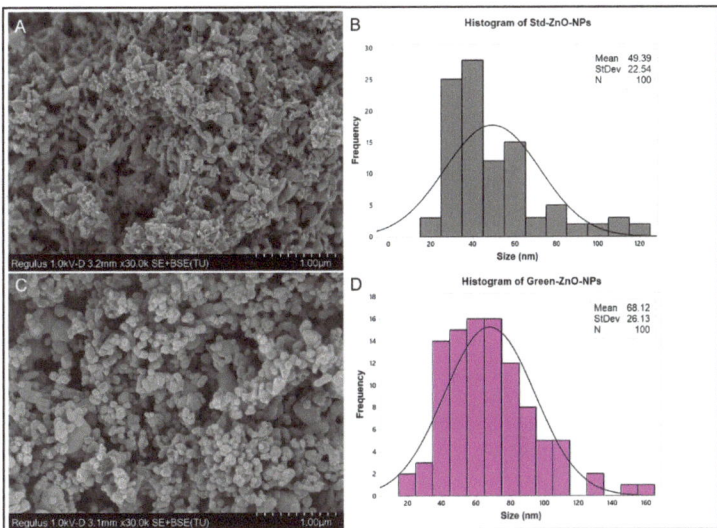

Figure 5. (**A**) Scanning electron microscopy images of Std-ZnO-NPs and (**B**) their corresponding histogram of particle size distribution ($n = 100$). (**C**) Scanning electron microscopy images of Green-ZnO-NPs and (**D**) their corresponding histogram of particle size distribution ($n = 100$).

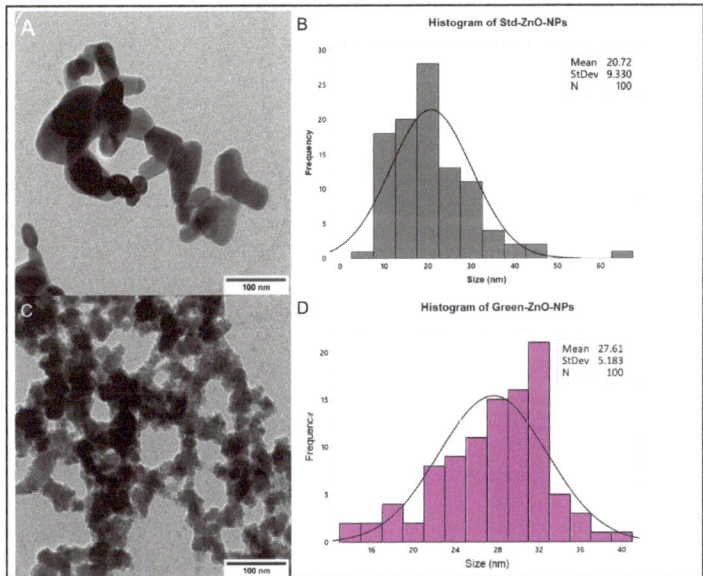

Figure 6. (**A**) Transmission electron microscopy images of Std-ZnO-NPs and (**B**) their corresponding histogram of particle size distribution ($n = 100$). (**C**) Transmission electron microscopy images of Green-ZnO-NPs and (**D**) their corresponding histogram of particle size distribution ($n = 100$).

2.2.5. Particle Size and Zeta Potential

The dynamic light scattering method was utilised to observe the zeta potential, median hydrodynamic size and the size distribution of Green-ZnO-NPs and Std-ZnO-NPs. Green-ZnO-NPs had a hydrodynamic size of 171.67 ± 45.83 nm, compared to 909 ± 65.18 nm for the Std-ZnO-NPs (Table 1). It is possible that the large size is related to particle aggregation. The size variations can also be attributed to the availability of curcumin molecules on the surface of the nanoparticles. Curcumin may improve the colloidal stability of Green-ZnO-NPs; however, the particles were colloidally unstable, as evidenced by zeta values [46]. Further, the zeta potential value of Std-ZnO-NPs has been recorded at +2.76 ± 0.20 mV, as the wurtzite structure of ZnO NPs possessed a positive charge [47]. The zeta potential value for Green-ZnO-NPs was −16.90 ± 0.26 mV which is attributed to the presence of negatively charged hydroxyl groups of curcumin on the surface of zinc oxide nanoparticles (curcumin zeta potential −3.82 ± 0.31). The polydispersity index (PDI) of Std-ZnO-NPs was lower than the value of Green-ZnO-NPs, at 0.412 ± 0.039 and 0.698 ± 0.271, respectively. The broad particle size distribution is mostly due to particle size aggregation, which is mainly related to the electrostatic attraction of zinc oxide nanoparticles [48]. It was reported that the biosynthesised zinc oxide nanoparticles from *Curcuma longa* rhizomes exhibited a spherical shape with a diameter of 25 nm [49]. Another study synthesised zinc oxide nanoparticles using casein as a capping agent and conjugated curcumin on their surfaces with a diameter of 12.8 nm and a zeta potential of −23.9 mV, and the particles remained stable in the solution [50].

Table 1. Median hydrodynamic size, zeta potential and polydispersity index values of Green-ZnO-NPs, Std-ZnO-NPs and curcumin. Tukey post hoc multiple comparison tests show a significant difference ($p < 0.05$) between samples with different superscript letters (mean ± SD; $n = 3$).

	Zeta Potential (mV)	PDI	Particle Size (nm)		
			DLS	SEM	TEM
Std-ZnO-NPs	+2.76 ± 0.20 [a]	0.412 ± 0.039 [a]	909 ± 65.18 [a]	48.98 ± 24.51 [a]	49.39 ± 22.54 [a]
Green-ZnO-NPs	−16.90 ± 0.26 [b]	0.698 ± 0.271 [a]	171.67 ± 45.83 [b]	68.12 ± 26.13 [a]	27.61 ± 5.18 [a]
Curcumin	−3.82 ± 0.31 [c]	-	-	-	-

2.3. Antioxidant Activity

The antiradical activity of Green-ZnO-NPs, Std-ZnO-NPs, and curcumin was determined using 2,2-diphenyl-1-picrylhydrazy (DPPH) radical savaging activity (Figure 7A). Curcumin and butylated hydroxyanisole (BHA) exhibited a concentration-dependent scanning activity, which was augmented significantly with an increase in their concentrations. Nevertheless, BHA generally exhibited a significantly higher activity than curcumin and the IC_{50} value of curcumin (33.97 ± 3.20 µg/mL) was significantly higher than the value of BHA (20.04 ± 2.01 µg/mL). Curcumin was significantly more effective as a radical scavenger compared to both zinc oxide nanoparticles at all concentrations. Both zinc oxide nanoparticles (Green-ZnO-NPs and Std-ZnO-NPs) showed no IC_{50} values at the studied concentration range (>250 µg/mL). The reaction of DPPH involves transferring a hydrogen atom to the odd electron of the radical, causing a change in the colour of the sample [51,52]. FTIR analysis demonstrated that Green-ZnO-NPs and Std-ZnO-NPs were not rich in hydrogen (Figure 3), explaining their low radical scavenging activity. Moreover, their low scavenging activity could probably be due to the lower specific surface area and large particle size. It has been reported that the scavenging activity of nanocomposite containing gold nanoparticles is insignificant due to their lower specific surface area [53]. According to Stan et al. [54], the scavenging activity of zinc oxide nanoparticles is size-dependent, where the smallest size displayed the highest antiradical activity [54]. Zinc oxide nanoparticles using *Curcuma longa* rhizomes exhibited good antiradical activity, almost 70% at

200 µg/mL [49]. The antioxidant activity of curcumin-ZnO NPs demonstrates moderate activity by scavenging 70% at 2 mg/mL [45].

The 2,2′-azino-bis(3-ethylbenzothiazoline-6-sulfonic acid (ABTS) test measures the antioxidant ability to scavenge ABTS and produce ABTS$^{•+}$. Radical scavenger acts as a representative for hydrogen donation [55]. Both BHA and curcumin showed a concentration-dependent ABTS inhibition effect (Figure 7B). BHA has shown considerably more efficacy in scavenging ABTS than curcumin at all studied concentrations, whereas ABTS inhibition is considerably increased at higher concentrations. Increasing the concentration from 3.9 to 250 µg/mL increased the scavenging activity of BHA and curcumin by 5.38- and 12.45-fold, respectively. Curcumin displayed an IC$_{50}$ of 66.93 ± 3.64 µg/mL, which was significantly higher compared to that of BHA (20.04 ± 1.70 µg/mL). Both zinc oxide nanoparticles showed an IC$_{50}$ > 250 µg/mL, and hence their antioxidant activity was significantly lower than that of curcumin.

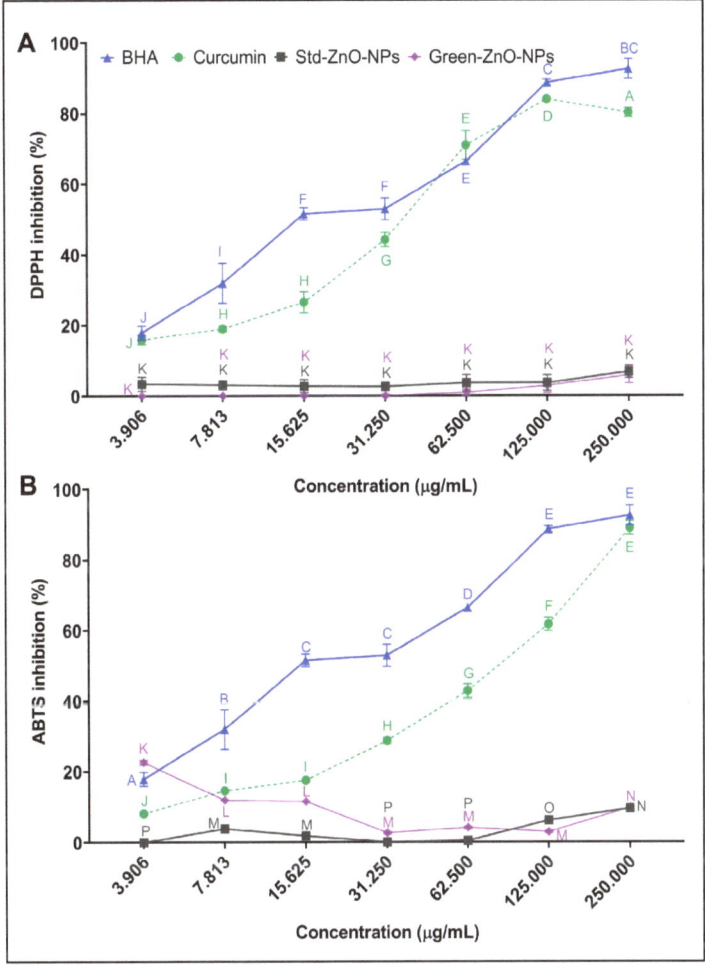

Figure 7. (**A**) DPPH and (**B**) ABTS antiradical activity of Green-ZnO-NPs, Std-ZnO-NPs and curcumin. Tukey post hoc multiple comparison tests show a significant difference ($p < 0.05$) between samples with different letters (mean ± SD; $n = 3$).

2.4. Antimicrobial Activity

The antibacterial properties of Green-ZnO-NPs, Std-ZnO-NPs, and curcumin against two Gram-negative [*Escherichia coli* (*E. coli*) and *Klebsiella pneumonia* (*K. pneumonia*)] and two Gram-positive [*Staphylococcus aureus* (*S. aureus*) and methicillin-resistant *S. aureus* (*MRSA*)] bacterial strains were measured as the diameter of zone of inhibition (ZOI), minimum inhibitory concentration (MIC), and minimum bactericidal concentration (MBC), using gentamicin as a positive control (Table 2). The ZOI varied based on the type of bacteria and the treatment (Figure 8). Gram-positive bacteria were more susceptible to Green-ZnO-NPs treatment than Gram-negative bacteria. The ZOI by Green-ZnO-NPs against *S. aureus* was 10.60 ± 0.10 mm, while no ZOI was observed against Gram-negative bacterial strains. Green-ZnO-NPs showed a greater ZOI compared to Std-ZnO-NPs against *S. aureus* (10.40 ± 0.15 mm), and their effect against *E. coli*, *K. pneumonia* and *MRSA* was significantly lower than that of gentamicin.

MIC is the lowest concentration that can reduce the growth of a microorganism after overnight incubation, whereas MBC is the lowest concentration that can prevent an organism from developing following a subculture of antibiotic-free media. MIC data showed that Green-ZnO-NPs exhibited bacteriostatic activity towards *E. coli*, *S. aureus* and *MRSA* at a concentration of 500 µg/mL; however, none of these concentrations demonstrated bactericidal activity (Table 2). Moreover, no MIC of Green-ZnO-NPs was observed against *K. pneumonia*. In addition, neither Std-ZnO-NPs nor curcumin showed antibacterial efficacy (MIC, MBC) against Gram-positive and Gram-negative bacteria.

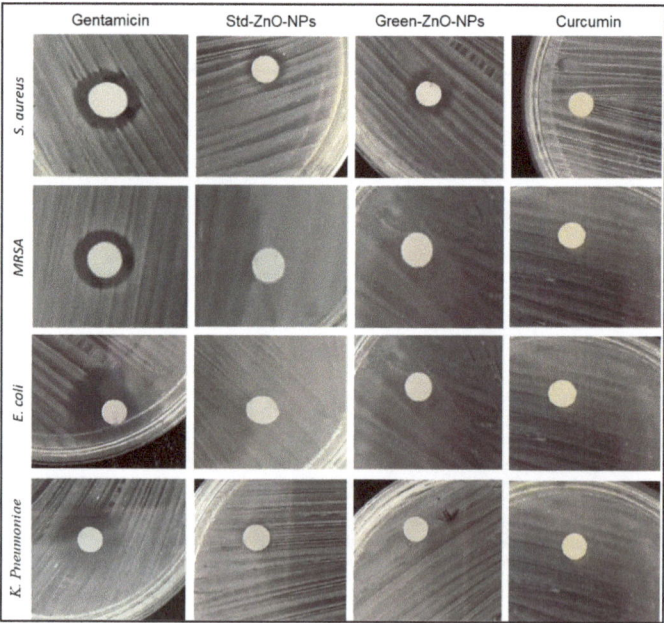

Figure 8. Zone of inhibitions of Gentamicin, Std-ZnO-NPs, Green-ZnO-NPs and curcumin against Gram-positive and Gram-negative bacteria.

The difference in the antibacterial activity between Green-ZnO-NPs and Std-ZnO-NPs could be due to the size of the nanoparticles. The activity of ZnO NPs is dependent on size and concentration. The concentration of ZnO NPs directly correlates with their antibacterial activity [56,57]. The higher concentration and smaller particle size are accountable for the higher antimicrobial activity of ZnO NPs [56,58]. Smaller ZnO NPs have a higher antibacterial efficacy owing to the large interfacial area that allows them to easily enter bacterial membranes. The MIC results revealed that the reduced size of the Green-ZnO-NPs displayed increased antibacterial propensity due to the large surface area to volume ratio, and subsequently, a high surface reactivity in comparison to Std-ZnO-NPs. Moreover, TEM analysis (Figure 6B,D) revealed more variability in the nanoparticle size distribution for Std-ZnO-NPs compared to Green-ZnO-NPs, which increases the probability of the Std-ZnO-NPs to congeal and form bigger particles, potentially reducing their antibacterial activity.

Moreover, this study found that *S. aureus* is more sensitive to ZnO NPs compared to *E. coli*, which is in accordance with a previous report by Reddy et al. [59]. Padmavathy and Vijayaraghavan [60] demonstrated that a higher degree of negatively charged free radicals caused cell damage and death in *S. aureus*. For Gram-negative bacteria strains, ZnO NPs must penetrate through the outer membrane alongside the peptidoglycan layer, while Gram-positive bacteria possess an outer membrane and a thick (30 μm) peptidoglycan layer [61]. Hence, Green-ZnO-NPs may function well as an antibacterial agent to combat both Gram-positive and Gram-negative bacteria.

Table 2. Zone of inhibitions, minimum inhibitory concentration, and minimum bactericidal concentration of Std-ZnO-NPs, Green-ZnO-NPs, and curcumin against Gram-positive and Gram-negative bacteria. Tukey post hoc multiple comparison tests show a significant difference ($p < 0.05$) between samples with different letters (mean ± SD; $n = 3$).

Microorganism	Gentamicin	Std-ZnO-NPs	Green-ZnO-NPs	Curcumin
		ZOI (mm)		
E. coli	22.87 ± 0.30 [a]	-	-	-
K. pneumonia	11.63 ± 0.10 [b]	-	-	-
MRSA	11.20 ± 0.06 [c]	-	-	-
S. aureus	15.7 ± 0.04 [d]	10.40 ± 0.15 [e]	10.60 ± 0.10 [e]	-
		MIC (μg/mL)		
E. coli	1.95	-	500	-
K. pneumonia	15.63	-	-	-
MRSA	7.81	-	500	-
S. aureus	0.98	-	500	-
		MBC (μg/mL)		
E. coli	7.81	-	-	-
K. pneumonia	31.25	-	-	-
MRSA	31.25	-	-	-
S. aureus	1.95	-	-	-
		Indicates no activity		

The main mechanism of the antimicrobial activity of ZnO NPs remains controversial. The proposed mechanisms are described as follows: direct interaction between ZnO NPs and the bacteria cell walls, consequently the destruction of the integrity of bacterial cell membrane [56,62,63], followed by liberation of Zn^{2+} [64–66], and generation of ROS [67–69]. In this context, the antibacterial mechanism of ZnO NPs could be hypothesised to be the production of ROS such as hydroxyl radicals, hydrogen peroxide (H_2O_2), singlet oxygen, and zinc ions (Zn^{2+}) released on the ZnO surface, which causes significant damage to the bacteria [57,70,71]. Bacterial growth is believed to be effectively inhibited by the production of H_2O_2 from the surface of ZnO [57]. According to certain reports, UV and visible light can activate ZnO, which results in the formation of electron–hole pairs (e^-/h^+). These holes break the H_2O molecule into OH^- and H^+ from the suspension of ZnO. Moreover, H^+ react with the dissolved oxygen molecules to generate superoxide radical anions (O_2^-), which are then converted into hydrogen peroxide anions (HO_2^-) radicals. These hydroxyl radicals will collide with electrons to form HO_2^-, and will then react with H to form H_2O_2

molecules. Consequently, produced H_2O_2 molecules can enter the cell membrane and kill the bacterium [72,73]. Lattice defects play a significant part in limiting the e^-/h^+ pair recombination process, which reduces the likelihood of ROS generation [74]. Biogenic ZnO made from aqueous extracts includes several defects that could serve as trapping centres and prevent photoinduced e^-/h^+ pair recombination [75] resulting in biogenic ZnO NPs having greater antibacterial activity compared to that of chemical ZnO NPs.

Moreover, several reports have demonstrated that the antibacterial property of zinc oxide nanoparticles is highly influenced by particle morphology [76–78]. It was revealed that the activity of nanoparticles is reliant on their shapes in terms of their active facets. Different synthesis techniques are involved in various active facets of the nanoparticle. ZnO nanorods have both (111) and (100) facets, while ZnO nanospheres only contain (100) facets. It is stated that higher antibacterial activity is exhibited by high-atom-density facets along with (111) facets [79]. Moreover, it has been stated that the enhanced internalisation of ZnO NPs nanostructures by the polar facets has contributed to the development of antibacterial effects and that a greater proportion of polar surfaces have a greater number of oxygen vacancies. ZnO morphologies having highly exposed (0001) Zn-terminated polar facets could provide higher antibacterial action [80].

2.5. Anticancer Activity

The anticancer effect of Green-ZnO-NPs was assessed against MCF-7 breast cancer cells by MTT assay for 24 and 48 h and was compared to Std-ZnO-NPs and curcumin (Figure 9). The results demonstrated a significant decline in MCF-7 cell viability upon increasing Green-ZnO-NPs concentration (3.125–200 µg/mL) for both treatment periods. However, Std-ZnO-NPs exhibited potential inhibiting activity against MCF-7 cells, which was higher than that of Green-ZnO-NPs at a concentration $\geq$ 12.5 µg/mL for both treatment periods. Std-ZnO-NPs showed a lower IC_{50} than Green-ZnO-NPs after 24 h of treatment (14.08 $\pm$ 0.91 µg/mL and 23.54 $\pm$ 0.04 µg/mL, respectively). However, extending the treatment time to 48 h enhanced the anticancer activity of Green-ZnO-NPs, while reducing the activity of Std-ZnO-NPs and Green-ZnO-NPs displayed IC_{50} values of 27.08 $\pm$ 0.91 µg/mL and 20.53 $\pm$ 5.12 µg/mL, respectively. This could be attributed to cell duplication, as the cells might double when the dose is decreased, allowing them to recover from a toxic shock and continue to proliferate. As Green-ZnO-NPs were substantially smaller than Std-ZnO-NPs, an improved anticancer effect was observed, supporting the claim of the particle size effect. Moreover, Green-ZnO-NPs exhibited a synergistic anticancer effect of curcumin and ZnO NPs.

Curcumin exhibited no anticancer activity before 24 h of treatment as the viability of curcumin-treated cells was >95% at all concentrations tested (3.125–200 µg/mL), whereas mild anticancer activity was obvious after prolongation of the treatment time to 48 h. Various studies have demonstrated that curcumin induces apoptosis in cancerous cells by inhibiting several intracellular transcription factors and secondary messengers [81–83]. Nevertheless, the reason for the low cytotoxicity could be related to the low solubility of curcumin. A low cytotoxicity of free curcumin against MCF-7 cell lines was observed by Chen et al., which is probably due to the low bioavailability caused by poor water solubility [84].

In addition, zinc oxide nanostructures could be used to attack tumour cells, providing a potential target for the development of an antitumour agent [85]. The toxic response to biological systems of zinc oxide nanoparticles is due to their catalytic activity and band gap [86,87]. Previous reports suggest that cytotoxicity depends on the size, shape and capping agent used to synthesise zinc oxide nanoparticles [88]. Although the actual mechanism of the cytotoxicity of zinc oxide nanoparticles is still unknown, various theories have been proposed. The intracellular release of Zn^{2+}, along with ROS generation, is the key mechanism driving zinc oxide nanoparticle cytotoxicity [8,89].

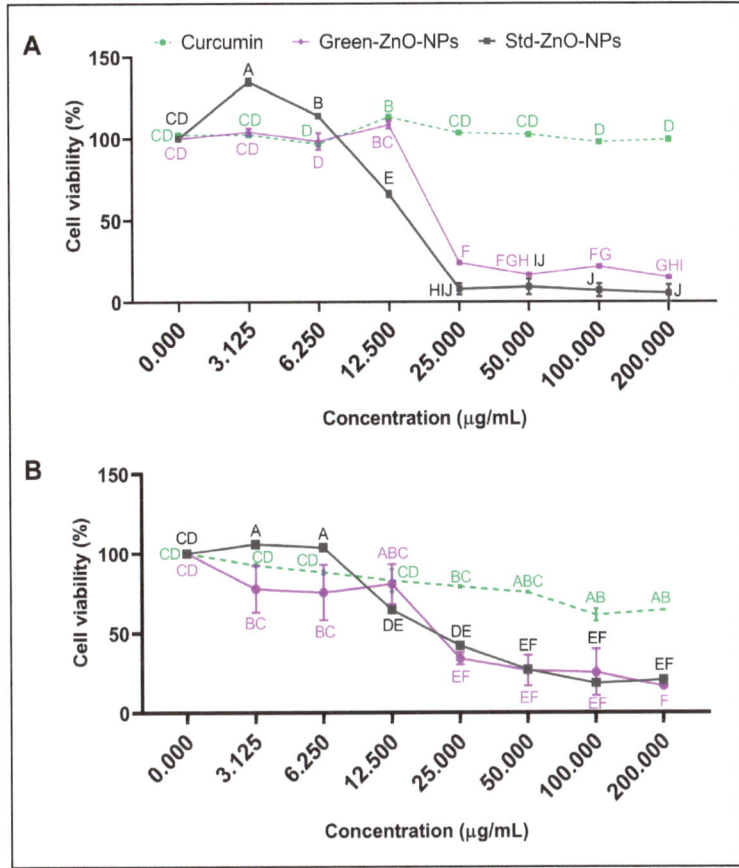

Figure 9. Anticancer activity of Std-ZnO-NPs, Green-ZnO-NPs and curcumin against MCF-7 human breast cancer cells after (**A**) 24 h and (**B**) 48 h of exposure. Tukey post hoc multiple comparison tests show a significant difference ($p < 0.05$) between samples with different letters (mean $\pm$ SD; $n = 3$).

2.6. Artemia Larvae Lethality Bioassay

Zero mortality was observed in the negative control, demonstrating that the deprivation of food had no lethal effect on *Artemia* larvae even after 24 h. The potassium dichromate showed a time-dependent effect, with no mortality observed after 4 h of exposure, while it showed a dose-dependent effect at 8 and 24 h (Figure 10). Although there was a substantial variation in mortality as the concentration increased (6.25 µg/mL–100 µg/mL), 100% mortality was reported using a concentration of 100 g/mL. However, approximately 30% of mortalities were observed at a concentration of 6.25 µg/mL after 8 h of exposure. The lethal effects were more apparent after extending the treatment time to 24 h. The mortality rate of larvae treated with 0.78 µg/mL was 69.05 $\pm$ 17.98%, while it increased to 100 $\pm$ 0.00% at 100 µg/mL, indicating that the LC_{50} concentration of potassium dichromate was 0.38 $\pm$ 0.27 µg/mL.

The mortalities of the larvae treated with Std-ZnO-NPs were raised by increasing the concentration of nanoparticles and increasing the incubation time ($p < 0.05$). The mortality rate between larvae treated with several concentrations of Std-ZnO-NPs did not change significantly after 4 and 8 h of exposure. The average mortality rate after 24 h of exposure to Std-ZnO-NPs ranged from 45.83 $\pm$ 9.79% (7.8 µg/mL) to 94.44 $\pm$ 9.62% (1000 µg/mL).

The LC$_{50}$ of Std-ZnO-NPs after 24 h of exposure was 11.96 ± 1.89 µg/mL. The mortality rate of larvae treated with Green-ZnO-NPs was lower than that of Std-ZnO-NPs. The lethal effects at 7.8 µg/mL were 0.00 ± 0.00%, 5.53 ± 4.79% and 46.44 ± 25.32% at 4, 8 and 24 h of exposure, respectively, and at 1000 µg/mL rose to 3.27 ± 5.66%, 13.33 ± 15.28% and 65.61 ± 1.72% at 4, 8, and 24 h of exposure, respectively. The LC$_{50}$ of ZnO-Cur-NPs at 24 h of exposure was 34.60 ± 9.45 µg/mL. At doses larger than 62.5 µg/mL, Green-ZnO-NPs had less fatal effects than Std-ZnO-NPs of identical concentrations ($p > 0.05$), even though the effects were not significantly different at 24 h exposure time at concentrations ≤ 62.5 µg/mL ($p < 0.05$). Curcumin's lethal effects followed the same temporal patterns as Std-ZnO-NPs, where the LC$_{50}$ of curcumin at 24 h of exposure was 7.30 ± 2.57 µg/mL. The mortalities of the curcumin treatment group recorded within 4 and 8 h were higher than those of Std-ZnO-NPs and Green-ZnO-NPs at the same concentration.

Although zinc is a versatile trace element for physical organisms, excessive quantities have been linked to cellular harm. Various studies on protozoa [90] and microalgae [91] have been undertaken on the harmful effects of ZnO NPs, where the toxicity is related to the release of Zn^{2+} into the solution from the nanomaterials. On the contrary, studies on the effect of ZnO NPs on various organisms, such as *Danio rerio* embryos [92], *Daphnia magna* [93], and *Tigriopus japonicus* [94], showed that the presence of zinc ions could not account for their toxicity.

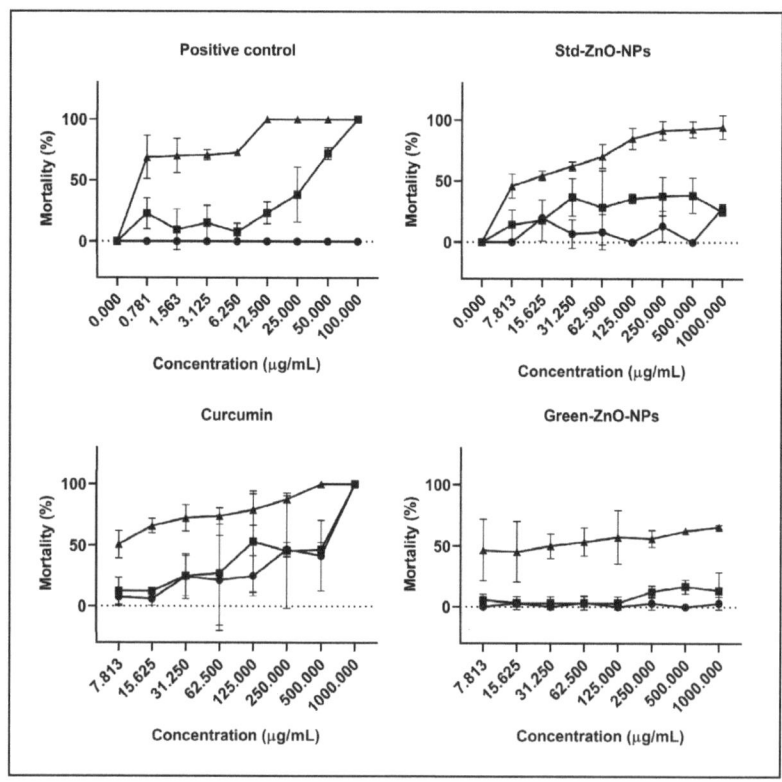

Figure 10. Mortality rates of *Artemia larvae* treated with potassium dichromate (positive control), Std-ZnO-NPs, Green-ZnO-NPs and curcumin at various concentrations after 4 (-●-), 8 (-■-), and 24 h (-▲-).

Furthermore, the *Artemia* larvae were imaged under the microscope after treatment with Green-ZnO-NPs, Std-ZnO-NPs and curcumin. Both Green-ZnO-NPs and Std-ZnO-

NPs aggregated inside the gut of *Artemia* larvae, as clearly observed in Figure 11 (red arrow). *Artemia* larvae have a nonselective filter-feeding behaviour, and it consumes particles smaller than 50 μm. The aggregation level is influenced not only by the concentration of the nanoparticles but also by the quantity consumed by each individual larva at different concentrations. The control group's guts were empty (the larvae did not exhibit any sign of aggregation, and the mouth and gut were transparent); however, the treatment group's guts were completely loaded with nanoparticles, specifically Green-ZnO-NPs (Figure 11). The images also show that the ingested nanoparticles were removed by *Artemia* larvae. Moreover, no significant difference in the size of treated larvae compared to the untreated ones was observed ($p > 0.005$).

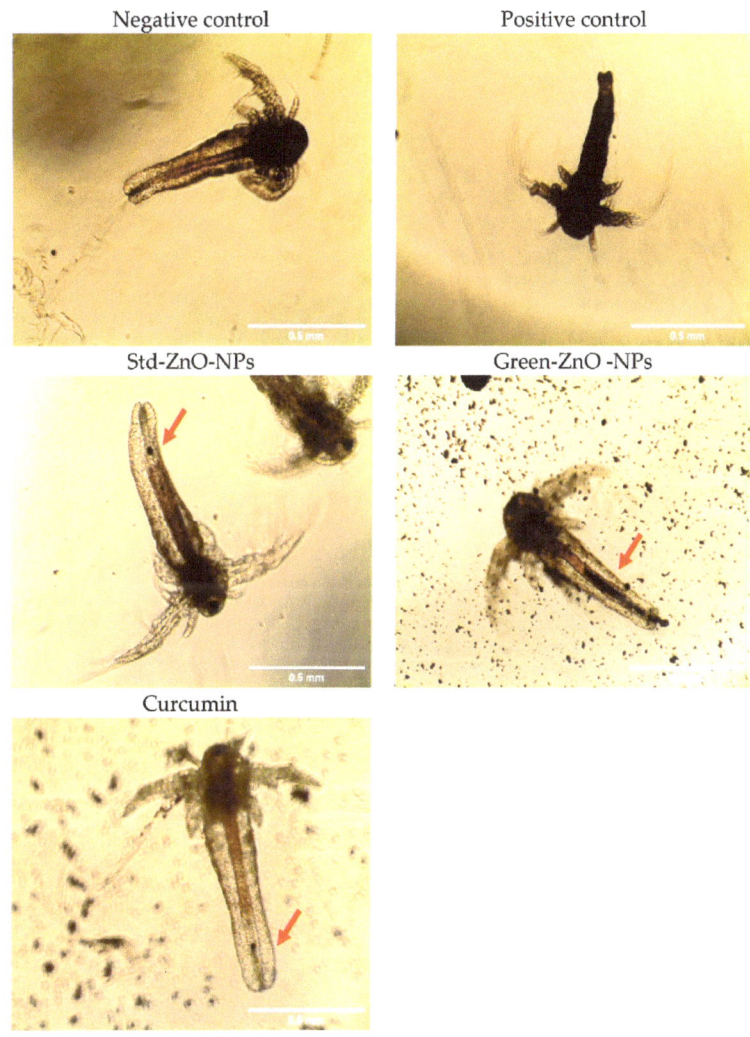

Figure 11. Morphology of treated (at their respective LC_{50}) and untreated Artemia larvae. The red arrows indicate the swallowed treatment by *Artemia* larvae.

3. Materials and Methods

3.1. Materials

Zinc acetate dihydrate, foetal bovine serum (FBS) and Dulbecco's modified eagle medium (DMEM) was purchased from Nacalai Tesque (Kyoto, Japan). Commercial zinc oxide nanoparticles (referred to as Std-ZnO-NPs in this study) with particle size < 100 nm, dimethyl sulfoxide (DMSO), 2,2-diphenyl-1-picrylhydrazyl (DPPH), 2,2'-azino-bis(3-ethylbenzothiazoline-6-sulfonic acid (ABTS) and 3-(4,5-dimethylthiazol-2-yl)-2,5-diphenyltetrazolium bromide (MTT) were received from Sigma Aldrich (Saint Louis, MO, USA). Curcumin (>97.0%) was received from Tokyo Chemical Industry (Tokyo, Japan). Bacterial culture media were purchased from Merck (Darmstadt, Germany). Gentamycin sulfate was received from Biobasic (Markham, ON, Canada). *Escherichia coli* [*E. coli* (ATCC 25922)], *Staphylococcus aureus* [*S. aureus* (ATCC 25923)], *Klebsiella pneumonia* [*k. pneumonia* (BAA-1705)] and methicillin-resistant *S. aureus* [*MRSA* (ATCC 33591)] were obtained from American type culture collection (ATCC).

3.2. Synthesis of Green-ZnO-NPs

Green-ZnO-NPs were synthesised following a method adopted from previous studies [95] with slight changes. Initially, a stock solution of curcumin was prepared using ethanol at 10 mM, and then it was diluted to 0.2 mM with ultrapure water. Zinc acetate was prepared as a stock solution (0.5 mM) using 20 mL of ultrapure water, and 20 mL of curcumin solution (0.2 mM) was added, followed by the mixing of these two solutions at room temperature (200 rpm, 2 h). Next, Green-ZnO-NPs were collected by centrifugation (3000× g, 3 min) and washed thrice with ultrapure water to eliminate the unreacted curcumin on the surface of zinc oxide, then dried at 70 °C for 24 h. Figure 1 illustrates the synthesis scheme of zinc oxide nanoparticles using pure curcumin.

3.3. Characterisation of Green-ZnO-NPs

3.3.1. UV–Vis

A 100 µg/mL aqueous suspension of Green-ZnO-NPs and Std-ZnO-NPs was prepared and homogenised in a sonicator for 5 min. Curcumin solution was prepared using absolute ethanol (10 µg/mL). The suspensions of Green-ZnO-NPs and Std-ZnO-NPs, as well as curcumin solution, were examined by UV–Vis spectrophotometer (Shimadzu, Japan) over the range from 300 to 700 nm.

3.3.2. ATR-FTIR Analysis

To evaluate the surface functionalisation, FTIR spectra of Green-ZnO-NPs, Std-ZnO-NPs, and curcumin were recorded using a Perkin Elmer FTIR spectrophotometer (Norwalk, CT, USA) at a wavelength of 4000 to 400 cm^{-1} [96].

3.3.3. XRD

The crystalline structure of Green-ZnO-NPs, Std-ZnO-NPs, and curcumin was characterised by an X-ray diffractometer using 40 kV/40 mA current with Co-Kα radiation. The samples were scanned in the 20° to 90° 2-theta range.

3.3.4. Surface Morphology Analysis

The primary size and morphology of Green-ZnO-NPs and Std-ZnO-NPs were evaluated using Libra 120 TEM (Zeiss, Oberkochen, Germany). Green-ZnO-NPs and Std-ZnO-NPs were dispersed at a concentration of 100 µg/mL in ultrapure water and homogenised in a sonicator for 5 min. A volume of 10 µL of Green-ZnO-NPs suspension was loaded onto a carbon-coated copper grid. The grid was dried for 10 min before it was examined using TEM. The histogram of particle size distribution was generated from three microscopy images by measuring the diameter of 100 nanoparticles using ImageJ software. Moreover, SEM (Hitachi-Regulus, Tokyo, Japan) was conducted to identify the surface morphology of Green-ZnO-NPs and it was compared to Std-ZnO-NPs. The SEM samples were prepared by placing the nanoparticles above the SEM carbon-coated stub, followed by removing the excessive nanoparticles with an air dust blower. The samples proceeded for imaging without coating.

3.3.5. Particle Size and Zeta Potential

Green-ZnO-NPs and Std-ZnO-NPs had their hydrodynamic particle size, size distribution, and zeta potential recorded by a Zetasizer Nano ZS (Malvern Instruments Ltd., Malvern, UK). The analysis was performed for a duration of 10 s, 12–15 times, at 25 °C. An aqueous suspension of Green-ZnO-NPs and Std-ZnO-NPs was prepared at a concentration of 100 µg/mL and was homogenised in the sonicator for 5 min. Curcumin solution was prepared using absolute ethanol at a stock concentration of 10 mg/mL, then it was diluted with ultrapure water to 10 µg/mL, and its zeta potential was recorded.

3.4. Antioxidant Activity

DPPH radical scavenging activity of the aqueous suspension of Green-ZnO-NPs was tested and compared with Std-ZnO-NPs and curcumin, following a previous report with minor modifications [97]. In brief, 150 µL of 100 µM DPPH (in methanol) was mixed with 50 µL of each concentration (3.906, 7.813, 31.625, 62.5, 125, 250, and 500 µg/mL) of Std-ZnO-NPs, Green-ZnO-NPs and curcumin (dissolved primarily in absolute ethanol at 10 mg/mL concentration then diluted in ultrapure water), and then incubated for 30 min. A plate reader was used to record the optical density at 517 nm. The percentage of DPPH inhibition was calculated by subtracting the sample absorbance from the absorbance of the control by dividing the control absorbance multiplied by 100. BHA and ultrapure water were utilised as positive and negative controls, respectively.

Moreover, ABTS radical scavenging activities of Green-ZnO-NPs, Std-ZnO-NPs and curcumin were determined based on a previous report with minor changes [97]. Briefly, the ABTS working solution was made by mixing a volume of ABTS solution (7 mM) with a volume of potassium persulfate (2.45 mM). The prepared solution was stored for 16 h at room temperature. The ABTS working solution was diluted with ethanol until reaching an absorbance of 0.7 at 734 nm. A volume of 50 µL for each concentration (3.906, 7.813, 31.625, 62.5, 125, 250, and 500 µg/mL) of Green-ZnO-NPs, Std-ZnO-NPs and curcumin was mixed with 150 µL of ABTS working solution, followed by 6 min of incubation. Then, the optical density was recorded at 734 nm. The ABTS inhibition percentage was determined by subtracting sample absorbance from the absorbance of control by dividing the control absorbance multiplied by 100. BHA and ultrapure water were utilised as positive and negative controls, respectively.

3.5. Antibacterial Activity

The antibacterial properties of Green-ZnO-NPs, Std-ZnO-NPs and curcumin were tested against two Gram-negative bacterial strains (*E. coli, K. pneumonia*) and two Gram-positive bacterial strains (*S. aureus* and *MRSA*) using disc diffusion and broth microdilution assays.

3.5.1. Preparation of Inoculum

A lawn culture prepared from each bacterial strain was prepared by subculturing a fresh 100 µL of bacterial solution (having 10^5 CFU/mL, complying with McFarland 0.5) on MHA, which was incubated overnight at 37 °C.

3.5.2. Disc Diffusion Method

The experiment was performed as described in a previous report by Chiu et al. [98]. The zones of inhibition of Green-ZnO-NPs were tested against the mentioned bacteria and compared with that of Std-ZnO-NPs and curcumin. Each bacterial strain was swabbed on the MHA plates. A volume of 30 µL of Green-ZnO-NPs and Std-ZnO-NPs suspensions (1 mg/mL), as well as curcumin solution, was applied to sterile discs with a diameter of 9 mm. Next, the discs were placed on swabbed plates. A clear zone of inhibition was measured after incubation and expressed in millimetres. Gentamicin solution (1 mg/mL) and ultrapure water were utilised as positive and negative controls, respectively.

3.5.3. Broth Microdilution Assay

The experiment was performed as mentioned by Chiu et al. [98]. To assess the minimum inhibitory concentration (MIC), 180 µL of bacterial inoculum suspension was mixed with 20 µL of the Green-ZnO-NPs, Std-ZnO-NPs and curcumin at various concentrations (3.906, 7.813, 31.625, 62.5, 125, 250, 500, and 1000 µg/mL) in a 96-well plate, followed by 24 h of incubation at 37 °C. Gentamicin solution (1 mg/mL) and ultrapure water were utilised as positive and negative controls, respectively. Afterwards, 50 µL of MTT solution (500 µg/mL) was introduced to each well, followed by 30 min of incubation. The existence of a purple colour indicated the presence of viable bacteria. To determine the minimum bactericidal concentration (MBC), 10 µL of the wells that did not have a purple colour were streaked on MHA plates, followed by incubation at 37 °C for 24 h.

3.6. Anticancer Activity

MCF-7 cells were maintained in a complete culture medium (DMEM supplemented with 10% FBS) in a 5% CO_2 incubator at 37 °C. The anticancer effect of Green-ZnO-NPs was assessed against MCF-7 cells according to a previous method [99] with minor changes and was compared to Std-ZnO-NPs and curcumin. Briefly, 1×10^4 cells/well were seeded in a 96-well plate, grown overnight, and then treated with various concentrations (3.125, 6.25, 12.5, 25, 50, 100, and 200 µg/mL) of Green-ZnO-NPs, Std-ZnO-NPs and curcumin. After 24 or 48 h treatment exposure, the media were replenished with 10 µL of MTT (500 µg/mL) reagent and 90 µL of a fresh medium and kept in the incubator for a further 4 h. The medium was replaced with 100 µL of DMSO in each well of the plate, and the optical densities were measured at 570 nm. The percent of cell viability was calculated by dividing the absorbance from the treated cell over the absorbance from the untreated cell after blank subtraction and multiplying by 100. The IC_{50} after treatment were calculated for both time periods.

3.7. Artemia Larvae Lethality Bioassay

The hydration of brine shrimp (*Artemia franciscana*) eggs was first undertaken in ultrapure water overnight at 4 °C, followed by the collection and washing of the sinking cysts. Deionised water was used to make 3% *w/v* saltwater (without iodine), which was then filtered through 30 µm Millipore cellulose filters. Approximately 2 g of previously cleansed cysts were added to 1 L of salt water and a steady fluorescent bulb (1500 lux daylight) at 30 ± 1 °C [100]. Artemia larvae hatched under these conditions in less than 24 h.

The toxic effect of Green-ZnO-NPs, Std-ZnO-NPs, and curcumin on larvae mortality was investigated as described by Ates et al. [100]. The experiment was carried out on a 12-well plate and lasted 4, 8, and 24 h. A volume of 1 mL of saltwater with the addition of the required concentration of Green-ZnO-NPs, Std-ZnO-NPs, and curcumin (7.813, 31.625, 62.5, 125, 250, 500, and 1000 µg/mL) with around 15 larvae (<24 h old) were transferred to each well. The Artemia larvae were incubated with the treatment for 24 h, and then the mortality rate and half maximum lethal concentration (LC_{50}) values were determined. Potassium dichromate at a concentration range of 0.781, 3.163, 6.250, 12.5, 25, 50, and 100 µg/mL was utilised as a positive control. The morphological variations in the treated and untreated brine shrimp larvae were observed using an inverted optical microscope at the treatment LC_{50} value (Kenis, 10×).

3.8. Statistical Analysis

All data in this research were collected from three independent biological replicates and presented as mean ± standard deviation (SD). Prism pad software was used to compute the IC_{50} and LC_{50} values. Significant differences between the means were analysed by one-way analysis of variance (ANOVA) in Minitab software, followed by Tukey post hoc multiple comparison tests. P less than 0.05 indicates significance.

4. Conclusions

In this research, the biosynthesis of ZnO NPs using curcumin was described, and their physicochemical properties were characterised. ATR-FTIR spectra have confirmed the role of curcumin in the formation of Green-ZnO-NPs. Moreover, Green-ZnO-NPs demonstrated a strong crystallinity property due to the hexagonal wurtzite structure. The produced NPs were grain-shaped in SEM and TEM microscopy images, with some of them having a spherical shape. They possessed a mean size of 27.62 ± 5.18 nm and a zeta potential of -16.90 ± 0.26 mV, respectively. Furthermore, the Green-ZnO-NPs showed a poor antioxidant effect using ABTS and DPPH tests. Even though Green-ZnO-NPs possessed weak antimicrobial activity, they exhibited high effectiveness in inhibiting MCF-7 breast cancer cells. MTT results suggest that Green-ZnO-NPs were more potent anticancer agents than chemically synthesised Std-ZnO-NPs and less toxic to *Artemia* larvae. Thus, it is envisaged that Green-ZnO-NPs could be a promising agent for anticancer applications.

Author Contributions: Conceptualization, V.L. and B.A.; methodology, B.A. and V.L.; software, B.A.; validation, B.A.; formal analysis, B.A. and M.A.; investigation, B.A.; resources, V.L.; data curation, B.A.; writing—original draft preparation, B.A.; writing—review and editing, B.A., M.A., A.A.D. and V.L.; visualization, V.L.; supervision, V.L.; project administration, V.L.; funding acquisition, V.L. and B.A. All authors have read and agreed to the published version of the manuscript.

Funding: This work was supported by the Research University Top-Down Grant Scheme, Universiti Sains Malaysia, with Project No: 1001/CIPPT/8070019, Project Code: NO0060 (Reference No: 2021/0318).

Institutional Review Board Statement: Not applicable.

Informed Consent Statement: Not applicable.

Data Availability Statement: All data is comprised within this manuscript.

Acknowledgments: Batoul Alallam would like to express appreciation to Universiti Sains Malaysia (USM) for providing her graduate fellowship scheme (GFUSM).

Conflicts of Interest: The authors declare no conflict of interest.

References

1. Jalal, M.Z.; John, A.; Rasheed, A.K.; Alallam, B.; Khalid, M.; Ismail, A.F.; Salleh, H. Earlier Denaturation of DNA By Using Novel Ternary Hybrid Nanoparticles. *IIUM Eng. J.* **2022**, *23*, 237–245. [CrossRef]
2. Nawaz, A.; Latif, M.S.; Alnuwaiser, M.A.; Ullah, S.; Iqbal, M.; Alfatama, M.; Lim, V. Synthesis and Characterization of Chitosan-Decorated Nanoemulsion Gel of 5-Fluorouracil for Topical Delivery. *Gels* **2022**, *8*, 412. [CrossRef] [PubMed]
3. Naz, F.F.; Shah, K.U.; Niazi, Z.R.; Zaman, M.; Lim, V.; Alfatama, M. Polymeric Microparticles: Synthesis, Characterization and In Vitro Evaluation for Pulmonary Delivery of Rifampicin. *Polymers* **2022**, *14*, 2491. [CrossRef] [PubMed]
4. Sabir, S.; Arshad, M.; Chaudhari, S.K. Zinc Oxide Nanoparticles for Revolutionizing Agriculture: Synthesis and Applications. *Sci. World J.* **2014**, *2014*, 925494. [CrossRef] [PubMed]
5. Rajendran, S.P.; Sengodan, K. Synthesis and Characterization of Zinc Oxide and Iron Oxide Nanoparticles Using *Sesbania grandiflora* Leaf Extract as Reducing Agent. *J. Nanosci.* **2017**, *2017*, 8348507. [CrossRef]
6. Saleemi, M.A.; Alallam, B.; Yong, Y.K.; Lim, V. Synthesis of Zinc Oxide Nanoparticles with Bioflavonoid Rutin: Characterisation, Antioxidant and Antimicrobial Activities and In Vivo Cytotoxic Effects on *Artemia* Nauplii. *Antioxidants* **2022**, *11*, 1853. [CrossRef]
7. Cross, S.E.; Innes, B.; Roberts, M.S.; Tsuzuki, T.; Robertson, T.A.; McCormick, P. Human Skin Penetration of Sunscreen Nanoparticles: In-vitro Assessment of a Novel Micronized Zinc Oxide Formulation. *Ski. Pharmacol. Physiol.* **2007**, *20*, 148–154. [CrossRef]
8. Rasmussen, J.W.; Martinez, E.; Louka, P.; Wingett, D.G. Zinc oxide nanoparticles for selective destruction of tumor cells and potential for drug delivery applications. *Expert Opin. Drug Deliv.* **2010**, *7*, 1063–1077. [CrossRef]
9. Jamdagni, P.; Khatri, P.; Rana, J. Green synthesis of zinc oxide nanoparticles using flower extract of Nyctanthes arbor-tristis and their antifungal activity. *J. King Saud Univ.-Sci.* **2018**, *30*, 168–175. [CrossRef]
10. Hasnidawani, J.; Azlina, H.; Norita, H.; Bonnia, N.; Ratim, S.; Ali, E. Synthesis of ZnO Nanostructures Using Sol-Gel Method. *Procedia Chem.* **2016**, *19*, 211–216. [CrossRef]

11. Mallikarjunaswamy, C.; Ranganatha, V.L.; Ramu, R.; Udayabhunu; Nagaraju, G. Facile microwave-assisted green synthesis of ZnO nanoparticles: Application to photodegradation, antibacterial and antioxidant. *J. Mater. Sci. Mater. Electron.* **2019**, *31*, 1004–1021. [CrossRef]
12. Nguyen, N.T.; Nguyen, V.A. Synthesis, Characterization, and Photocatalytic Activity of ZnO Nanomaterials Prepared by a Green, Nonchemical Route. *J. Nanomater.* **2020**, *2020*, 1768371. [CrossRef]
13. Kunnumakkara, A.B.; Sailo, B.L.; Banik, K.; Harsha, C.; Prasad, S.; Gupta, S.C.; Bharti, A.C.; Aggarwal, B.B. Chronic diseases, inflammation, and spices: How are they linked? *J. Transl. Med.* **2018**, *16*, 14. [CrossRef]
14. Santini, A.; Tenore, G.C.; Novellino, E. Nutraceuticals: A paradigm of proactive medicine. *Eur. J. Pharm. Sci.* **2017**, *96*, 53–61. [CrossRef]
15. Das, T.; Sa, G.; Saha, B.; Das, K. Multifocal signal modulation therapy of cancer: Ancient weapon, modern targets. *Mol. Cell. Biochem.* **2009**, *336*, 85–95. [CrossRef]
16. Tung, B.T.; Nham, D.T.; Hai, N.T.; Thu, D.K. Curcuma longa, the Polyphenolic Curcumin Compound and Pharmacological Effects on Liver. In *Dietary Interventions in Liver Disease: Foods, Nutrients and Dietary Supplements*; Academic Press: Cambridge, MA, USA, 2019; pp. 125–134. [CrossRef]
17. Anand, P.; Kunnumakkara, A.B.; Newman, R.A.; Aggarwal, B.B. Bioavailability of curcumin: Problems and promises. *Mol. Pharm.* **2007**, *4*, 807–818. [CrossRef]
18. Hassani, A.; Mahmood, S.; Enezei, H.H.; Hussain, S.A.; Hamad, H.A.; Aldoghachi, A.F.; Hagar, A.; Doolaanea, A.A.; Ibrahim, W.N. Formulation, Characterization and Biological Activity Screening of Sodium Alginate-Gum Arabic Nanoparticles Loaded with Curcumin. *Molecules* **2020**, *25*, 2244. [CrossRef]
19. Goel, A.; Kunnumakkara, A.B.; Aggarwal, B.B. Curcumin as "Curecumin": From kitchen to clinic. *Biochem. Pharmacol.* **2007**, *75*, 787–809. [CrossRef]
20. Verma, A.; Jain, N.; Singha, S.K.; Quraishi, M.A.; Sinha, I. Green synthesis and catalytic application of curcumin stabilized silver nanoparticles. *J. Chem. Sci.* **2016**, *128*, 1871–1878. [CrossRef]
21. Khalil, M.I.; Al-Qunaibit, M.M.; Al-Zahem, A.M.; Labis, J.P. Synthesis and characterization of ZnO nanoparticles by thermal decomposition of a curcumin zinc complex. *Arab. J. Chem.* **2014**, *7*, 1178–1184. [CrossRef]
22. Jayarambabu, N.; Rao, K.V.; Prabhu, Y.T. Beneficial Role of Zinc Oxide Nanoparticles on Green Crop Production Effects of Temperature, Deposition Time and Catalyst Loading on the Synthesis of Carbon Nanotubes in a Fixed Bed Reactor View Project Phytochemical Screening and Evaluation of In Vitro Antioxidant and Antimicrobial Activities of the Indigenous Medicinal Plant Albizia Odoratissima View Project. 2015. Available online: https://www.researchgate.net/publication/301541596 (accessed on 4 January 2023).
23. El-Kattan, N.; Emam, A.N.; Mansour, A.S.; Ibrahim, M.A.; El-Razik, A.B.A.; Allam, K.A.M.; Riad, N.Y.; Ibrahim, S.A. Curcumin assisted green synthesis of silver and zinc oxide nanostructures and their antibacterial activity against some clinical pathogenic multi-drug resistant bacteria. *RSC Adv.* **2022**, *12*, 18022–18038. [CrossRef] [PubMed]
24. Perera, W.P.T.D.; Dissanayake, R.K.; Ranatunga, U.I.; Hettiarachchi, N.M.; Perera, K.D.C.; Unagolla, J.M.; De Silva, R.T.; Pahalagedara, L.R. Curcumin loaded zinc oxide nanoparticles for activity-enhanced antibacterial and anticancer applications. *RSC Adv.* **2020**, *10*, 30785–30795. [CrossRef] [PubMed]
25. Facile Synthesis of Silver-Zinc Oxide Nanocomposites Using Curcuma Longa Extract and Its In Vitro Antimicrobial Efficacy against Multi-Drug Resistant Pathogens of Public Health Importance—Google Search. Available online: https://www.google.com/search?q=Facile+synthesis+of+silver-zinc+oxide+nanocomposites+using+Curcuma+longa+extract+and+its+in+vitro+antimicrobial+efficacy+against+multi-drug+resistant+pathogens+of+public+health+importance&oq=Facile+synthesis+of+silver-zinc+oxide+nanocomposites+using+Curcuma+longa+extract+and+its+in+vitro+antimicrobial+efficacy+against+multi-drug+resistant+pathogens+of+public+health+importance&aqs=chrome..69i57j69i61l3.201j0j4&sourceid=chrome&ie=UTF-8 (accessed on 4 January 2023).
26. Khalil, M.I.; Al-Zahem, A.; Qunaibit, M.M. Synthesis, characterization, and antitumor activity of binuclear curcumin-metal(II) hydroxo complexes. *Med. Chem. Res.* **2014**, *23*, 1683–1689. [CrossRef]
27. Rajapriya, M.; Sharmili, S.A.; Baskar, R.; Balaji, R.; Alharbi, N.S.; Kadaikunnan, S.; Khaled, J.M.; Alanzi, K.F.; Vaseeharan, B. Synthesis and Characterization of Zinc Oxide Nanoparticles Using Cynara scolymus Leaves: Enhanced Hemolytic, Antimicrobial, Antiproliferative, and Photocatalytic Activity. *J. Clust. Sci.* **2019**, *31*, 791–801. [CrossRef]
28. Wang, Y.-J.; Pan, M.-H.; Cheng, A.-L.; Lin, L.-I.; Ho, Y.-S.; Hsieh, C.-Y.; Lin, J.-K. Stability of curcumin in buffer solutions and characterization of its degradation products. *J. Pharm. Biomed. Anal.* **1997**, *15*, 1867–1876. [CrossRef]
29. Payton, F.; Sandusky, P.; Alworth, W.L. NMR study of the solution structure of curcumin. *J. Nat. Prod.* **2007**, *70*, 143–146. [CrossRef]
30. Menon, V.P.; Sudheer, A.R. Antioxidant and anti-inflammatory properties of curcumin. *Adv. Exp. Med. Biol.* **2007**, *595*, 105–125. [CrossRef]
31. Jovanovic, S.V.; Steenken, S.; Boone, C.W.; Simic, M.G. H-Atom Transfer Is a Preferred Antioxidant Mechanism of Curcumin. *J. Am. Chem. Soc.* **1999**, *121*, 9677–9681. [CrossRef]
32. Dobrucka, R.; Dlugaszewska, J.; Kaczmarek, M. Cytotoxic and antimicrobial effects of biosynthesized ZnO nanoparticles using of Chelidonium majus extract. *Biomed. Microdevices* **2017**, *20*, 5. [CrossRef]

33. Zak, A.K.; Majid, W.A.; Mahmoudian, M.; Darroudi, M.; Yousefi, R. Starch-stabilized synthesis of ZnO nanopowders at low temperature and optical properties study. *Adv. Powder Technol.* **2013**, *24*, 618–624. [CrossRef]
34. Kim, H.J.; Kim, D.J.; Karthick, S.N.; Hemalatha, K.V.; Raj, C.J.; Ok, S.; Choe, Y. Curcumin Dye Extracted from *Curcuma longa* L. Used as Sensitizers for Efficient Dye-Sensitized Solar Cells. *Int. J. Electrochem. Sci.* **2013**, *8*, 8320–8328.
35. Das, R.K.; Pachapur, V.L.; Lonappan, L.; Naghdi, M.; Pulicharla, R.; Maiti, S.; Cledon, M.; Dalila, L.M.A.; Sarma, S.J.; Brar, S.K. Biological synthesis of metallic nanoparticles: Plants, animals and microbial aspects. *Nanotechnol. Environ. Eng.* **2017**, *2*, 18. [CrossRef]
36. Xiong, H.-M.; Ma, R.-Z.; Wang, S.-F.; Xia, Y.-Y. Photoluminescent ZnO nanoparticles synthesized at the interface between air and triethylene glycol. *J. Mater. Chem.* **2011**, *21*, 3178–3182. [CrossRef]
37. Umar, A.; Rahman, M.; Vaseem, M.; Hahn, Y.-B. Ultra-sensitive cholesterol biosensor based on low-temperature grown ZnO nanoparticles. *Electrochem. Commun.* **2009**, *11*, 118–121. [CrossRef]
38. Kwon, Y.J.; Kim, K.H.; Lim, C.S.; Shim, K.B. Characterization of ZnO nanopowders synthesized by the polymerized complex method via an organochemical route. *J. Ceram. Process. Res.* **2002**, *3*, 146–149.
39. Kolev, T.M.; Velcheva, E.A.; Stamboliyska, B.A.; Spiteller, M. DFT and experimental studies of the structure and vibrational spectra of curcumin. *Int. J. Quantum Chem.* **2005**, *102*, 1069–1079. [CrossRef]
40. Priyadarsini, K.I. The Chemistry of Curcumin: From Extraction to Therapeutic Agent. *Molecules* **2014**, *19*, 20091–20112. [CrossRef]
41. Ciszewski, A.; Milczarek, G.; Lewandowska, B.; Krutowski, K. Electrocatalytic Properties of Electropolymerized Ni(II)curcumin Complex. *Electroanalysis* **2003**, *15*, 518–523. [CrossRef]
42. Tayyari, S.F.; Rahemi, H.; Nekoei, A.R.; Zahedi-Tabrizi, M.; Wang, Y.A. Vibrational assignment and structure of dibenzoylmethane. A density functional theoretical study. *Spectrochim. Acta-Part A Mol. Biomol. Spectrosc.* **2007**, *66*, 394–404. [CrossRef]
43. Krishnankutty, K.; John, V.D. Synthesis, Characterization, and Antitumour Studies of Metal Chelates of Some Synthetic Curcuminoids. *Synth. React. Inorganic, Met. Nano-Metal Chem.* **2003**, *33*, 343–358. [CrossRef]
44. Rajalaxshmi, A.; Clara Jeyageetha, J. Green Syntheses and Characterization of Zinc Oxide and Cerium Ion Doped Zinc Oxide Nanoparticles Assisted by Mangifera Indica. *Eur. J. Pharm. Med. Res.* **2018**, *4*, 712–717.
45. Nasrallah, O.; El Kurdi, R.; Mouslmani, M.; Patra, D. Doping of ZnO Nanoparticles with Curcumin: pH Dependent Release and DPPH Scavenging Activity of Curcumin in the Nanocomposites. *Curr. Nanomater.* **2019**, *3*, 147–152. [CrossRef]
46. Joseph, E.; Singhvi, G. Multifunctional nanocrystals for cancer therapy: A potential nanocarrier. In *Nanomaterials for Drug Delivery and Therapy*; William Andrew Publishing: Norwich, NY, USA, 2019; pp. 91–116.
47. An, S.S.A.; Kim, K.; Choi, M.; Lee, J.-K.; Jeong, J.; Kim, Y.-R.; Kim, M.-K.; Paek, S.-M.; Shin, J.-H. Physicochemical properties of surface charge-modified ZnO nanoparticles with different particle sizes. *Int. J. Nanomed.* **2014**, *9*, 41–56. [CrossRef] [PubMed]
48. Sirelkhatim, A.; Mahmud, S.; Seeni, A.; Kaus, N.H.M.; Ann, L.C.; Bakhori, S.K.M.; Hasan, H.; Mohamad, D. Review on Zinc Oxide Nanoparticles: Antibacterial Activity and Toxicity Mechanism. *Nano-Micro Lett.* **2015**, *7*, 219–242. [CrossRef] [PubMed]
49. Jacob, V.; P, R. In vitro analysis: The antimicrobial and antioxidant activity of zinc oxide nanoparticles from curcuma longa. *Asian J. Pharm. Clin. Res.* **2019**, *12*, 200–204. [CrossRef]
50. Somu, P.; Paul, S. A biomolecule-assisted one-pot synthesis of zinc oxide nanoparticles and its bioconjugate with curcumin for potential multifaceted therapeutic applications. *New J. Chem.* **2019**, *43*, 11934–11948. [CrossRef]
51. Huang, D.; Ou, B.; Prior, R.L. The Chemistry behind Antioxidant Capacity Assays. *J. Agric. Food Chem.* **2005**, *53*, 1841–1856. [CrossRef]
52. Kumar, V.; Mohan, S.; Singh, D.K.; Verma, D.K.; Singh, V.K.; Hasan, S.H. Photo-mediated optimized synthesis of silver nanoparticles for the selective detection of Iron(III), antibacterial and antioxidant activity. *Mater. Sci. Eng. C* **2017**, *71*, 1004–1019. [CrossRef]
53. Yakimovich, N.O.; Ezhevskii, A.A.; Guseinov, D.V.; Smirnova, L.A.; Gracheva, T.A.; Klychkov, K.S. Antioxidant properties of gold nanoparticles studied by ESR spectroscopy. *Russ. Chem. Bull.* **2008**, *57*, 520–523. [CrossRef]
54. Stan, M.; Popa, A.; Toloman, D.; Silipas, T.-D.; Vodnar, D.C. Antibacterial and Antioxidant Activities of ZnO Nanoparticles Synthesized Using Extracts of *Allium sativum*, *Rosmarinus officinalis* and *Ocimum basilicum*. *Acta Metall. Sin.* **2016**, *29*, 228–236. [CrossRef]
55. Prior, R.L.; Wu, X.; Schaich, K. Standardized Methods for the Determination of Antioxidant Capacity and Phenolics in Foods and Dietary Supplements. *J. Agric. Food Chem.* **2005**, *53*, 4290–4302. [CrossRef]
56. Zhang, L.; Jiang, Y.; Ding, Y.; Povey, M.; York, D. Investigation into the antibacterial behaviour of suspensions of ZnO nanoparticles (ZnO nanofluids). *J. Nanoparticle Res.* **2007**, *9*, 479–489. [CrossRef]
57. Yamamoto, O. Influence of particle size on the antibacterial activity of zinc oxide. *Int. J. Inorg. Mater.* **2001**, *3*, 643–646. [CrossRef]
58. Peng, X.; Palma, S.; Fisher, N.S.; Wong, S.S. Effect of morphology of ZnO nanostructures on their toxicity to marine algae. *Aquat. Toxicol.* **2011**, *102*, 186–196. [CrossRef]
59. Reddy, K.M.; Feris, K.; Bell, J.; Wingett, D.G.; Hanley, C.; Punnoose, A. Selective toxicity of zinc oxide nanoparticles to prokaryotic and eukaryotic systems. *Appl. Phys. Lett.* **2007**, *90*, 213902–2139023. [CrossRef]
60. Padmavathy, N.; Vijayaraghavan, R. Enhanced bioactivity of ZnO nanoparticles—An antimicrobial study. *Sci. Technol. Adv. Mater.* **2008**, *9*, 035004. [CrossRef]
61. Feng, Q.L.; Wu, J.; Chen, G.; Cui, F.; Kim, T.; Kim, J.O. A mechanistic study of the antibacterial effect of silver ions on Escherichia coli and Staphylococcus aureus. *J. Biomed. Mater. Res.* **2000**, *52*, 662–668. [CrossRef]

62. Brayner, R.; Ferrari-Iliou, R.; Brivois, N.; Djediat, S.; Benedetti, M.F.; Fiévet, F. Toxicological Impact Studies Based on *Escherichia coli* Bacteria in Ultrafine ZnO Nanoparticles Colloidal Medium. *Nano Lett.* **2006**, *6*, 866–870. [CrossRef]
63. Adams, L.K.; Lyon, D.Y.; Alvarez, P.J. Comparative eco-toxicity of nanoscale TiO_2, SiO_2, and ZnO water suspensions. *Water Res.* **2006**, *40*, 3527–3532. [CrossRef]
64. Li, M.; Zhu, L.; Lin, D. Toxicity of ZnO Nanoparticles to *Escherichia coli*: Mechanism and the Influence of Medium Components. *Environ. Sci. Technol.* **2011**, *45*, 1977–1983. [CrossRef]
65. Brunner, T.J.; Wick, P.; Manser, P.; Spohn, P.; Grass, R.N.; Limbach, L.K.; Bruinink, A.; Stark, W.J. In Vitro Cytotoxicity of Oxide Nanoparticles: Comparison to Asbestos, Silica, and the Effect of Particle Solubility. *Environ. Sci. Technol.* **2006**, *40*, 4374–4381. [CrossRef] [PubMed]
66. Kasemets, K.; Ivask, A.; Dubourguier, H.-C.; Kahru, A. Toxicity of nanoparticles of ZnO, CuO and TiO_2 to yeast Saccharomyces cerevisiae. *Toxicol. Vitr.* **2009**, *23*, 1116–1122. [CrossRef] [PubMed]
67. Lipovsky, A.; Nitzan, Y.; Gedanken, A.; Lubart, R. Antifungal activity of ZnO nanoparticles—The role of ROS mediated cell injury. *Nanotechnology* **2011**, *22*, 105101. [CrossRef] [PubMed]
68. Zhang, L.; Ding, Y.; Povey, M.; York, D. ZnO nanofluids—A potential antibacterial agent. *Prog. Nat. Sci.* **2008**, *18*, 939–944. [CrossRef]
69. Jalal, R.; Goharshadi, E.K.; Abareshi, M.; Moosavi, M.; Yousefi, A.; Nancarrow, P. ZnO nanofluids: Green synthesis, characterization, and antibacterial activity. *Mater. Chem. Phys.* **2010**, *121*, 198–201. [CrossRef]
70. Huh, A.J.; Kwon, Y.J. "Nanoantibiotics": A new paradigm for treating infectious diseases using nanomaterials in the antibiotics resistant era. *J. Control. Release* **2011**, *156*, 128–145. [CrossRef]
71. Feris, K.; Otto, C.; Tinker, J.; Wingett, D.; Punnoose, A.; Thurber, A.; Kongara, M.; Sabetian, M.; Quinn, B.; Hanna, C.; et al. Electrostatic Interactions Affect Nanoparticle-Mediated Toxicity to Gram-Negative Bacterium *Pseudomonas aeruginosa* PAO1. *Langmuir* **2009**, *26*, 4429–4436. [CrossRef]
72. Shah, A.; Manikandan, E.; Ahamed, M.B.; Mir, D.A.; Mir, S. Antibacterial and Blue shift investigations in sol–gel synthesized $CrxZn1-xO$ Nanostructures. *J. Lumin.* **2014**, *145*, 944–950. [CrossRef]
73. Da Silva, B.L.; Abuçafy, M.P.; Manaia, E.B.; Junior, J.A.O.; Chiari-Andréo, B.G.; Pietro, R.C.L.R.; Chiavacci, L.A. Relationship Between Structure And Antimicrobial Activity Of Zinc Oxide Nanoparticles: An Overview. *Int. J. Nanomed.* **2019**, *14*, 9395. [CrossRef]
74. Yıldırım, Ö.A.; Unalan, H.E.; Durucan, C. Highly Efficient Room Temperature Synthesis of Silver-Doped Zinc Oxide (ZnO:Ag) Nanoparticles: Structural, Optical, and Photocatalytic Properties. *J. Am. Ceram. Soc.* **2013**, *96*, 766–773. [CrossRef]
75. Zhao, J.; Wang, L.; Yan, X.; Yang, Y.; Lei, Y.; Zhou, J.; Huang, Y.; Gu, Y.; Zhang, Y. Structure and photocatalytic activity of Ni-doped ZnO nanorods. *Mater. Res. Bull.* **2011**, *46*, 1207–1210. [CrossRef]
76. Ma, J.; Liu, J.; Bao, Y.; Zhu, Z.; Wang, X.; Zhang, J. Synthesis of large-scale uniform mulberry-like ZnO particles with microwave hydrothermal method and its antibacterial property. *Ceram. Int.* **2013**, *39*, 2803–2810. [CrossRef]
77. Talebian, N.; Amininezhad, S.M.; Doudi, M. Controllable synthesis of ZnO nanoparticles and their morphology-dependent antibacterial and optical properties. *J. Photochem. Photobiol. B Biol.* **2013**, *120*, 66–73. [CrossRef]
78. Stanković, A.; Dimitrijević, S.; Uskoković, D. Influence of size scale and morphology on antibacterial properties of ZnO powders hydrothemally synthesized using different surface stabilizing agents. *Colloids Surfaces B Biointerfaces* **2013**, *102*, 21–28. [CrossRef]
79. Vennilaraj, R.; Palanisamy, K.; Arthanareeswari, M.; Bitragunta, S. Green synthesis of silver nanoparticles from Cleistanthus Collinus leaf extract and their biological effects. *Int. J. Chem.* **2022**, *34*, 1103–1107.
80. Tong, G.-X.; Du, F.-F.; Liang, Y.; Hu, Q.; Wu, R.-N.; Guan, J.-G.; Hu, X. Polymorphous ZnO complex architectures: Selective synthesis, mechanism, surface area and Zn-polar plane-codetermining antibacterial activity. *J. Mater. Chem. B* **2012**, *1*, 454–463. [CrossRef]
81. Kurita, T.; Makino, Y. Novel curcumin oral delivery systems. *Anticancer Res.* **2013**, *33*, 2807–2822.
82. Kundu, M.; Sadhukhan, P.; Ghosh, N.; Chatterjee, S.; Manna, P.; Das, J.; Sil, P. pH-responsive and targeted delivery of curcumin via phenylboronic acid-functionalized ZnO nanoparticles for breast cancer therapy. *J. Adv. Res.* **2019**, *18*, 161–172. [CrossRef]
83. Bansal, S.S.; Goel, M.; Aqil, F.; Vadhanam, M.V.; Gupta, R.C. Advanced Drug Delivery Systems of Curcumin for Cancer Chemoprevention. *Cancer Prev. Res.* **2011**, *4*, 1158–1171. [CrossRef]
84. Wang, J.; Wang, Y.; Liu, Q.; Yang, L.; Zhu, R.; Yu, C.; Wang, S. Rational Design of Multifunctional Dendritic Mesoporous Silica Nanoparticles to Load Curcumin and Enhance Efficacy for Breast Cancer Therapy. *ACS Appl. Mater. Interfaces* **2016**, *8*, 26511–26523. [CrossRef]
85. Moghaddam, A.B.; Moniri, M.; Azizi, S.; Rahim, R.A.; Bin Ariff, A.; Navaderi, M.; Mohamad, R. Eco-Friendly Formulated Zinc Oxide Nanoparticles: Induction of Cell Cycle Arrest and Apoptosis in the MCF-7 Cancer Cell Line. *Genes* **2017**, *8*, 281. [CrossRef]
86. Punnoose, A.; Dodge, K.; Rasmussen, J.W.; Chess, J.; Wingett, D.; Anders, C. Cytotoxicity of ZnO Nanoparticles Can Be Tailored by Modifying Their Surface Structure: A Green Chemistry Approach for Safer Nanomaterials. *ACS Sustain. Chem. Eng.* **2014**, *2*, 1666–1673. [CrossRef] [PubMed]
87. Sindhura, K.S.; Prasad, T.N.V.K.V.; Selvam, P.P.; Hussain, O.M. Synthesis, characterization and evaluation of effect of phytogenic zinc nanoparticles on soil exo-enzymes. *Appl. Nanosci.* **2013**, *4*, 819–827. [CrossRef]
88. Bharathi, D.; Bhuvaneshwari, V. Synthesis of zinc oxide nanoparticles (ZnO NPs) using pure bioflavonoid rutin and their biomedical applications: Antibacterial, antioxidant and cytotoxic activities. *Res. Chem. Intermed.* **2019**, *45*, 2065–2078. [CrossRef]

89. Bisht, G.; Rayamajhi, S. ZnO Nanoparticles: A Promising Anticancer Agent. *Nanobiomedicine* **2016**, *3*, 9. [CrossRef]
90. Mortimer, M.; Kasemets, K.; Kahru, A. Toxicity of ZnO and CuO nanoparticles to ciliated protozoa Tetrahymena thermophila. *Toxicology* **2010**, *269*, 182–189. [CrossRef]
91. Franklin, N.M.; Rogers, N.J.; Apte, S.C.; Batley, G.E.; Gadd, G.E.; Casey, P.S. Comparative Toxicity of Nanoparticulate ZnO, Bulk ZnO, and $ZnCl_2$ to a Freshwater Microalga (*Pseudokirchneriella subcapitata*): The Importance of Particle Solubility. *Environ. Sci. Technol.* **2007**, *41*, 8484–8490. [CrossRef]
92. Zhu, X.; Wang, J.; Zhang, X.; Chang, Y.; Chen, Y. The impact of ZnO nanoparticle aggregates on the embryonic development of zebrafish (*Danio rerio*). *Nanotechnology* **2009**, *20*, 195103. [CrossRef]
93. Poynton, H.C.; Lazorchak, J.M.; Impellitteri, C.A.; Smith, M.E.; Rogers, K.; Patra, M.; Hammer, K.A.; Allen, H.J.; Vulpe, C.D. Differential Gene Expression in *Daphnia magna* Suggests Distinct Modes of Action and Bioavailability for ZnO Nanoparticles and Zn Ions. *Environ. Sci. Technol.* **2010**, *45*, 762–768. [CrossRef]
94. Wang, H.; Wick, R.L.; Xing, B. Toxicity of nanoparticulate and bulk ZnO, Al_2O_3 and TiO_2 to the nematode Caenorhabditis elegans. *Environ. Pollut.* **2009**, *157*, 1171–1177. [CrossRef]
95. Abinaya, C.; Devi, R.M.; Suresh, P.; Balasubramanian, N.; Muthaiya, N.; Kannan, N.D.; Annaraj, J.; Shanmugaiah, V.; Pearce, J.M.; Shanmugapriya, P.; et al. Antibacterial and anticancer activity of hydrothermally-synthesized zinc oxide nanomaterials using natural extracts of neem, pepper and turmeric as solvent media. *Nano Express* **2020**, *1*, 010029. [CrossRef]
96. Oo, M.K.; Alallam, B.; Doolaanea, A.A.; Khatib, A.; Mohamed, F.; Chatterjee, B. Exploring the Effect of Glycerol and Hydrochloric Acid on Mesoporous Silica Synthesis: Application in Insulin Loading. *ACS Omega* **2022**, *7*, 27126–27134. [CrossRef]
97. Rahim, R.A.; Jayusman, P.A.; Lim, V.; Ahmad, N.H.; Hamid, Z.A.A.; Mohamed, S.; Muhammad, N.; Ahmad, F.; Mokhtar, N.; Mohamed, N.; et al. Phytochemical Analysis, Antioxidant and Bone Anabolic Effects of *Blainvillea acmella* (L.) Philipson. *Front. Pharmacol.* **2022**, *12*, 796509. [CrossRef]
98. Chiu, H.I.; Mood, C.N.A.C.; Zain, N.N.M.; Ramachandran, M.R.; Yahaya, N.; Kamal, N.N.S.N.M.; Tung, W.H.; Yong, Y.K.; Lee, C.K.; Lim, V. Biogenic Silver Nanoparticles of Clinacanthus nutans as Antioxidant with Antimicrobial and Cytotoxic Effects. *Bioinorg. Chem. Appl.* **2021**, *2021*, 9920890. [CrossRef]
99. Yaseen, M.R.; Faisal, G.G.; Fuaat, A.A.; Affandi, K.A.; Alallam, B.; Nasir, M.H.M. Preparation of Euyrycoma Longifolia Jack (E.L) Tongkat Ali (Ta) Root Extract Hydrogel for Wound Application. *Pharmacogn. J.* **2021**, *13*, 1456–1463. [CrossRef]
100. Ates, M.; Daniels, J.; Arslan, Z.; Farah, I.O.; Rivera, H.F. Comparative evaluation of impact of Zn and ZnO nanoparticles on brine shrimp (Artemia salina) larvae: Effects of particle size and solubility on toxicity. *Environ. Sci. Process. Impacts* **2012**, *15*, 225–233. [CrossRef]

Disclaimer/Publisher's Note: The statements, opinions and data contained in all publications are solely those of the individual author(s) and contributor(s) and not of MDPI and/or the editor(s). MDPI and/or the editor(s) disclaim responsibility for any injury to people or property resulting from any ideas, methods, instructions or products referred to in the content.

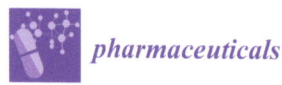 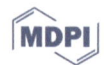

Article

Antihyperglycemic Effects of *Annona cherimola* Miller and the Flavonoid Rutin in Combination with Oral Antidiabetic Drugs on Streptozocin-Induced Diabetic Mice

Miguel Valdes [1,*], Fernando Calzada [2,*], Jesús Martínez-Solís [1,2] and Julita Martínez-Rodríguez [1,2]

1. Instituto Politécnico Nacional, Sección de Estudios de Posgrado e Investigación, Escuela Superior de Medicina, Plan de San Luis y Salvador Díaz Mirón S/N, Col. Casco de Santo Tomás, Miguel Hidalgo, Mexico City CP 11340, Mexico
2. Unidad de Investigación Médica en Farmacología, UMAE Hospital de Especialidades 2° Piso CORSE Centro Médico Nacional Siglo XXI, Instituto Mexicano del Seguro Social, Av. Cuauhtémoc 330, Col. Doctores, Mexico City CP 06720, Mexico
* Correspondence: valdesguevaramiguel@gmail.com (M.V.); fercalber10@gmail.com (F.C.); Tel.: +52-5627-6900 (ext. 21567) (M.V. & F.C.)

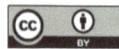

Citation: Valdes, M.; Calzada, F.; Martínez-Solís, J.; Martínez-Rodríguez, J. Antihyperglycemic Effects of *Annona cherimola* Miller and the Flavonoid Rutin in Combination with Oral Antidiabetic Drugs on Streptozocin-Induced Diabetic Mice. *Pharmaceuticals* 2023, 16, 112. https://doi.org/10.3390/ph16010112

Academic Editor: Chung-Yi Chen

Received: 6 December 2022
Revised: 2 January 2023
Accepted: 9 January 2023
Published: 12 January 2023

Copyright: © 2023 by the authors. Licensee MDPI, Basel, Switzerland. This article is an open access article distributed under the terms and conditions of the Creative Commons Attribution (CC BY) license (https://creativecommons.org/licenses/by/4.0/).

Abstract: Ethanolic extract obtained from *Annona cherimola* Miller (EEAc) and the flavonoid rutin (Rut) were evaluated in this study to determine their antihyperglycemic content, % HbA1c reduction, and antihyperlipidemic activities. Both treatments were evaluated separately and in combination with the oral antidiabetic drugs (OADs) acarbose (Aca), metformin (Met), glibenclamide (Gli), and canagliflozin (Cana) in acute and subchronic assays. The evaluation of the acute assay showed that EEAc and Rut administered separately significantly reduce hyperglycemia in a manner similar to OADs and help to reduce % HbA1c and hyperlipidemia in the subchronic assay. The combination of EEAc + Met showed the best activity by reducing the hyperglycemia content, % HbA1c, Chol, HDL-c, and LDL-c. Rutin in combination with OADs used in all treatments significantly reduced the hyperglycemia content that is reflected in the reduction in % HbA1c. In relation to the lipid profiles, all combinate treatments helped to avoid an increase in the measured parameters. The results show the importance of evaluating the activity of herbal remedies in combination with drugs to determine their activities and possible side effects. Moreover, the combination of rutin with antidiabetic drugs presented considerable activity, and this is the first step for the development of novel DM treatments.

Keywords: *Annona cherimolla* Miller; diabetes mellitus; flavonoids; rutin; oral antidiabetic drugs

1. Introduction

Diabetes Mellitus (DM) is a chronic disease characterized by high blood glucose levels as a consequence of resistance or lack of insulin secretion from the pancreas [1]. This disease affected 463 million people worldwide in 2019 [2]. DM caused 1.6 million deaths in 2016 and is considered as one of the main causes of deaths globally [3]. DM type 2 accounts for 90 to 95% of all diabetes cases and its specific etiology remains unknown [4].

The pathophysiology of DM type 2 consists of a heterogeneous field where progression can considerably vary. The changes occurring in the metabolism of carbohydrates and proteins are a consequence of several disturbances defined as ominous octets [5]. The excess quantity of glucose in the blood stream causes micro- and macrovascular damage as a result of the increase in free radicals [6] that react with tissue proteins via a non-enzymatic oxidation process in the hemoglobin and explains the synthesis of many advanced glycation end-products (AGEs) as glycated hemoglobin (HbA1c) [7]. HbA1c values reflect the average values of fasting blood glucose levels [8] and are used as parameters to continuously monitor patients with this disease [9,10]. Moreover, hyperglycemia is related to the changes occurring in the lipid metabolism process characterized by hypertriglyceridemia, high levels of cholesterol, and the alteration between low-density (LDLs) and high-density (HDLs) lipoproteins [11] that are associated with an increase in mortality rates.

The management of DM is a standing problem that requires a continued search of the possible alternatives. Numerous attempts have been made to address this situation and, at present, there several oral antidiabetic drugs exist [12], which are classified according to their mechanism of action into secretagogues, such as glibenclamide, which joins the cell receptor SUR1 and causes insulin release. Sensitizers, such as metformin, which improve the consumption rate of glucose, and antihyperglycemics, such as acarbose or canagliflozin, which can avoid the absorption of glucose or stimulation of urinary glucose excretion, thus reducing high blood glucose levels, have also been considered in the literature. However, the goal of glycemic control has not yet been achieved in the research due to the limitations induced by their use for a long period of time [13,14]. In this sense, the search for more effective treatments is urgent [15]. Medicinal plants are the main ingredients that have been used in traditional medicine [16]; in this sense, medicinal plants can be used to complement treatments to achieve improved glycemia control. *Annona* genera include several species that have presented antidiabetic properties [17,18]. *Annona cherimola* Miller (*A. cherimola*) is a fruit tree that belongs to the annonaceae family [19] and is a perennial species showing the presence of its leaves almost all year round, and it is widely cultivated and distributed in subtropical areas around the world [20], mostly for its fruit known as "annona" or "cherimoya" [20,21]. Local populations also use its leaves as a remedy to treat several illnesses, such as gastrointestinal disorders, worms, and diarrhea [22]. Studies have proved that the leaves of this species have antidepressant [23] and pro-apoptotic [24] activities. In respect to the toxicity of *Annona cherimola*, it has been evaluated according to the OCDE procedure in a mouse model, and the results presented a median lethal dose (LD$_{50}$) higher than 3000 mg/kg; these results suggest that it is safe to use [25].

All the compounds present in the leaves of *Annona cherimola* have recently been listed in the literature [26]. Flavonoids are highlighted due to their wide-ranging properties [27]. Moreover, previous studies indicated the presence of antihyperglycemic components in polar fractions [28], such as the flavonoid rutin, one of the principal secondary metabolites responsible for the antihyperglycemic activity of *A. cherimola*. Rutin is present in higher quantities compared to other flavonoids in leaf extracts and exerts antioxidant effects and lowers glucose diffusion properties [29]. This effect can be enhanced by its structure that provides it with α-glucosidase inhibitory activity [30], as well as other activities [31], whose mechanisms are already known in the field [32] and contribute to the antihyperlipidemic activity [33] of this species. Although the antihyperglycemic effect of ethanolic extract obtained from *A. cherimola* and rutin administrated alone has already been studied, there are no acute or subchronic studies that evaluate their combination with oral antidiabetic agents. Thus, the aim of the present study is to assess the effect of *A. cherimola* ethanolic extract and the flavonoid rutin administered alone and in combination with oral antidiabetic drugs on hyperglycemic states in acute and subchronic studies in animals and its effects on other parameters, such as HbA1c and lipid profiles.

2. Results

2.1. Acute Antihyperglycemic Effects of Ethanolic Extract from Annona cherimola, Rutin, and Oral Antidiabetic Drugs on SIT2D Mice Model

First, the acute effect of ethanolic extract obtained from *Annona cherimola* Miller (EEAc), rutin, and oral antidiabetic drugs (OADs) were measured in SIT2D mice following the administration of treatments separately. We observed that the groups treated with EEAc or glibenclamide showed a significant decrease in blood glucose levels at 2 h of treatment, the group treated with the flavonoid rutin presented a significant decrease at 4 h of treatment, and the group treated with canagliflozin showed a significant decrease at 2 and 4 h of treatment (Table 1).

Table 1. Blood glucose levels of normoglycemic mice (NM) and streptozocin induced type 2 diabetic mice (SIT2D) at 0, 2, and 4 h, on the acute antihyperglycemic test.

Treatment	Glycemia (mg/dL)		
	0 h	2 h	4 h
NM Control	119 ± 5.2	132 ± 3.8	135 ± 4.1
SIT2D Control	385.7 ± 28.4	404.3 ± 15.3	404.7 ± 9.6
EEAc	368.3 ± 16	230 ± 15.9 *,ψ	342 ± 3.3 ψψ
Rut	358 ± 7.9	323 ± 6.6 *,ψ	266.3 ± 14.4 *,ψψ
Aca	365.7 ± 15	302.6 ± 21.9 *,ψ	283.7 ± 10.3 *
Met	368 ± 14.3	388 ± 15.9 *	363.6 ± 12.6
Gli	373.7 ± 11.4	267.5 ± 30.3 *,ψ	353 ± 3.4 ψψ
Cana	412.3 ± 2.2	242 ± 28.5 *,ψ	257.3 ± 46.3 *,ψψ
EEAc + Aca	350.7 ± 14.9	212.9 ± 36.7 *,ψ	219.4 ± 35.9 *,ψψ
EEAc + Met	353 ± 9.3	178.3 ± 12.7 *,ψ	156 ± 6 *,ψψ
EEAc + Glib	339.3 ± 14.2	145.7 ± 24.3 *,ψ	202 ± 42.3 *,ψψ
EEAc + Cana	348 ± 6.5	140 ± 48.5 *,ψ	135.3 ± 51 *,ψψ
Rut + Aca	340 ± 13.4	311.2 ± 19.4	250.7 ± 28.9 *,ψψ
Rut + Met	326 ± 8.4	366.7 ± 38.3	327.7 ± 34.7 ψψ
Rut + Glib	316.3 ± 5.2	317.7 ± 9.1	272.4 ± 9.8 *,ψψ
Rut + Cana	337 ± 17.3	103.7 ± 9.4 *,ψ	117.7 ± 2.5 *,ψψ

Data are expressed as means ± SEM, n = 6; * $p < 0.05$ vs. initial values; ψ $p < 0.05$ vs. SIT2D control for 2 h; ψψ $p < 0.05$ vs. SIT2D control for 4 h SEM: standard error of the mean; NM: normoglycemic mice; SITD2: streptozocin-induced diabetes 2 mice; EEAc: ethanolic extract of *Annona cherimola* Miller; Rut: flavonoid rutin; Aca: acarbose; Met: metformin; Gli: glibenclamide; Cana: canaglifozin.

When the OADs were combined with the EEAc, all treatments presented better effects on the hyperglycemia rather than separately; all combinations with EEAc showed a significant decrease at 2 and 4 h of treatment (Table 1).

On the other hand, when the OADs were combined with rutin, the combination of rutin + acarbosa and rutin + glibenclamide showed a significant decrease at 4 h of treatment; in the case of the treatment of rutin + canagliflozin, a significant decrease was presented at 2 and 4 h of treatment (Table 1).

2.2. Subchronic Effects of Ethanolic Extract from Annona cherimola, Rutin, and Oral Antidiabetic Drugs on SIT2D Mice Model

Once we demonstrated the acute activity over hyperglycemia of the treatments alone or in combination, we decided to perform a chronic evaluation for 8 weeks.

Following the chronic administration of the treatments, we observed that the group treated with EEAc showed a significant reduction in hyperglycemic values at weeks 1 and 2; however, the animals returned to their previous hyperglycemic values in week 3 and these values were maintained, similar to the SIT2D control, for the rest of the treatment (Figure 1A). The group treated with rutin showed a significant reduction in hyperglycemic values at weeks 3 to 7 (Figure 1B). In the case of the OADs, the group treated with acarbose presented a significant reduction in hyperglycemic values in weeks 3 and 5 to 7; however, during week 8 of the treatment, the glycemic values increased, reaching SIT2D control values (Figure 1C). The group treated with metformin presented a significant reduction in its hyperglycemic values in week 1 only; during the rest of the weeks, glycemic values similar to the SIT2D control were presented (Figure 1D). The group treated with glibenclamide did not present significant activity exceeding the hyperglycemic values (Figure 1E). The group treated with canagliflozin presented a significant reduction in hyperglycemic values from the first week until the end of the treatment (Figure 1F).

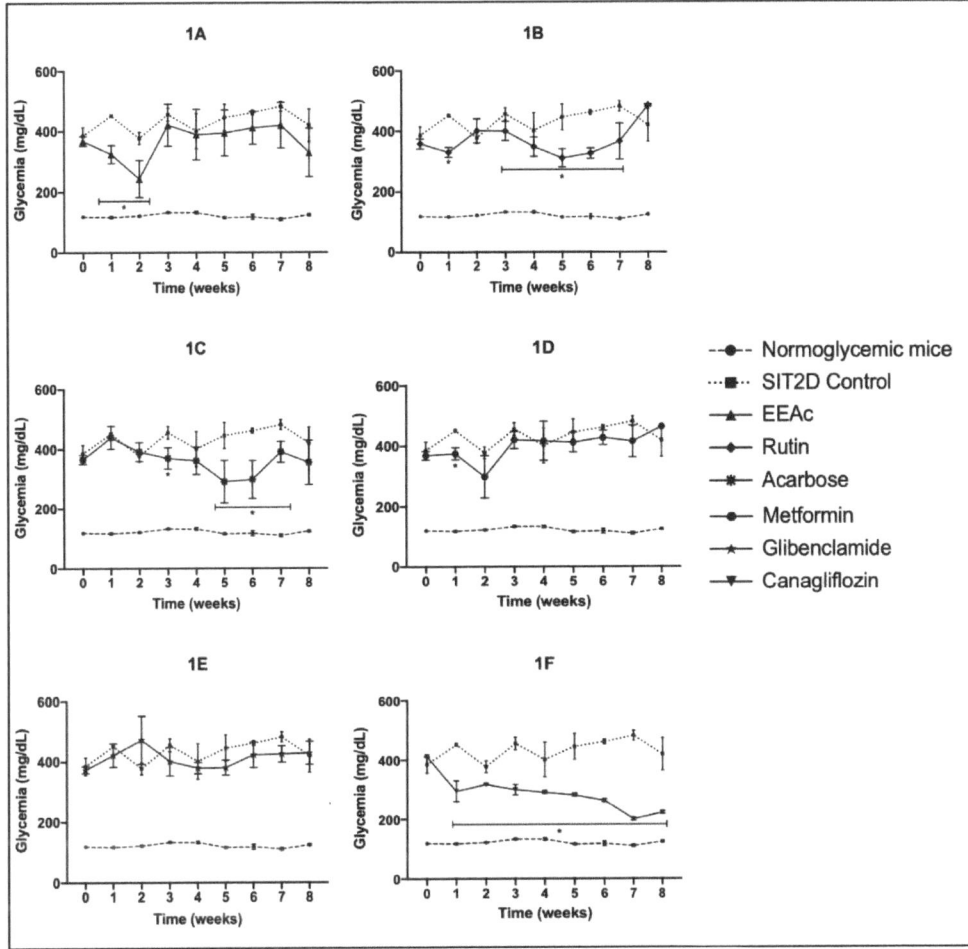

Figure 1. Effect over glycemic values of separate administration of the treatments in SIT2D mice compared with SIT2D and normoglycemic control groups. Groups treated with EEAc 300 mg/kg (**1A**), rutin 50 mg/kg (**1B**), acarbose 50 mg/kg (**1C**), metformin 850 mg/kg (**1D**), glibenclamide 5 mg/kg (**1E**), and canagliflozin 50 mg/kg (**1F**). Results are expressed as the mean + SEM, $n = 6$, * $p < 0.05$ vs. SIT2D control at same week of treatment.

When the OADs were chronically administered in combination with the EEAc, we observed that EEAc + acarbose reduced hyperglycemia from the first week; however, in week 4, we observed the death of all the treated animals (Figure 2A) and the mean value of the blood glucose levels for the dead animals was 43.5 ± 13.8 mg/dL. The group treated with EEAc + metformin presented a significant reduction in its hyperglycemic values from the first week and this was maintained until the end of the treatment, close to the normoglycemic values (Figure 2B). The group treated with EEAc + glibenclamide did not present a reduction in its blood glucose levels (Figure 2C); finally, the group treated with EEAc + canagliflozin presented a significant reduction in its hyperglycemic values from the first week; however, at week 4, we observed the death of all the animals treated with this combination (Figure 2D)—the mean value of the blood glucose levels for the dead animals was 100.5 ± 15.1 mg/dL.

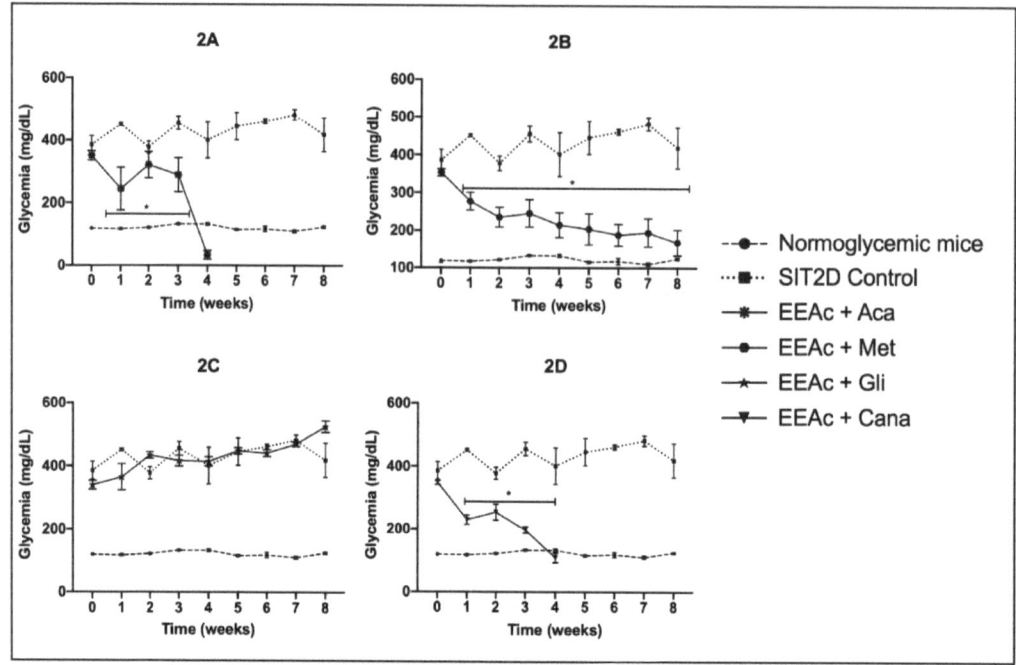

Figure 2. Effect over glycemic values of combined administration of the oral antidiabetic drugs with EEAc in SIT2D mice compared with SIT2D and normoglycemic control groups. Groups treated with EEAc 300 mg/kg + acarbose 50 mg/kg (**2A**), EEAc 300 mg/kg + metformin 850 mg/kg (**2B**), EEAc 300 mg/kg + glibenclamide 5 mg/kg (**2C**), EEAc 300 mg/kg + canagliflozin 50 mg/kg (**2D**). Results are expressed as the mean ± SEM, $n = 6$, * $p < 0.05$ vs. SIT2D control at same week of treatment.

When the OADs were chronically administered in combination with rutin, we observed that the group treated with rutin + acarbose presented a significant reduction in its hyperglycemic values during the first week of treatment and during the fourth week until the end of the treatment (Figure 3A). The group treated with rutin + metformin presented a significant reduction in its hyperglycemic values from the third until the seventh week; the glycemic values began to increase until achieving hyperglycemic values similar to the SIT2D control (Figure 3B). The group treated with rutin + glibenclamide showed a significant decrease in its blood glucose levels in the third until the seventh week (Figure 3C). In the case of the group treated with rutin + canagliflozin, this treatment generated a significant reduction in the hyperglycemic values from the first week until the end of the treatment, attaining values almost similar to the normoglycemic values obtained during the fourth week of treatment (Figure 3D).

2.3. Effects over Glycated Hemoglobin Levels after Chronical Administration of Ethanolic Extract from Annona cherimola, Rutin, and Oral Antidiabetic Drugs on SIT2D Mice Model

The subchronic administration of the individual treatments generated a significant decrease in the percentage of glycated hemoglobin (% HbA1c) at weeks four and eight in the groups treated with rutin, acarbose, and canaglifozin, in comparison with the SIT2D group (Figure 4A), when the OADs were administered in combination with EEAc. The combination of EEAc + acarbose and EEAc + canagliflozin caused the death of the animals in week four, due to the fact that % HbA1c could not be measured in both groups. The administration of the combination of EEAc + glibenclamide did not generate a significant reduction in % HbA1c (Figure 4B).

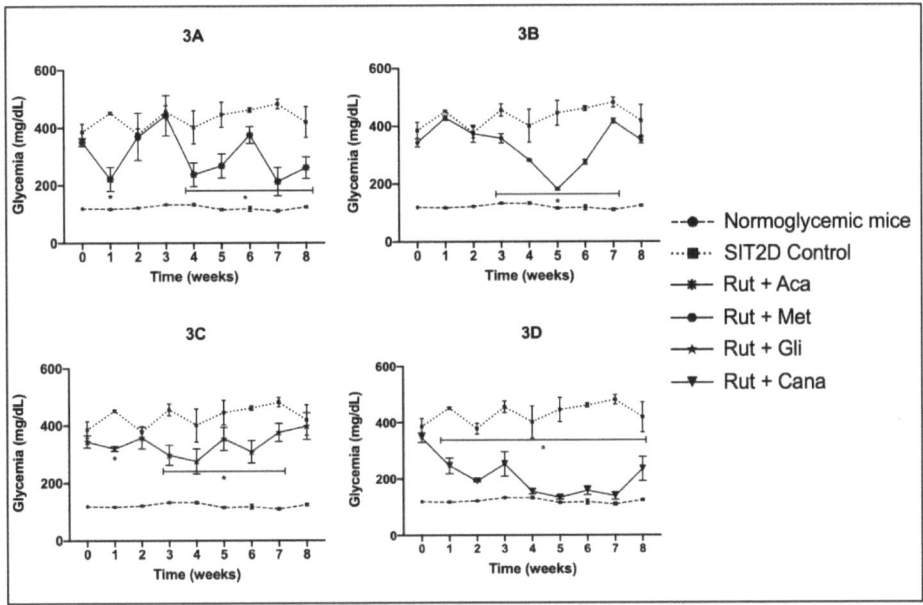

Figure 3. Effect over glycemic values of combined administration of the oral antidiabetic drugs with rutin in SIT2D mice compared with SIT2D and normoglycemic control groups. Groups treated with rutin 50 mg/kg + acarbose 50 mg/kg (**3A**), rutin 50 mg/kg + metformin 850 mg/kg (**3B**), rutin 50 mg/kg + glibenclamide 5 mg/kg (**3C**), rutin 50 mg/kg + canagliflozin 50 mg/kg (**3D**). Results are expressed as the mean ± SEM, $n = 6$, * $p < 0.05$ vs. SIT2D control at same week of treatment.

In the case of the combination of OADs with rutin, we observed a significant reduction in % HbA1c following the administration of rutin + acarbose in weeks four and eight. In the case of rutin + canalgiflozin, a significant reduction in the % of HbA1c was observed at weeks four and eight, achieving normoglycemic % HbA1c values in week eight. It is important to mention that the groups treated with rutin in combination with OADs did not kill the animals when compared to the mortality rates resulting from the combinations of EEAc + Aca and EEAc + Cana. On the other hand, for the groups treated with rutin + metformin and rutin + glibenclamide, we did not observe a significant reduction in % HbA1c (Figure 4C) during the administration of the treatments.

2.4. Effects over Lipid Profile Levels after Chronical Administration of Ethanolic Extract from Annona cherimola, Rutin, and Oral Antidiabetic Drugs on SIT2D Mice Model

At the end of the treatment, lipid profiles were measured for all the study groups. We observed that the SIT2D control group significantly increased the values of Chol, Tri, and LDL-c in comparison with the NM control. In the case of HDL-c, these values were significantly reduced in comparison with the NM control and the atherogenic index plasma (AIP); this index was significantly increased in comparison with the NM control index. In the case of the treatments, we observed that the groups treated with EEAc, rutin, and canagliflozin presented lower values with significant differences, in comparison with the SIT2D control group, these values being similar to the NM control group. The group treated with acarbose presented a significant increase in Tri values in comparison with the SIT2D and NM control groups; the remaining parameters were similar to the NM control group. In the case of the groups treated with metformin and glibenclamide, they did not show a difference in comparison to the SIT2D group; moreover, the AIP calculated showed a significant increase in comparison with the AIP of the NM control group (Table 2).

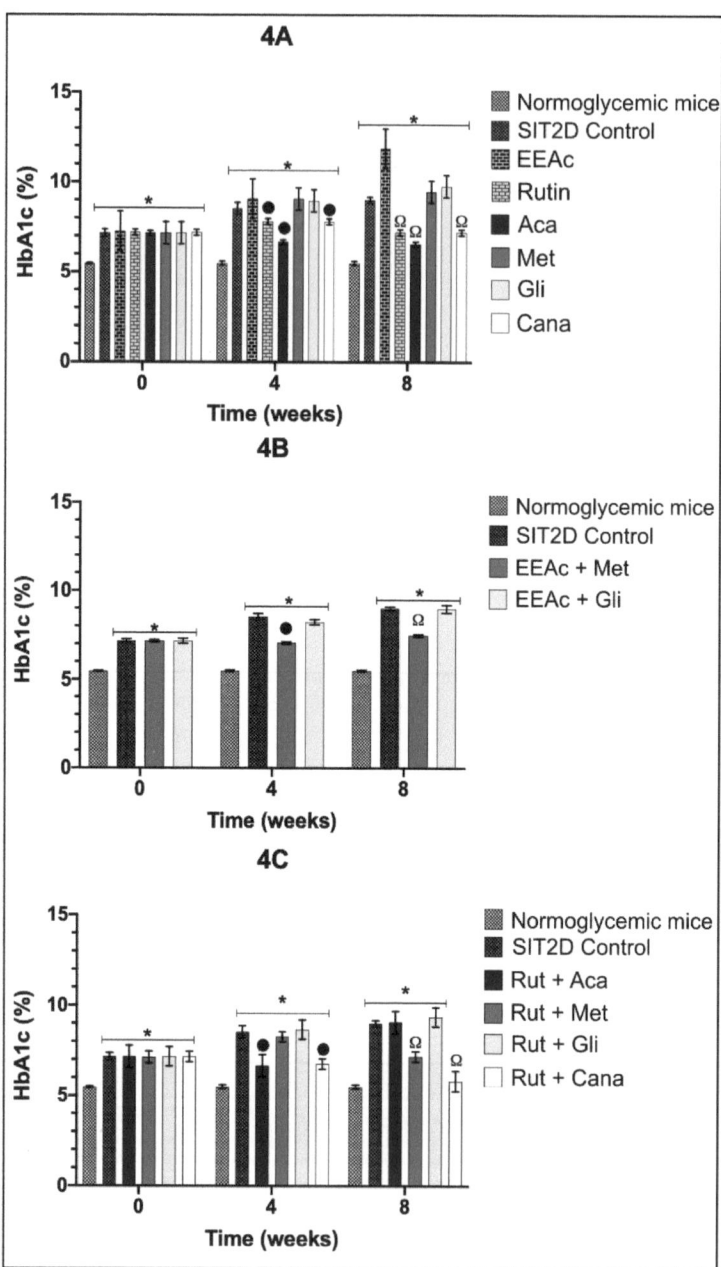

Figure 4. Effect over % glycated hemoglobin (% HbA1c), values after administration of the treatments separately and in combination. Groups administrated with treatments separately (**4A**), groups administrated with the combination of oral antidiabetic drugs and EEAc (**4B**), groups administrated with the combination of oral antidiabetic drugs and rutin (**4C**). Results are expressed as the mean ± SEM, n = 6, * $p < 0.05$ vs. Normoglycemic mice at same week of treatment; • $p < 0.05$ vs. SIT2D control in week 4; Ω $p < 0.05$ vs. SIT2D in week 8.

Table 2. Lipid profile values of groups treated with EEAc, rutin and oral antidiabetic drugs separately.

Treatment	Parameter				
	Chol (mg/dL)	Tri (mg/dL)	HDL-c (mg/dL)	LDL-c (mg/dL)	AIP
NM Control	92 ± 1 ♦	88.9 ± 0.2 ♦	62.9 ± 0.7 ♦	79.4 ± 1.1	1.46 ± 0.02
SIT2D Control	163.7 ± 7.1 *	127 ± 5.5 *	29.9 ± 1 *	157.7 ± 6.9 *	5.4 ± 0.04 *
EEAc	113 ± 8.8 ♦	65.9 ± 4.6 ♦	111 ± 9.5 *,♦	90.7 ± 6.9 ♦	1.02 ± 0.008 *,♦
Rut	125 ± 3.3 *,♦	118 ± 8 ♦	91.9 ± 6.4 *,♦	107.4 ± 2 *,♦	1.3 ± 0.06 ♦
Aca	80.7 ± 2.1 ♦	201.7 ± 23.4 *,♦	78.9 ± 6.4 *,♦	64.9 ± 1.6 ♦	1.04 ± 0.07 ♦
Met	171 ± 9 *	203.7 ± 18.1 *,♦	77.9 ± 7.3 *,♦	155.4 ± 7.6 *	2.2 ± 0.09 *,♦
Gli	160 ± 4 *	87 ± 7.5 ♦	86 ± 6.2 *,♦	142.6 ± 5.2 *	1.8 ± 0.1 *,♦
Cana	98.9 ± 3 ♦	84.3 ± 2.6 ♦	64.9 ± 3.9 ♦	85.9 ± 2.2 ♦	1.5 ± 0.04 ♦

* $p < 0.05$ vs. NM Control; ♦ $p < 0.05$ vs. SIT2D Control.

The subchronic administration of OADs in combination with EEAc resulted in the death of the animals treated with EEAc + Aca and EEAc + Cana; thus, the lipid profile could not be measured. In the case of EEAc + Met, the parameters Chol, HDL-c, and LDL-c were maintained in a manner similar to the NM control group; however, the Tri values significantly increased in comparison to the NM and SIT2D controls. The group treated with EEAc + Gli presented similar behavior to the SIT2D control with a significant increase in the AIP in comparison to the NM control (Table 3). Finally, the combination of OADs with rutin showed that Rut + Aca, Rut + Gli, and Rut + Cana maintained the values of Chol, Tri, LDL-c, and AIP in a manner similar to the NM control and showed a significant increase in the HDL-c value in comparison to the NM control. The group treated with Rut + Met presented activity similar to the SIT2D control with a significant increase in the AIP value (Table 4).

Table 3. Lipid profile values of groups treated with oral antidiabetic drugs in combination with EEAc.

Treatment	Parameter				
	Chol (mg/dL)	Tri (mg/dL)	HDL-c (mg/dL)	LDL-c (mg/dL)	AIP
NM Control	92 ± 1 ♦	88.9 ± 0.2 ♦	62.9 ± 0.7 ♦	79.4 ± 1.1	1.46 ± 0.02
SIT2D Control	163.7 ± 7.1 *	127 ± 5.5 *	29.9 ± 1 *	157.7 ± 6.9 *	5.4 ± 0.04 *
EEAc + Met	77 ± 2.4 ♦	240 ± 26.8 *,♦	78.6 ± 4.6 ♦	62.2 ± 1.5 ♦	0.99 ± 0.02 *,♦
EEAc + Gli	208 ± 13.2 *,♦	102 ± 5.9 *,♦	38.9 ± 9.8 *	184 ± 11.2 *,♦	1.7 ± 0.03 *,♦

* $p < 0.05$ vs. NM Control; ♦ $p < 0.05$ vs. SIT2D Control.

Table 4. Lipid profile values of groups treated with oral antidiabetic drugs in combination with rutin.

Treatment	Parameter				
	Chol (mg/dL)	Tri (mg/dL)	HDL-c (mg/dL)	LDL-c (mg/dL)	AIP
NM Control	92 ± 1 ♦	88.9 ± 0.2 ♦	62.9 ± 0.7 ♦	79.4 ± 1.1	1.46 ± 0.02
SIT2D Control	163.7 ± 7.1 *	127 ± 5.5 *	29.9 ± 1 *	157.7 ± 6.9 *	5.4 ± 0.04 *
Rut + Aca	88.9 ± 1.1 ♦	81.9 ± 3.8 ♦	79.5 ± 3.8 *,♦	73 ± 0.6 ♦	1.1 ± 0.04 ♦
Rut + Met	163 ± 7.3 *	69.9 ± 2.1 ♦	39.9 ± 3.3	155 ± 6.6 *	4.1 ± 0.1 *,♦
Rut + Gli	114 ± 2.3 ♦	91.9 ± 5.3 ♦	72.9 ± 4.1 *,♦	99.3 ± 1.5 ♦	1.5 ± 0.05 ♦
Rut + Cana	110 ± 1.7 ♦	107 ± 3.9 ♦	94.9 ± 6.7 *,♦	90.9 ± 0.3 ♦	1.1 ± 0.06 ♦

* $p < 0.05$ vs. NM Control; ♦ $p < 0.05$ vs. SIT2D Control.

3. Discussion

Diabetes mellitus (DM) is one of the most prevalent chronic diseases worldwide; thus, its management requires new alternatives that will help to control the hyperglycemia levels of patients with DM [1,3]. To date, a wide variety of drugs are used to control hyperglycemia; nevertheless, prolonged use can result in adverse effects [12]. One of the principal approaches towards the use of oral antidiabetic drugs (OADs) is to reduce hyperglycemia values; in this sense, the correct management of hyperglycemia can be reflected in the adequate good control of the percentage of glycated hemoglobin (% HbA1c); however, not all OADs have good control of this parameter. In the long term, the increase in % HbA1c is related to an elevated cardiovascular risk [4], such as diabetic nephropathy and glaucoma, among the other DM complications [34–36]. Furthermore, some of the most common diseases that accompany patients with DM are dyslipidemias; if they are not adequately controlled, they can generate vascular complications as well as acute myocardial infarctions that can cause the death of the patient [37]. In patients with DM, it has been demonstrated in the research that the administration of sulfonylureas as well as thiazolidinediones may help to reduce the values of hyperlipidemia [38]. In addition to % HbA1c, several treatments performed on patients with DM2 help to reduce dyslipidemias; however, in the long term, all of them did not adequately control this problem. As a result, it is important to search for new treatments that can help to reduce and control the complications implicated by DM.

The aim of this study was to determine the effects of hyperglycemia, % HbA1c, and hyperlipidemic values following the chronic administration of ethanolic extract obtained from the leaves of *A. cherimola* and the flavonoid rutin, a compound isolated from *A. cherimola* that has been demonstrated to be one of the metabolites present in the plant that is responsible, in part, for their antihyperglycemic activity [28], as well as OADs commonly used in therapy. All the treatments were first administered alone and the combination of antidiabetic drugs with the extract and antidiabetic drugs with rutin was used to evaluate their activity.

First, all the treatments were evaluated separately. It is important to mention that the doses evaluated in the study were selected according to the posology of every OAD; in the case of EEAc and rutin, both doses were selected as reported in previous studies [25]. The reduction in the hyperglycemia observed was consistent with the results reported by other authors [26–28]. In the case of the OADs, the values obtained following the administration of acarbose were similar to those obtained for the evaluation of rutin; this can be explained by the fact that both molecules share a similar action mechanism to reduce the hyperglycemia mediated by the inhibition of α–glucosidase enzymes [28]. Moreover, rutin is a glucoside conformed by quercetin linked to rutinoside disaccharide; this disaccharide is structurally similar to acarbose, and it has been described as helping the interaction with the a-glucosidase enzyme inhibiting it [25,28]. In the case of metformin and glibenclamide, they presented poor activity over the hyperglycemia values. Perhaps, in the case of metformin, a daily administration is needed to achieve good control of hyperglycemia; in the case of glibenclamide, this can be explained due to the destruction of β cells following the administration of streptozocin to induce the SIT2D model [39,40]. Perhaps, there are not enough β cells to generate an adequate acute secretion of insulin to reduce the hyperglycemic values. In all cases, the combination of EEAc with antidiabetic drugs reduces hyperglycemia in the treated animals; it is possible that the pharmacological effect of each antidiabetic drug was favored as a synergism with some of the metabolites present in the EEAc. Several products have been isolated from *A. cherimola*, such as flavonoids, alkaloids, acetogenins, sterols, and sesquiterpenes, among others [17]; it is possible that the combination of antidiabetic drugs with one or more of the products present in the extract helps to reduce hyperglycemia in the treated animals.

Flavonoids have been widely reported in the literature as molecules presenting antihyperglycemic activity in vivo and in vitro [41–43]. Considering the abovementioned issues and that a bio-guided phytochemical study conducted by our research group led to the isolation of rutin as one of the products with antidiabetic effects present in *A. cherimola* [26,28], we decided to evaluate the activity of this flavonoid in combination with antidiabetic drugs. The combination of rutin with acarbose and canagliflozin was the treatment with the greatest reduction in the hyperglycemic values. We suggested that this was due to the combination of the mechanism of action. Rutin and acarbose have been commonly described as α-glucosidase inhibitors [28,44]; it is possible that the combination of these two compounds in the doses administered were enough to generate a greater reduction in the α-glucosidase enzyme. On the other hand, canagliflozin is a sodium glucose co-transporter-2 (SGLT2) inhibitor [45]; we suggested that the combination of rutin with a SGLT2 inhibitor, such as canagliflozin, may help to completely reduce the postprandial peak of glucose following food intake due to the combination of both mechanisms of action [46]. The reduction in the complex carbohydrates' hydrolysis combined with the inhibition of glucose absorption may result in the significant reduction in hyperglycemia. The combination of rutin with glibenclamide and metformin did not generate a significant reduction in the hyperglycemic values in acute evaluation; however, we attributed this result to the necessary long-time administration of the treatments to achieve a reduction in the hyperglycemic values. Considering our results, the subchronic evaluations of all treatments previously described were performed with the aim to observe the effect of the hyperglycemic values on the long-time administration as well as the effect on the % HbA1c and hyperlipidemic values.

The subchronic evaluation of the separate treatments showed that the subchronic administration of EEAc, rutin, acarbose, and canagliflozin significantly reduced hyperglycemia in the treated animals; in the case of EEAc, the effect was maintained from weeks 1 to 4, and this was consistent with the activity demonstrated in previous subchronic studies [28]. However, after the fourth week, antihyperglycemic activity was lost; this may have been due to the dose of 300 mg/kg not being adequate to achieve normoglycemic values in a subchronic evaluation; thus, we propose the consideration of future experiments with the evaluation of EEAc at higher doses to observe the acute and chronic antihyperglycemic activities. The significant reduction in hyperglycemia following the administration of rutin is similar to that observed in the group treated with acarbose; this result is consistent with the result obtained in the acute evaluation of both treatments, and we attribute this result to the similar mechanism of action that has been described for rutin, an α-glucosidase inhibitor [28]. In the case of the group treated with canagliflozin, it achieved considerable control of the hyperglycemic values; we attribute this result to the mechanism of action of this drug, an SGLT2 inhibitor, and it has also been reported in the literature that monotherapy performed with canagliflozin lowers blood glucose levels independently from insulin and, with SGLT2 inhibition, reduces the renal glucose absorption of glucose and increases the excretion of glucose in the urine [45]. The previously noted effects on hyperglycemia were reflected in % HbA1c; in the case of EEAc, the inadequate diminution of hyperglycemic values at weeks 4 and 8 significantly increased % HbA1c in a manner similar to the SITD2 control. On the other hand, in the groups treated with rutin, acarbose, and canagliflozin, the reduction in the hyperglycemia values was reflected in the significant reduction in % HbA1c. We propose that the effective reduction in high blood glucose levels is related to the decrease in % HbA1c due to the fact that a high concentration of glucose in the bloodstream does not exist; thus, the reduction in glucose to form Schiff bases and Amadori products to produce advanced glycation end-products (AGEs) cannot be performed [47,48]. In respect to the lipid profile, EEAc, rutin, acarbose, and canagliflozin showed a significant reduction in Chol, Tri, and LDL-c with an increase in HDL-c values; in the cases of EEAc and rutin, our results are similar to those reported in the previous studies [26,49]. Studies of *A. cherimola* reported that subchronic treatment performed with an infusion from this plant helped to reduce cholesterol and triglycerides in diabetic mice and led an increase in HDL values, this activity being attributed to phenolic compounds [25]. In respect to rutin, it has been demonstrated in the literature that flavonoids can also reduce hepatic peroxidation and lead to a decrease in the synthesis of cholesterol. This is partly mediated by the regulation of fatty acid and cholesterol metabolism, affecting the gene expression of regulatory enzymes [25,50]. In respect to the atherogenic index plasma (AIP), the values calculated for the animals treated with EEAc, rutin, acarbose, and canagliflozin were similar to the NM control; we associated our results with these treatments possibly reducing the chance of increased cardiovascular risk, vascular damage, and mortality risk, which are some of the most common complications associated with secondary diabetes [4]; however, there is a need to conduct further experiments to confirm our hypothesis.

When the OADs were administered in combination with EEAc, we observed that the groups treated with acarbose and canagliflozin showed a reduction in hyperglycemia from the first week of treatment; however, all the animals died in week four. We discarded the possibility that the mortality observed after four weeks of treatment were possibly due to the toxicity generated for the administration of the extract since there are experiments that demonstrate the toxicity of the ethanolic extract obtained from the leaves of *A. cherimola*, categorized as number 5 in the safe or not label >2000 mg/kg [25]. According to our observations, we suggest that the death of the animals was due to the possible hypoglycemic activity after the repeated administration of both combinations; this could have been due to the quantity of drugs or EEAc administered in combination to the animals. We propose further experiments in the future to determine the correct doses to reduce hypoglycemia and to obtain normoglycemic values, avoiding the possible mortality rate increase as a result of the treatments. The group treated with the combination of EEAc + glibenclamide did not generate a significant reduction in hyperglycemic values; this could have been due to the principal effect of STZ to generate experimental diabetes mellitus in the β cells' destruction [46]. In this sense, the molecular mechanism of glibenclamides is insulin secretion following the β cells' stimulation [51]. In consideration of the abovementioned factors, if no β cells are present, the secretion of insulin and, consequently, the reduction in hyperglycemia cannot be achieved. In the case of the combination of EEAc + metformin, we observed a progressive reduction in the hyperglycemic values reaching the normoglycemic control group values; in comparison with the separate administration of metformin, the control of hyperglycemia was enhanced. We propose that the effect observed was due to EEAc generating a reduction in complex disaccharides mediated by the inhibition of the α-glucosidase enzyme, and this effect was attached to the hepatic uptake of glucose and the inhibition of gluconeogenesis generated by the action of metformin [44], which helped to reduce hyperglycemia in the animals treated with this combination. In respect to % HbA1c, the decrease in the hyperglycemic values was consistent with the HbA1c quantity; this was probably due to the correct utilization of the glucose that did not allow the production of AGEs [47]. In respect to the lipid profile, the parameters obtained after the administration of EEAc + glibenclamide indicate that this combination helps to delay the chronic incrementation of the parameters measured in comparison with the SIT2D control; however, considering the previous results, this combination is not a candidate for future investigations in our research group. In the case of the combination of EEAc + metformin, we observed a reduction in Chol and LDL-c with an increase in the LDL-c values; when the AIP was calculated, we observed a significant reduction in this value. Metformin has been described in the literature as a first-line treatment for DM type 2, being a primary pharmacological effect to control disturbed glucose metabolism; however, the completed mechanism of action of this drug is controversial due to metformin also influencing lipid/cholesterol pathways [52]. Several studies have reported the effects of metformin on atherosclerotic vascular disease in people with type 2 diabetes [52]; our results agree with the previous results presented for metformin, and in combination with EEAc in the doses administered, it is possible to achieve a correct reduction in hyperglycemia, % HbA1c, and lipid profile values, and considering the calculated AIP, the possibility of developing cardiovascular risks, vascular damage, among other mortal complications [4], can be reduced.

Finally, following the administration of OADs in combination with rutin, we observed in all the treatments a significant reduction in the hyperglycemic values during treatment. We propose that the combination of rutin with control drugs helped us achieve a significant reduction in hyperglycemia, as rutin was the only compound that was combined with the control drug, and there were also only two mechanisms of action that were involved in the reduction in hyperglycemia [25,28,43] in comparison with the combination with EEAc, which contained a higher number of compounds [21,23] that could produce other types of interactions to reduce the hyperglycemic values [14,16]. Additionally, it is important to mention that in this case, the subchronic combination of rutin with acarbose and canagliflozin did not generate the death of animals. This can be due to the possibility that in the EEAc there are more compounds [21,23] that can generate hypoglycemia, and their combination with control drugs at the doses administered in this study generated a mortal hypoglycemic effect. In respect to % HbA1c, the adequate control of hyperglycemia mediated after the subchronic administrations of rutin + acarbose, rutin + metformin, and rutin + canagliflozin were reflected in the reduction in % HbA1c. Our principal theory is that the subchronic administration of these combinations helps to reduce the concentration of glucose in the bloodstream and this reduction may help to avoid the generation of AGEs [53]. In respect to the lipid profile, the combinations of rutin + acarbosa and rutin + canagliflozin were the treatments with the greatest reductions in the parameters measured. We observed a significant reduction in Chol, Tri, and LDL-c with a significant increase in HDL-c values. Consequently, the AIPs calculated for these treatments were significantly lower than the SIT2D control; our results suggest that these combinations may help to significantly reduce the possibility of producing alterations of lipid metabolism, hypertriglyceridemia, high levels of cholesterol, and alterations between low-density lipoproteins (LDLs) and high-density lipoproteins (HDLs) [4], which are associated with an increase in mortality rates and other DM secondary complications, such as cardiovascular risk, vascular damage, diabetic nephropathy, and glaucoma, among others [34–36]. It is important to mention that the combination of rutin + canagliflozin was the only treatment that obtained normoglycemic values during all the treatments with the reduction in %HbA1c in all the treatments and with an important reduction in the lipid parameters measured. We propose that this combination helps to present one of the principal approaches in the management of DM, that is, the reduction in postprandial hyperglycemia in patients mediated by the prevention of hydrolysis (α-glucosidase) and the absorption of carbohydrates (SGLT-2) after food intake. The effective control of blood glucose levels being a key step in the prevention or reversion of diabetic complications, such as dyslipidemias, and other DM mortality complications, helps to improve the quality of life in diabetic patients [54].

According to the manuscript, the treatments used in this investigation showed good activity for the control of hyperglycemia, the combination of the extract obtained from the leaves of *A. cherimola* Miller, and the flavonoid rutin in combination with antidiabetic drugs showed an important improvement in the control of high blood glucose levels that is reflected in % HbA1c and the control of the lipid profile; however, further studies are necessary on the treatments with the best activity in order to determine their possible toxicity, and to reproduce our results in other experimental models to confirm the activity presented on this study.

4. Materials and Methods

4.1. Chemicals, Reagents and Drugs

Streptozocin ($\geq$75% α-anomer basis, PN: S0130-5G), nicotinamide ($\geq$99.5%, PN: 47865-U), sucrose ($\geq$99.5% GC, PN: S9378-1Kg), acarbose (PN: PHR1253-500MG), canagliflozin (95%, PN: 721174-1G), glibenclamide (PN: PHR1287-1G), metformin (PN: PHR1084-500MG) were purchased from Sigma-Aldrich® (Sigma®, Saint Louis, MO, USA). Buffer solution (citric acid/sodium hydroxide/hydrogen chloride, pH 4.00, CC: 109445) was purchased from Merck® (Merck®, Darmstadt, Germany).

4.2. Plant Material

Annona cherimola Miller leaves were collected by Dr. Fernando Calzada in December 2019 at San Jose, Tláhuac, Mexico (19°16′32.6″ N 99°00′07.1″ W). The plant material was authenticated by Santiago Xolalpa of the Herbarium IMSSM of Mexican Institute of Social Security (IMSS) where the voucher specimen is conserved under reference number: 15,795.

4.3. Ethanolic Extract Preparation

The air-dried and finely powdered leaves (2.9 kg) were extracted by maceration at room temperature with EtOH (2 times × 10 L). After filtration, the extract was combined and evaporated in vacuum to yield 131 g (yield 4.5%) of green residue. The chemical characterization of rutin and other compounds was made (see Supplementary Material).

4.4. Animals

For the biological tests, male BALB/c strain mice 8 to 10 weeks of age (20 ± 5 g) were obtained from the Animal Facility of the Centro Médico Nacional "Siglo XXI" of the Instituto Mexicano del Seguro Social (IMSS). The mice were maintained at room temperature (22 ± 2 °C) in a natural 12-h light–dark cycle and fed with laboratory rodent diet 5001 (Lab Diet ®, Saint Louis, MO, USA) and water ad libitum. All research with experimental animals was conducted in accordance with the Mexican Official Norm NOM-062-ZOO-1999 [54] for Animal Experimentation and Care. All research was performed with the approval of the Hospital Ethics Committee of Specialties of the National Medical Center "Siglo XXI" of the IMSS (registration: R-2015-3601-211 and R-2019-3601-004).

4.5. Induction of Experimental Type 2 Diabetes

The experimental diabetes mellitus was induced according to the streptozocin-induced type 2 (SIT2D) model described by Valdes et al. [39]. Mice fasted for 16 h before receiving treatment (day 0). Streptozocin (STZ) was dissolved in a cold pH 4 buffer solution, then it was administered at 100 mg/kg intraperitoneally (IP) on days 1 and 3. Nicotinamide (NA) was dissolved in a cold saline solution and administered at 240 mg/kg IP 30 min after STZ treatment only on day 1. At the end of the treatment on day 3, a 10% sucrose solution was used ad libitum over two days. On day 5, the sucrose solution was withdrawn and substituted with water ad libitum. Then, 24 h later, the development of SIT2D was determined by measuring postprandial blood glucose levels using a conventional glucometer (ACCU-CHECK® Performa Blood Glucose Systems, Roche®, DC, Basel, Switzerland). Additionally, to confirm the SIT2D model, β-cell function was evaluated with the administration of 5 mg/kg glibenclamide orally and measuring the decrease in glucose values 2 and 4 h after administration; according to the results, there can be confirmed the existence of functional β-cell [39,40], therefore, the generated model was classified as an experimental type 2 diabetes mellitus model.

4.6. Grouping

For acute and subchronic evaluations, mice were randomly divided into 14 groups (n = 6 each) as follows: ethanolic extract of A. cherimola (EEAc) at a dose of 300 mg/kg, rutin (Rut) 50 mg/kg, oral antidiabetic drugs metformin (Met) 850 mg/kg, glibenclamide (Gli) 5 mg/kg, acarbose (Aca) 50 mg/kg, and canagliflozin (Cana) 50 mg/kg. The combinations with EEAc were: EEAc + Met 300/850 mg/kg, EEAc + Cana (300/50 mg/kg), EEAc + Gli (300/5 mg/kg), and EEAc + Aca (300/50 mg/kg). The combinations with rutin were Rut + Aca (50/50 mg/kg), Rut + Cana (50/50 mg/kg), Rut + Met (50/850 mg/kg), and Rut+ Gli (50/5 mg/kg). All samples were dissolved in 2% Tween 80 in water as a vehicle. The normoglycemic and SIT2D control groups were treated with the vehicle (2% Tween 80 in water); all treatments were administered orally with a gavage at a volume of 0.5 mL for each animal [38].

4.6.1. Acute Evaluation of Ethanolic Extract from *Annona cherimola*, Rutin, and Oral Antidiabetic Drugs on SIT2D Mice Model

Animals with blood glucose levels between 250–380 mg/dL were used for this study. The treatments described above were administered orally, once administered the treatments, the blood samples were collected from the tail vein at the beginning (0 h), 2 and 4 h after administration using a conventional glucometer (ACCU-CHECK® Performa Blood Glucose Systems, Roche®, DC, Basel, Switzerland) [46].

4.6.2. Subchronic Evaluation of Ethanolic Extract from *Annona cherimola*, Rutin, and Oral Antidiabetic Drugs on SIT2D Mice Model

Animals from the acute test continued to be used for the subchronic evaluation, all the treatments were administered daily for 8 weeks, doses are described above. Blood glucose levels were measured weekly as previously described. Additionally, lipid profile and glycated hemoglobin (HbA1c) measurement were carried out every 2 weeks.

4.6.3. % HbA1c Measurement

For the measurement of glycated hemoglobin (HbA1c), blood sample were collected from the tail vein of the animals treated and were analyzed using the system automated boronate affinity assay for the determination of the percentage of Hemoglobin A1c (HbA1c%) in whole blood, Clover HbA1c reader, Infopía® (Anyang, Korea).

4.6.4. Lipid Profile Measurement

After eight weeks of treatment, a lipid profile was created for the study groups; to perform the measurements, blood samples were obtained from the tail vein of the animals and analyzed using VERI-Q® monitoring equipment. The parameters measured were cholesterol (Chol), triglycerides (TRIGs), high-density lipoprotein cholesterol (HDL-c), low-density lipoprotein cholesterol (LDL-c), and atherogenic index of plasma (AIP).

For the atherogenic index calculation the next formula was used:

$$\text{Atherogenic index of plasma (AIP)} = \frac{\text{Chol}}{\text{HDL-c}}$$

4.7. Statistical Analysis

All the results are expressed as mean values ± standard error of the mean (SEM). All statistical analyses were performed using GraphPad Prism version 8.02 (GraphPad Software Inc., San Diego, CA, USA). The statistical evaluation was conducted through an analysis of variance followed by a Tukey test for multiple comparisons. $p \leq 0.05$ was considered a statistically significant difference.

5. Conclusions

The complete analysis of the results performed showed the adequate management of hyperglycemia, % HbA1c, and lipid profile following the administration of ethanolic extract obtained from the leaves of *A. cherimola* and the flavonoid rutin. Additionally, for the first time, we presented the activity of ethanolic extract in combination with oral antidiabetic drugs. Our results demonstrate the importance of evaluating the activity of herbal remedies in combination with common oral drugs, as in some cases, these combinations can generate side effects in the patients. Finally, it was shown that the administration of rutin at doses of 50 mg/kg in combination with oral antidiabetic drugs helps to reduce hyperglycemia, % HbA1c, and lipid profiles, being considered as a first step to develop new treatments focusing on the control of DM and its complications.

Supplementary Materials: The following supporting information can be downloaded at: https://www.mdpi.com/article/10.3390/ph16010112/s1, HPLC-DAD analysis at 254 nm of the ethanol extract of the leaves of *Annona cherimola* Miller, rutin, nicotiflorin, and narcissin; Ultraviolet spectra obtained from HPLC-DAD: rutin, nicotinflorin, and narcissin; ^{1}H-NMR of rutin, nicotiflorin, and narcissin; ^{13}C-NMR of rutin, nicotiflorin, and narcissin.

Author Contributions: Conceptualization, M.V. and F.C.; Formal analysis, J.M.-S. and J.M.-R.; Funding acquisition, F.C.; Investigation, J.M.-R.; Project administration, F.C.; Resources, F.C.; Supervision, F.C.; Writing—original draft, M.V., J.M.-S. and J.M.-R.; Writing—review & editing, M.V. and F.C. All authors have read and agreed to the published version of the manuscript.

Funding: This research was supported by grants from Instituto Mexicano del Seguro Social (IMSS): FIS/IMSS/PROT/PRIO/19/110 and FIS/IMSS/PROT/G17-2/1722. Awarded to F.C.

Institutional Review Board Statement: The study was conducted according to the guidelines of the 18 Declaration of Helsinki and the Official Mexican Regulations to animal care and experimental manage 19 NOM-062-ZOO-1999. This study was approved by the Local Ethics Committee of CMN SXXI in the 20 Instituto Mexicano del Seguro Social under protocol code R-2020-3601-038 and R-2019-3601-004.

Informed Consent Statement: Not applicable.

Data Availability Statement: The data presented in this article are available on request from the corresponding authors.

Acknowledgments: This work is the bachelor's thesis of Julita Martínez Rodríguez. We would like to thank IMSS for the contract grant sponsor FIS/IMSS/PROT/PRIO/19/110 and FIS/IMSS/PROT/G17-2/1722.

Conflicts of Interest: The authors declare no conflict of interest.

References

1. Guthrie, R.; Guthrie, D. Pathophysiology of diabetes mellitus. *Crit. Care Nurs. Q.* **2004**, *27*, 113–125. [CrossRef]
2. International Diabetes Federation (IDF). Diabetes Atlas 9th Edition. Available online: https://www.diabetesatlas.org/en/ (accessed on 18 August 2022).
3. World Health Organization. Diabetes. Available online: https://www.who.int/news-room/fact-sheets/detail/diabetes (accessed on 22 August 2022).
4. American Diabetes Association. Classification and diagnosis of diabetes: Standards of Medical Care in Diabetes 2020. *Diabetes Care* **2021**, *43*, S14–S31.
5. DeFronzo, R. From the Triumvirate to the Ominous Octet: A New Paradigm for the Treatment of Type 2 Diabetes Mellitus. *Diabetes* **2009**, *58*, 773–795. [CrossRef]
6. Strain, W.; Paldánius, P. Diabetes, cardiovascular disease and the microcirculation. *Cardiovasc. Diabetol.* **2018**, *17*, 57. [CrossRef]
7. Maritin, A.; Sanders, R.; Watkins, J. Diabetes, oxidative stress, and antioxidants: A review. *J. Biochem. Mol. Toxicol.* **2003**, *17*, 24–38. [CrossRef]
8. Gan, T.; Liao, B.; Xu, G. The clinical usefulness of glycated albumin in patients with diabetes and chronic kidney disease: Progress and challenges. *J. Diabetes Complicat.* **2018**, *32*, 876–884. [CrossRef]
9. Kovatchev, B. Metrics for glycaemic control—From HbA1c to continuous glucose monitoring. *Nat. Rev. Endocrinol.* **2017**, *13*, 425–436. [CrossRef]
10. Wong, N.; Nicholls, S.; Tan, J.; Bursill, C. The Role of High-Density Lipoproteins in Diabetes and Its Vascular Complications. *Int. J. Mol. Sci.* **2018**, *19*, 1680. [CrossRef]
11. Association, A. Standards of Medical Care in Diabetes-2020. *Diabetes Care* **2020**, *43*, S7–S13. [CrossRef]
12. Tan, S.; Mei, J.; Sim, Y. Type 1 and 2 diabetes mellitus: A review on current treatment approach and gene therapy as potential intervention. *Diabetes Metab. Syndr.* **2019**, *13*, 364–372. [CrossRef]
13. Khursheed, R.; Singh, S.; Wadhwa, S. Treatment strategies against diabetes: Success so far and challenges ahead. *Eur. J. Pharmacol.* **2019**, *862*, 172625. [CrossRef] [PubMed]
14. El-Tantawy, W.; Temraz, A. Management of diabetes using herbal extracts: Review. *Arch. Physiol. Biochem.* **2018**, *124*, 383–389. [CrossRef] [PubMed]
15. Giovannini, P.; Howes, M.; Edwards, S. Medicinal plants used in the traditional management of diabetes and its sequelae in Central America: A review. *J. Ethnopharmacol.* **2016**, *184*, 58–71. [CrossRef] [PubMed]
16. Choudhury, H.; Pandey, M.; Hua, C. An update on natural compounds in the remedy of diabetes mellitus: A systematic review. *J. Tradit. Complement. Med.* **2017**, *8*, 361–376. [CrossRef] [PubMed]
17. Quilez, A.M.; Fernández-Arche, M.A.; García-Giménez, M.M.; De la Puerta, R. Potential therapeutic applications of the genus *Annona* Local and traditional uses and pharmacology. *J. Ethnopharmacol.* **2018**, *225*, 244–270. [CrossRef] [PubMed]
18. Pineda-Ramírez, N.; Calzada, F.; Alquisiras-Burgos, I. Antioxidant Properties and Protective Effects of Some Species of the Annonaceae, Lamiaceae, and Geraniaceae Families against Neuronal Damage Induced by Excitotoxicity and Cerebral Ischemia. *Antioxidants* **2020**, *9*, 253. [CrossRef] [PubMed]
19. Larranaga, N.; Albertazzi, F.; Fontecha, G. A Mesoamerican origin of cherimoya (*Annona cherimola* Mill.): Implications for the conservation of plant genetic resources. *Mol. Ecol.* **2017**, *26*, 4116–4130. [CrossRef]
20. Andrade-Cetto, A.; Heinrich, M. Mexican plants with hypoglycaemic effect used in the treatment of diabetes. *J. Ethnopharmacol.* **2005**, *99*, 325–348. [CrossRef]
21. González, M. Chirimoya (*Annona cherimola* Miller), fruit-bearing tropical and sub-tropical of promissory values. *Cul. Trop* **2012**, *34*, 52–63.
22. Calzada, F.; Correa-Basurto, J.; Barbosa, E.; Mendez-Luna, D.; Yepez-Mulia, L. Antiprotozoal Constituents from *Annona cherimola* Miller, a Plant Used in Mexican Traditional Medicine for the Treatment of Diarrhea and Dysentery. *Pharmacogn. Mag.* **2017**, *13*, 148–152.

23. Martínez-Vázquez, M.; Estrada-Reyes, R.; Araujo, A. Antidepressant-like effects of an alkaloid extract of the aerial parts of Annona cherimolia in mice. *J. Ethnopharmacol.* **2012**, *139*, 164–170. [CrossRef]
24. Ammoury, C.; Younes, M.; El-Khoury, M. The pro-apoptotic effect of a Terpene-rich *Annona cherimola* leaf extract on leukemic cell lines. *BMC Complement. Altern. Med.* **2019**, *19*, 365. [CrossRef] [PubMed]
25. Martínez-Solís, J.; Calzada, F.; Barbosa, E.; Valdés, M. Antihyperglycemic and Antilipidemic Properties of a Tea Infusion of the Leaves from *Annona cherimola* Miller on Streptozocin-Induced Type 2 Diabetic Mice. *Molecules* **2021**, *9*, 2408. [CrossRef]
26. Díaz-de-Cerio, E.; Aguilera-Saez, L.; Gómez-Caravaca, A. Characterization of bioactive compounds of *Annona cherimola* L. leaves using a combined approach based on HPLC-ESI-TOF-MS and NMR. *Anal. Bioanal. Chem.* **2018**, *410*, 3607–3619. [CrossRef] [PubMed]
27. Mannino, G.; Gentile, C.; Porcu, A.; Agliassa, C.; Caradonna, F.; Bertea, C. Chemical Profile and Biological Activity of Cherimoya (*Annona cherimola* Mill.) and Atemoya (*Annona atemoya*) Leaves. *Molecules* **2020**, *25*, 2612. [CrossRef] [PubMed]
28. Calzada, F.; Solares-Pascasio, J.I.; Ordoñez-Razo, R.M.; Velázquez, C.; Barbosa, E.; García-Hernández, N. Antihyperglucemic Activity of the leaves from *Annona chermiola* Miller on Alloxan-induced Diabetic Rats. *Pharmacogn. Res.* **2017**, *9*, 1–6. [CrossRef] [PubMed]
29. Asgharpour, F.; Pouramir, M.; Khalilpour, A.; Asgharpour, A.; Rezaei, M. Antioxidant activity and glucose diffusion relationship of traditional medicinal antihyperglycemic plant extracts. *Int. J. Mol. Cell Med.* **2013**, *2*, 169–176. [PubMed]
30. Jo, S.; Ka, E.; Lee, H.; Apostolidis, E.; Jang, H.-D.; Kwon, Y.-I. Comparison of Antioxidant Potential and Rat intestinal α-Glucosidases inhibitory Activities of Quercetin, Rutin, and Isoquercetin. *Int. J. Appl. Res. Nat. Prod.* **2009**, *2*, 52–60.
31. Sharma, S.; Ali, A.; Ali, J.; Sahni, J.; Baboota, S. Rutin: Therapeutic potential and recent advances in drug delivery. *Expert Opin. Investig. Drugs* **2013**, *22*, 1063–1079. [CrossRef]
32. Ghorbani, A. Mechanisms of antidiabetic effects of flavonoid rutin. *Biomed Pharmacother.* **2017**, *96*, 305–312. [CrossRef]
33. Verma, A.; Kumar, A.; Shekar, R.; Kumar, K.; Chakrapani, R. Pharmacological Screening of *Annona cherimola* for Antihyperlipidemic Potential. *J. Basic Clin. Pharm.* **2011**, *2*, 63–69. [PubMed]
34. Wada, J.; Makino, H. Inflammation and the pathogenesis of diabetic nephropathy. *Clin. Sci.* **2013**, *124*, 139–152. [CrossRef] [PubMed]
35. Robert, N.; Aung, T.; Madeiros, F. The Pathophysiology and Treatment of Glaucoma. *JAMA* **2014**, *18*, 1901–1911.
36. Brajendra, K.; Arvind, K. Diabetes mellitus: Complications and therapeutics. *Med. Sci. Monit* **2006**, *7*, RA130–RA147.
37. Oki, J. Dyslipidemias in Patients with Diabetes Mellitus: Classification and Risks and Benefits of Therapy. *Pharmacotherapy* **1995**, *3*, 317–337.
38. Valdés, M.; Calzada, F.; Mendieta-Wejebe, J. Structure-activity relationship study of acyclic terpenes in blood glucose levels: Potential α-glucosidase and sodium glucose cotransporter (SGLT-1) inhibitors. *Molecules* **2019**, *24*, 4020. [CrossRef]
39. Hsu, J.; Wu, C.; Hung, C.; Wang, C.; Huang, H. *Myrciaria cauliflora* extract improves diabetic nephropathy via suppression of oxidative stress and inflammation in streptozotocin-nicotinamide mice. *J. Food Drug Anal.* **2016**, *24*, 730–737. [CrossRef]
40. Mata, R.; Sol, C.; Sonia, E.; Krzkaya, J.; Rivero, C. Mexican antidiabetic herbs: Valuable sources of inhibitors of a-glucosidases. *J. Nat. Prod.* **2013**, *3*, 468–483. [CrossRef]
41. Kanter, M.; Aktas, C.; Erborga, M. Protective effects of quercetin against apoptosis and oxidative stress in streptozocin-induced diabetic rat testis. *Food Chem. Toxicol.* **2012**, *50*, 719–725. [CrossRef] [PubMed]
42. Chua, L.S. A review on plant-based rutin extraction methods and its pharmacological activities. *J. Ethnopharmacol.* **2013**, *150*, 805–817. [CrossRef]
43. Chaudhury, A.; Duvoor, C.; Reddy, V.; Kraleti, S.; Chada, A.; Ravilla, R.; Marco, A.; Shekhawat, N.; Montales, M.; Kuriakose, K.; et al. Clinical Review of Antidiabetic Drugs: Implications for Type 2 diabetes Mellitus Management. *Front. Endocrinol.* **2017**, *8*, 1–12. [CrossRef] [PubMed]
44. Deeks, E.; Schen, J. Canagliflozin: A Review in Type 2 Diabetes *Adis Drug Eval.* **2017**, *77*, 1577–1592. [CrossRef] [PubMed]
45. Valdés, M.; Calzada, F.; Mendieta-Wejebe, J.; Merlín-Lucas, V.; Velázquez, C.; Barbosa, E. Antihyperglycemic Effects of *Annona diversifolia* Safford and Its Acyclic Terpenoids: α-Glucosidase and Selective SGLT1 Inhibitors. *Molecules* **2020**, *25*, 3361. [CrossRef] [PubMed]
46. Singh, R.; Barden, A.; Mori, T.; Bellin, L. Advanced glycation end-products: A review. *Diabetologia* **2001**, *44*, 129–146. [CrossRef]
47. Snelson, M.; Coughlan, M. Dietary Advanced Glycation End Products: Digestion, Metabolism and Modulation of Gut Microbial Ecology. *Nutrients* **2019**, *2*, 215. [CrossRef]
48. Falé, P.; Ferreira, C.; Maruzzella, F.; Florêncio, M.; Farazão, F.; Serralheiro, M. Evaluation of cholesterol absorption and biosynthesis by decoctions of Annona cherimola leaves. *J. Ethnopharmacol.* **2013**, *150*, 718–723. [CrossRef]
49. Miranda-Pérez, M.; Ortega-Camarillo, C.; Escobar-Villanueva, M.; Blancas-Flores, G.; Alarcon-Aguilar, F. *Cucurbita fiicifolia* Bouché increases insulin secretion in RINm5F cells through an influx of Ca^{2+} from the endoplasmic reticulum. *J. Ethnopharmacol.* **2016**, *188*, 159–166. [CrossRef]
50. Un, J.; Mi-Kyung, L.; Yong, B.; Mi, A.; Myung-Sook, C. Effect of citrus flavonoids on lipid metabolism and glucose-regulating enzyme mRNA levels in type-2 diabetic mice. *Int. Biochem. Cell Biol.* **2006**, *38*, 1134–1145.
51. Stee, M.; Graaf, A.; Groen, A. Actions of Metformin and statins on lipid and glucose metabolism and possible benefit of combination therapy. *Cardiovasc. Diabetol.* **2018**, *17*, 94. [CrossRef]

52. Duncan, M.; Alkizim, F. Complementary and alternative medicine for type 2 diabetes mellitus: Role of medicinal herbs. *J. Diabetes Endocrinol.* **2012**, *3*, 44–56.
53. Calzada, F.; Valdés, M.; García-Hernández, N.; Velázquez, C.; Barbosa, E.; Bustos-Brito, C.; Quijano, L.; Pina-Jimenez, E.; Mendieta-Wejebe, J. Antihyperglycemic activity of the leaves from *Annona diversifolia* Safford. and farnesol on normal and alloxan-induced diabetic mice. *Phcog. Mag.* **2019**, *15*, S5–S11.
54. Norma Oficial Mexicana (NOM). Especificaciones Técnicas Para la Producción, Cuidado y Uso de los Animales de Laboratorio. Available online: https://www.fmvz.unam.mx/fmvz/principal/archivos/062ZOO.PDF (accessed on 12 July 2022).

Disclaimer/Publisher's Note: The statements, opinions and data contained in all publications are solely those of the individual author(s) and contributor(s) and not of MDPI and/or the editor(s). MDPI and/or the editor(s) disclaim responsibility for any injury to people or property resulting from any ideas, methods, instructions or products referred to in the content.

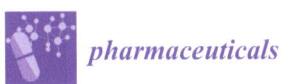

Article

A Mechanism of Isoorientin-Induced Apoptosis and Migration Inhibition in Gastric Cancer AGS Cells

Tong Zhang [1,†], Yun-Hong Xiu [2,†], Hui Xue [1], Yan-Nan Li [1], Jing-Long Cao [1], Wen-Shuang Hou [1], Jian Liu [1], Yu-He Cui [1], Ting Xu [1], Ying Wang [3,4,*] and Cheng-Hao Jin [1,3,4,*]

1. College of Life Science & Technology, Heilongjiang Bayi Agricultural University, Daqing 163319, China
2. Hemodialysis Center, Daqing Oilfield General Hospital, Daqing 163001, China
3. National Coarse Cereals Engineering Research Center, Daqing 163319, China
4. College of Food Science & Technology, Heilongjiang Bayi Agricultural University, Daqing 163319, China
* Correspondence: wychen156@163.com (Y.W.); jinchenghao3727@byau.edu.cn (C.-H.J.)
† These authors contributed equally to this work.

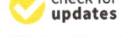

Citation: Zhang, T.; Xiu, Y.-H.; Xue, H.; Li, Y.-N.; Cao, J.-L.; Hou, W.-S.; Liu, J.; Cui, Y.-H.; Xu, T.; Wang, Y.; et al. A Mechanism of Isoorientin-Induced Apoptosis and Migration Inhibition in Gastric Cancer AGS Cells. *Pharmaceuticals* 2022, 15, 1541. https://doi.org/10.3390/ph15121541

Academic Editors: Fernando Calzada and Miguel Valdes

Received: 15 November 2022
Accepted: 6 December 2022
Published: 12 December 2022

Publisher's Note: MDPI stays neutral with regard to jurisdictional claims in published maps and institutional affiliations.

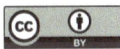

Copyright: © 2022 by the authors. Licensee MDPI, Basel, Switzerland. This article is an open access article distributed under the terms and conditions of the Creative Commons Attribution (CC BY) license (https://creativecommons.org/licenses/by/4.0/).

Abstract: Isoorientin (ISO) is a flavonoid compound containing a luteolin structure, which can induce autophagy in some tumor cells. This study investigated the impact of ISO in gastric cancer AGS cells, and performed an experimental analysis on the main signaling pathways and transduction pathways it regulates. CCK–8 assay results showed that ISO reduced the survival rate of gastric cancer AGS cells, but the toxicity to normal cells was minimal. Hoechst 33342/PI double staining assay results showed that ISO induced apoptosis in gastric cancer AGS cells. Further analysis by flow cytometry and Western blot showed that ISO induced apoptosis via a mitochondria-dependent pathway. In addition, the level of reactive oxygen species (ROS) in gastric cancer AGS cells also increased with the extension of the ISO treatment time. However, cell apoptosis was inhibited by preconditioning cells with N–acetylcysteine (NAC). Moreover, ISO arrested the cell cycle at the G2/M phase by increasing intracellular ROS levels. Cell migration assay results showed that ISO inhibited cell migration by inhibiting the expression of p–AKT, p–GSK–3β, and β–catenin and was also related to the accumulation of ROS. These results suggest that ISO-induced cell apoptosis by ROS–mediated MAPK/STAT3/NF–κB signaling pathways inhibited cell migration by regulating the AKT/GSK–3β/β–catenin signaling pathway in gastric cancer AGS cells.

Keywords: isoorientin; gastric cancer; cell apoptosis; cell cycle; cell migration; reactive oxygen species

1. Introduction

Globally, gastric cancer ranks third in terms of prevalence and death rates after lung cancer [1,2]. In China, gastric cancer is more common in people over 50 years of age [3,4]. In the present day, gastric cancer can be treated primarily through surgery and chemotherapy. Chemotherapy drugs, as the primary means of treatment after surgery, have an inhibitory effect on cancer cells, but they often destroy healthy normal cells, leading to the disorder of immune metabolism in the human body, with great side effects on the body [5,6]. There is, therefore, a need for a drug that is highly efficient and has a low risk of side effects. There are a number of natural products that have potential therapeutic effects on cancer cells while causing few side effects on other cells, so they have been subjected to intense research [7–9].

Isoorientin (ISO) is a flavonoid compound widely found in *Polygonum orientale* L., *Patrinia*, *Phyllostachys edulis* leaf, passionflower, and other plants [10–12]. ISO possesses a range of pharmacological actions, including anti–inflammatory, antiviral, and antibacterial activity, as well as weakening the development of liver fibrosis [13–16]. In addition, studies have shown that ISO has superior anticancer activity against breast cancer cells, hepatoblastoma, and other tumor cells [17–20]. The anticancer mechanism of ISO on stomach cancer cells, however, is unknown. In this study, ISO was examined for its effects on the apoptosis, proliferation, and migration of stomach cancer cells.

Apoptosis induction is currently one of the main ways to treat cancer cells. A high level of reactive oxygen species (ROS) promotes mitochondrial membrane potential reversal by activating mitogen–activated protein kinase (MAPK), leading to cytochrome c release and caspase–3 activation, ultimately resulting in apoptosis [21,22]. In addition, ROS can also regulate the STAT3 and NF–κB signaling pathways and cooperate with the MAPK signaling pathway to promote cell apoptosis [23].

By contrast, inhibiting tumor cell growth and metastasis play a critical role in cancer treatment. Glycogen synthase kinase 3β (GSK–3β) is the main intracellular serine/threonine kinase and has a bidirectional regulatory effect on the growth and development of tumor cells. When it is inhibited as a cancer–promoting factor, it promotes β–catenin entry into the nucleus, thereby activating the β–catenin signaling pathway and inhibiting the spread of tumor cells [24].

The effect of ISO on the apoptosis and migration of gastric cancer AGS cells was explored in this study, and its probable mechanism was found.

2. Results

2.1. Isoorientin Reduces the Viabilities of Gastric Cancer Cells

As shown in Figure 1A,B, ISO reduced the viability of twelve typical gastric cancer cell lines in a dose-dependent manner with a toxic effect higher than 5–FU, and ISO had a lower cytotoxic effect on normal cells. The IC_{50} values of each cell treated for this drug are summarized (Table 1). As shown in Figure 1C,D, ISO produced similar results in a time-dependent manner at a specific dose. Among the above gastric cancer cells, with an IC_{50} value of 36.54 μM, AGS cells had the highest sensitivity to ISO.

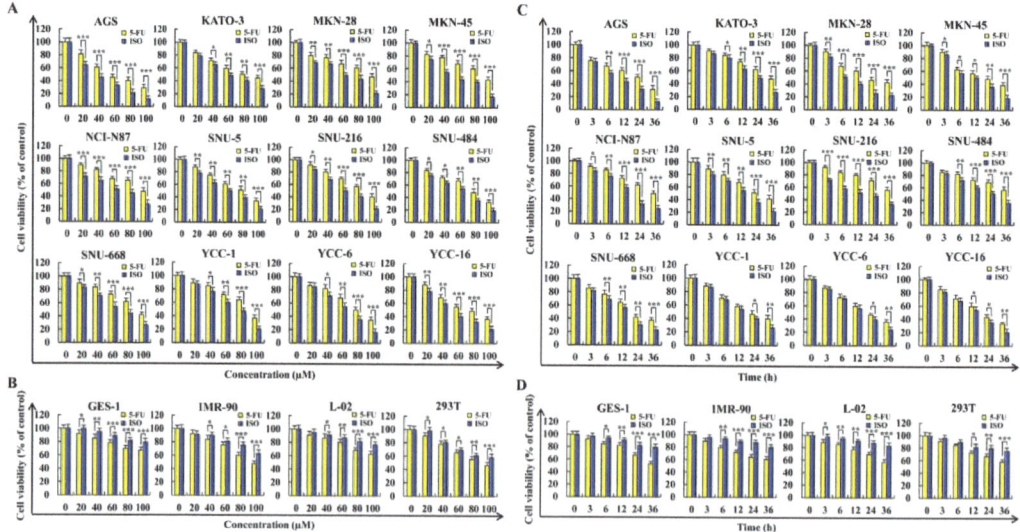

Figure 1. The cytotoxic effect of ISO. The CCK-8 assay was used to determine if cells had survived after being exposed to various doses or time of 5–FU or ISO. (**A**) Survival rate of gastric cancer cells. (**B**) Survival rate of normal cells. (**C**) Survival rate of gastric cancer cells. (**D**) Survival rate of normal cells. * $p < 0.05$, ** $p < 0.01$ and *** $p < 0.001$ vs. 5–FU.

Table 1. IC$_{50}$ values of ISO and 5–FU in gastric cancer cells.

Cell Line	5–FU (μM)	ISO (μM)
AGS	56.27 ± 2.04	36.54 ± 1.93
KATO-3	81.11 ± 1.28	60.28 ± 1.21
MKN-28	98.12 ± 1.87	61.31 ± 2.42
MKN-45	89.67 ± 2.26	49.77 ± 2.18
NCI-N87	99.37 ± 1.98	68.16 ± 2.38
SNU-5	80.97 ± 2.01	62.21 ± 1.73
SNU-216	86.35 ± 2.84	59.57 ± 1.66
SNU-484	78.38 ± 1.76	65.59 ± 2.44
SNU-668	90.63 ± 1.57	71.74 ± 2.75
YCC-1	91.37 ± 1.03	78.62 ± 1.24
YCC-6	82.47 ± 1.63	66.83 ± 2.68
YCC-16	80.16 ± 2.72	56.72 ± 2.62

2.2. Isoorientin Induces AGS Cell Apoptosis

As shown in Figure 2A,B, the edge of the AGS cells shrank after treatment with ISO. At 24 h, fluorescence intensity reached its maximum, which was higher than that of the 5–FU treatment group over the same period. Figure 2C illustrates the findings of flow cytometry, which demonstrated that the apoptosis of AGS cells treated with ISO increased over time and reached 35.76% of apoptotic cells at 24 h. As shown in Figure 2D, the AGS cells' mitochondrial membrane potential fluctuation trend was inversely associated with the length of time they underwent ISO treatment. As seen in Figure 2E, ISO markedly lowered the protein expression level of Bcl–2 while dramatically increasing the protein expression levels of Bad, cyto–c, cle–caspase–3, and cle–PARP. The mitochondrial apoptotic pathway was involved in ISO–induced AGS cell apoptosis, according to our findings.

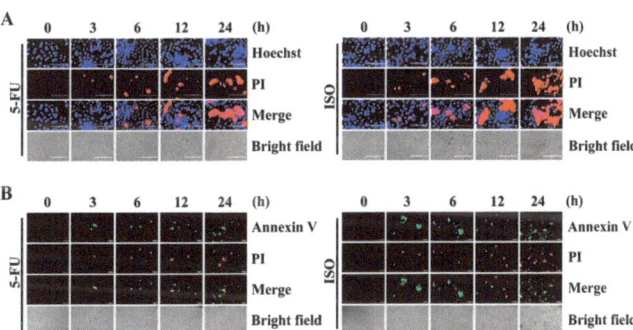

Figure 2. *Cont.*

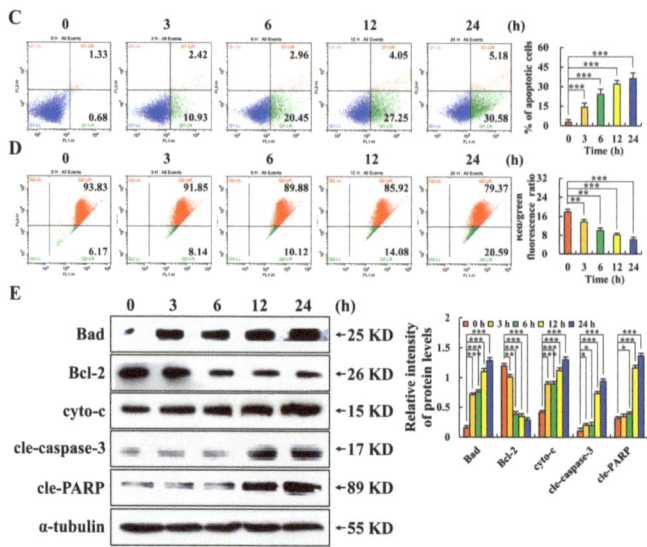

Figure 2. Apoptotic effects of ISO in AGS cells. A total of 36.54 μM ISO was applied to AGS cells from 0 to 24 h. (**A**) AGS cells after Hoechst and PI staining were observed by fluorescence microscope (original magnification, ×200). (**B**) AGS cells after Annexin V and PI staining were observed by fluorescence microscope (original magnification, ×400). (**C**) Apoptosis rate of AGS cells. (**D**) Flow cytometry was used to calculate the mitochondrial membrane potential. (**E**) Expression levels of apoptosis–related proteins in AGS cells treated with ISO. The α–tubulin was used as an internal reference protein. * $p < 0.05$, ** $p < 0.01$ and *** $p < 0.001$ vs. 0 h.

2.3. Isoorientin Regulates MAPK/STAT3/NF–κB Signaling Pathways

As seen in Figure 3A, ISO considerably decreased the expression levels of p–ERK, p–STAT3, and NF–κB while significantly upregulating the expression levels of p–JNK, p–p38, and IκBα in a time-dependent way. Then, we tested several nuclear proteins and found that ISO significantly reduced the levels of STAT3, NF–κB, and p–IκBα (Figure 3B). As seen in Figure 3C–E, compared with the ISO alone treatment groups, FR180204, SP600125, and SB203580 inhibited the expression of p–ERK, p–JNK, and p–p38 in AGS cells, respectively. Meanwhile, pretreatment with ERK inhibitors enhanced the decrease in p–STAT3 and Bcl–2 protein expression levels and inhibited the increase in cle–caspase–3 protein expression, while the level of p–STAT3 after pretreatment with the JNK inhibitor or p38 inhibitor was higher than that of ISO treatment alone. The above results indicate that the MAPK–dominated ISO–induced AGS cell apoptosis is an upstream signaling pathway.

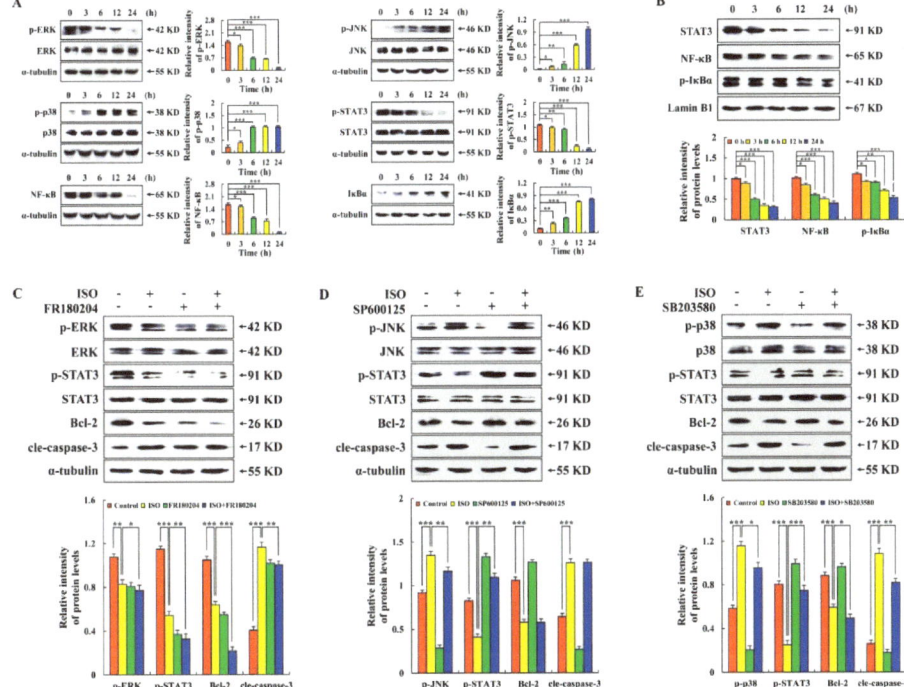

Figure 3. Regulation of ISO on the MAPK/STAT3/NF–κB signaling pathway in AGS cells. A total of 36.54 μM ISO was applied to AGS cells from 0 to 24 h. (**A**) MAPK/STAT3/NF–κB signaling pathway related protein expression level. (**B**) Nuclear protein expression level. (**C**) Expression levels of p–ERK, p–STAT3, Bcl-2, and cle–caspase–3 proteins in AGS cells treated with ISO (36.54 μM) and/or an ERK inhibitor (10 μM). (**D**) Expression levels of p–JNK, p–STAT3, Bcl-2, and cle–caspase–3 proteins in AGS cells treated with ISO (36.54 μM) and/or a JNK inhibitor (10 μM). (**E**) Expression levels of p–p38, p–STAT3, Bcl-2 and cle–caspase–3 proteins in AGS cells treated with ISO (36.54 μM) and/or a p38 inhibitor (10 μM). Lamin B1 and α–tubulin were used as an internal reference protein. * $p < 0.05$, ** $p < 0.01$ and *** $p < 0.001$ vs. 0 h or ISO + MAPK inhibition.

2.4. Isoorientin Regulates the MAPK/STAT3/NF–κB Signaling Pathways That Are Mediated by ROS

As shown in Figure 4A, in a time-dependent way, ISO dramatically increased the accumulation of ROS in AGS cells, reaching 83.42% after 24 h of treatment. However, ISO reduced ROS accumulation in normal gastric GES–1 cells (Figure 4B). As shown in Figure 4C, ISO–induced AGS cell apoptosis was inhibited by NAC treatment. As shown in Figure 4D,E, the expression levels of p–JNK, p–p38, IκBα, cle–caspase–3, and cle–PARP regulated by ISO was decreased by NAC treatment. ISO-regulated expression levels of p–ERK, p–STAT3, NF–κB, nuclear protein STAT3, NF–κB, and p–IκBα were increased by NAC treatment. These results suggest that ISO induces AGS cell apoptosis by promoting ROS accumulation.

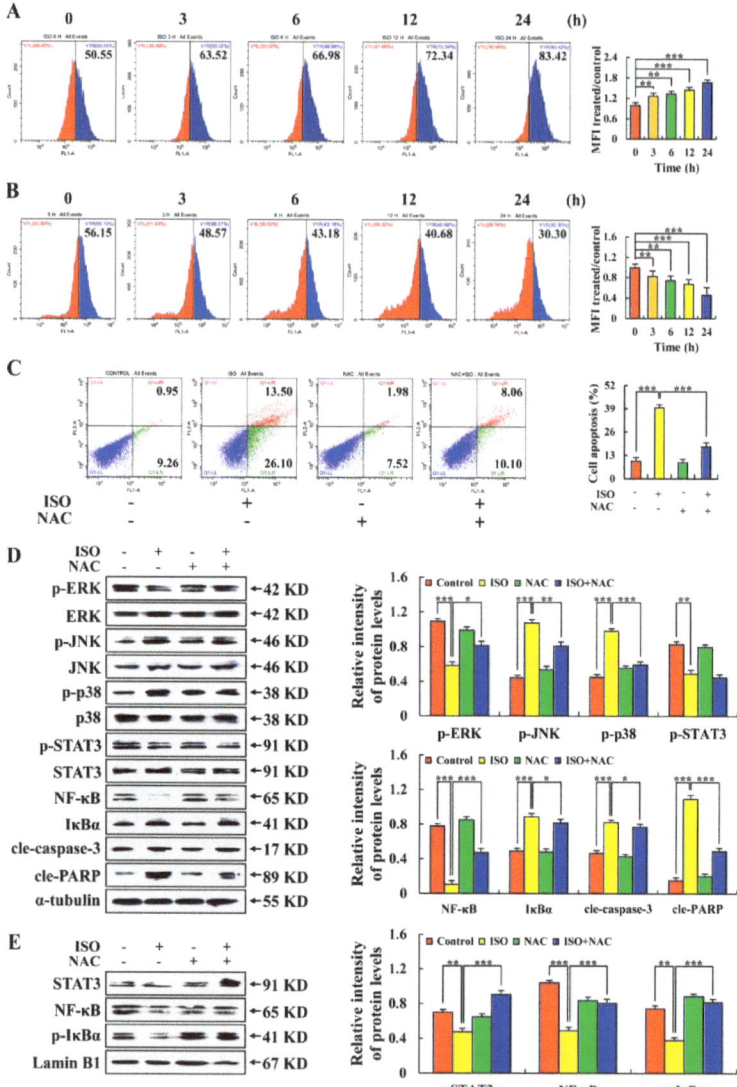

Figure 4. The promoting effects of ISO on ROS levels in AGS cells. A total of 36.54 μM ISO was applied to cells from 0 to 24 h. (**A**) AGS cell levels of ROS. (**B**) GES-1 cell levels of ROS. (**C**) Apoptosis rate of AGS cells treated with ISO (36.54 μM) and/or NAC (10 mM). (**D**) Expression levels of related signaling pathway proteins in AGS cells treated with ISO (36.54 μM) and/or NAC (10 mM). (**E**) Expression levels of nuclear proteins in AGS cells treated with ISO (36.54 μM) and/or NAC (10 mM). Lamin B1 and α–tubulin were used as an internal reference protein. * $p < 0.05$, ** $p < 0.01$ and *** $p < 0.001$ vs. 0 h or NAC + ISO.

2.5. Isoorientin Arrested the AGS Cell Cycle at the G2/M Phase

As seen in Figure 5A,B, following ISO treatment, fewer cells were in the G0/G1 phase (down from 64.64% to 47.69%), but more cells were in the G2/M phase. ISO decreased expression levels of p–AKT, CDK1/2, and Cyclin B, and increased expression levels of p21 and p27. As seen in Figure 5C,D, when NAC was added before ISO treatment, the number of G0/G1 cells increased from 61.76% to 70.12%, and ISO–induced expression of the above proteins was similarly reversed. The above results indicate that ISO could arrest the AGS cell cycle in the G2/M phase by up–regulating ROS.

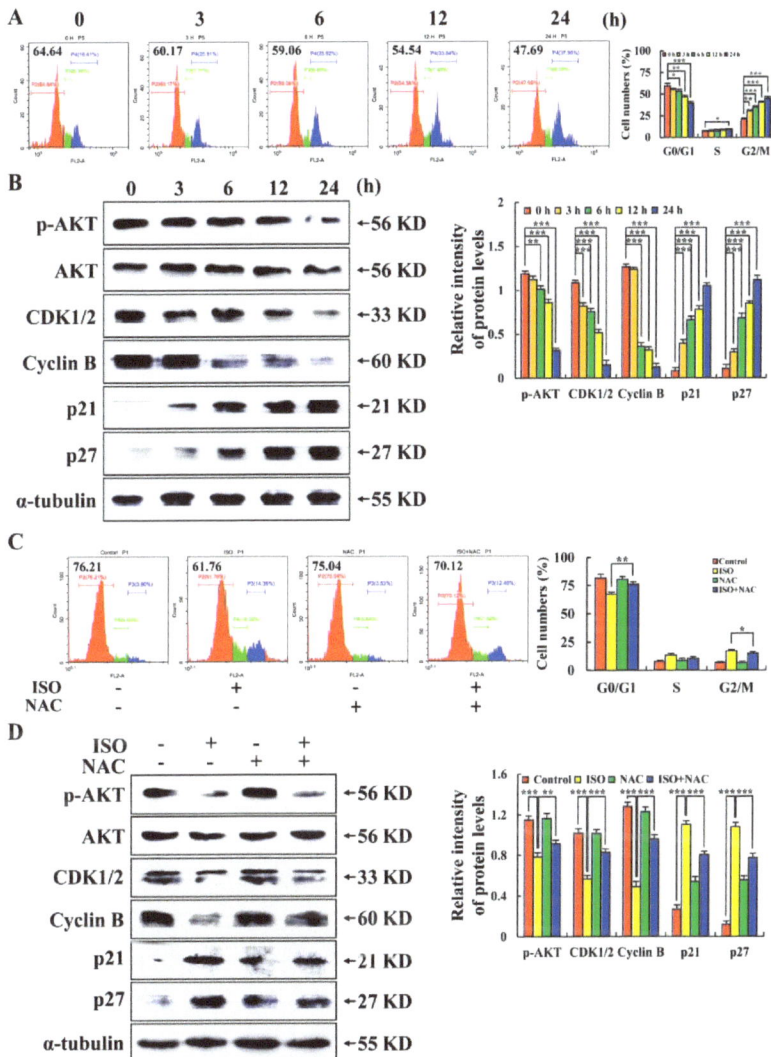

Figure 5. The arresting effects of ISO on the cell cycle in AGS cells. A total of 36.54 µM ISO was applied to AGS cells from 0 to 24 h. (A) Percentage of cell cycle number of AGS cells. (B) Expression of proteins involved in the G2/M cell cycle. (C) Percentage of cell cycle number of AGS cells treated with ISO (36.54 µM) and/or NAC (10 mM). (D) Expression of proteins involved in the G2/M cell cycle of AGS cells treated with ISO (36.54 µM) and/or NAC (10 mM), and α–tubulin was used as an internal reference protein. * $p < 0.05$, ** $p < 0.01$ and *** $p < 0.001$ vs. 0 h or NAC + ISO.

2.6. Isoorientin Inhibited AGS Cell Migration via the AKT/GSK–3β/β–catenin Signaling Pathways

As seen in Figure 6A,B, ISO reduced the AGS cell migration area and the number of AGS cells, demonstrating that ISO had the ability to inhibit the migration of AGS cells. As seen in Figure 6C,D, we further detected migration-related proteins and found that the expression levels of p–AKT, p–GSK–3β, Twist, ZEB1, N–cadherin, and β–catenin were all decreased, while the expression levels of E-cadherin were increased. These protein expression levels were reversed after NAC pretreatment. The above results indicate that ISO inhibited AGS cell migration via the ROS–mediated AKT/GSK–3β/β–catenin signaling pathways.

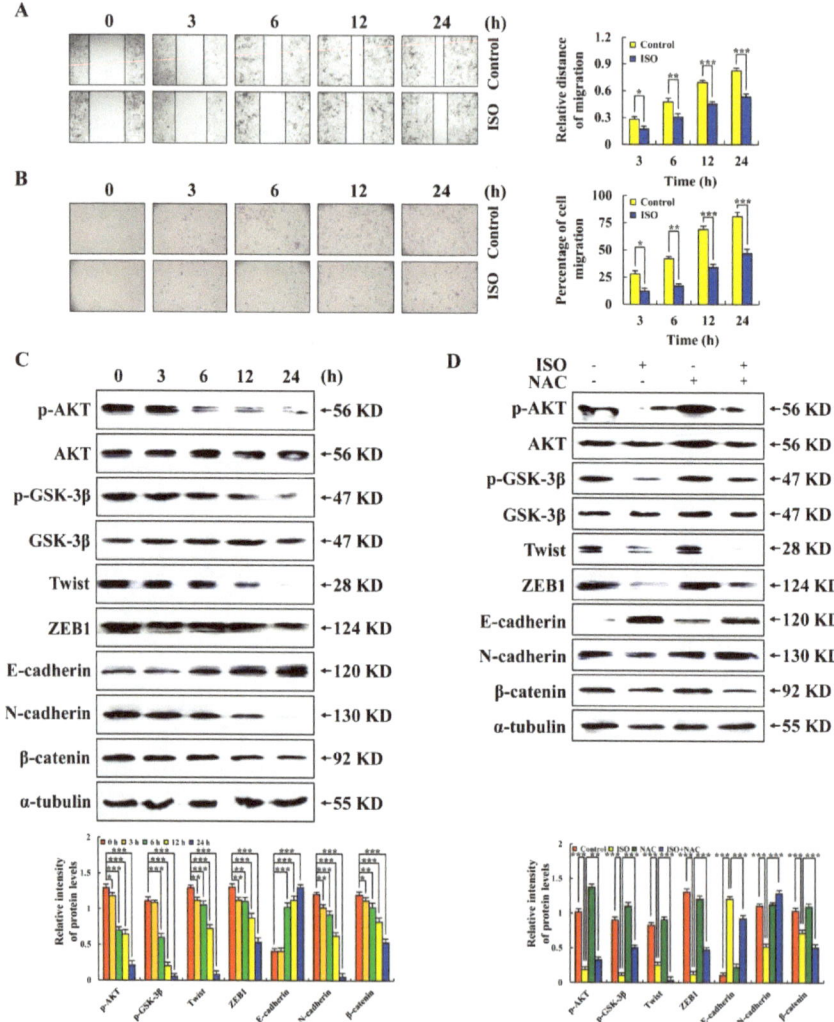

Figure 6. The inhibiting effects of ISO on migration in AGS cells. A total of 36.54 µM ISO was applied to AGS cells from 0 to 24 h. (**A**) Migration changes in AGS cells were observed by fluorescence microscope (original magnification, ×200). (**B**) The number of AGS cell migration was observed by fluorescence microscope (original magnification ×400). (**C**) Migration related protein expression level. (**D**) Expression of migration related proteins of AGS cells treated with ISO (36.54 µM) and/or NAC (10 mM), and α–tubulin was used as an internal reference protein. * $p < 0.05$, ** $p < 0.01$ and *** $p < 0.001$ vs. 0 h or NAC + ISO.

3. Discussion

Numerous studies have revealed that Chinese herbal medicines can replace certain chemicals due to their mild effects and low toxicity. In terms of inhibiting tumor growth and inducing tumor cell apoptosis, higher concentrations of traditional Chinese medicine extracts have been shown to have good biological activities [25–27]. Isoorientin (ISO), a flavonoid compound, has been demonstrated to decrease growth and induce apoptosis in some tumor cells. In the preliminary experiment of this study, it was found that under the same conditions, the killing effect of 5–FU on most of the gastric cancer cells from 12 different sources was better than that of other chemotherapy drugs. So, we selected 5–FU as the positive control in our subsequent research on ISO. In this study, ISO was used to treat 12 kinds of gastric cancer cells, and the analysis showed that ISO had excellent killing effects on these gastric cancer cells, and the effect was better than 5–FU. While inhibiting the growth of tumor cells, ISO was significantly less harmful to normal cells than 5–FU in the control group (Figure 1).

In this study, the CCK–8 assay results show that the effect of ISO on AGS cells was the most significant among these gastric cancer cells. AGS cells came from human gastric adenocarcinoma epithelial cell lines. Some studies have shown that gastric cancer cells from different sources have different biomarkers, different cell metabolites, and different drug sensitivity. In addition, the occurrence of gastric cancer is not only related to genetic susceptibility but also related to genetic mutations. Both KRAS and CTNNB1 genes were mutated in AGS cells. KRAS regulates downstream effectors of the MAPK pathway through phosphorylation. CTNNB1 can encode β–catenin and play a role in regulating cell migration [28]. In this study, we found that ISO can induce the apoptosis of AGS cells through the MAPK pathway and inhibit the migration of AGS cells by regulating β–catenin. We speculate that the origin of AGS cells and the mutated genes may be the reason why AGS cells are most affected by ISO. AGS cells were finally selected in this study to prove the anticancer effect of ISO.

In the process of apoptosis, Bcl-2 family proteins dominate the changes in mitochondrial membrane permeability [19,29]. This study has shown that ISO can reduce the expression of Bcl-2 and increase the expression of Bax by blocking the PI3K/Akt pathway, thus inducing the apoptosis of HepG2 cells [30]. Similarly, this study found that ISO up–regulated the expression of pro–apoptotic protein Bad and down–regulated the expression of anti-apoptotic protein Bcl-2, resulting in a decrease in the mitochondrial membrane potential and ultimately leading to AGS cell apoptosis (Figure 2). We found that when the ISO treatment time of cells was more than 24 h or close to 48 h, the cells basically lost their original form and were not enough for research. Therefore, when exploring the anti–tumor effects of ISO on AGS cells, 24 h of ISO treatment was selected as the last time point. In addition, in order to confirm the molecular mechanism of ISO–induced AGS cell apoptosis. Through the analysis of signal pathways, this study found that in the ISO–induced apoptosis of AGS cells, the ISO–regulated MAPK signaling pathway and STAT3 signaling pathway, together with the NF–κB signaling pathway, play an anti–cancer role (Figure 3).

Flavonoids are often used as antioxidants because of their ability to scavenge oxygen–free radicals [31]. However, it has been shown that their antioxidant effects depend on the cells being treated [32]. This study has shown that the ISO treatment of HepG2 cells significantly increased intracellular ROS levels, which were 33.58% higher than normal liver cells HL–7702 [33]. In tumor and normal cell lines of the same organ, different concentrations of one flavonoid are commonly observed to induce oxidative stress and have antioxidant effects. However, our aim was to explore the effects of ISO on ROS in different cell types. Therefore, we analyzed the regulatory effects of ISO on ROS levels in gastric cancer cells and normal cells under the same ISO treatment concentration. This study found that with the same ISO treatment concentration, decreased ROS accumulation in normal gastric GES–1 cells as ISO treatment time increased, but ROS accumulation in AGS cells continued to increase. This study also found that ISO induced AGS cell apoptosis by the up–regulation of ROS, activated p38 and JNK signaling pathways, and inhibited ERK, STAT3, and NF–κB signaling pathways (Figure 4).

When a cell becomes cancerous, the host loses control of the cell cycle. Therefore, the principle of cell cycle regulation can be used in tumor treatment to block the cycling of cancer cells, thereby preventing the metastasis and spread of cancer cells and, at the same time, inducing tumor cell apoptosis [34]. RT–PCR analysis showed that ISO significantly reduced gene transcription and Cyclin D, Cyclin E, and CDK 2 expression levels in HepG2 cells [19]. This study analyzed the cycle of AGS cells after ISO treatment by flow cytometry. It was found that ISO led to the G2/M cycle arrest of AGS cells through the accumulation of ROS (Figure 5).

The development of cancer is usually accompanied by rapid spread and invasion. Studies have shown that after the ISO treatment of pancreatic cancer cells, the expression levels of VEGF, MMP2, and MMP9 decreased, but the expression level of E–cadherin increased [35]. However, this study discovered that ISO inhibits AGS cell migration via modulating the AKT/GSK–3β/β–catenin signaling pathway and through regulating ROS generation (Figure 6).

In summary, through the ROS–mediated MAPK/STAT3/NF–κB and AKT signaling pathways, ISO triggered apoptosis and cell cycle arrest in AGS cells. ISO, on the other hand, reduced cell migration via ROS–mediated GSK–3β signaling pathways (Figure 7). Furthermore, ISO has the advantage of being less toxic to normal cells. Therefore, this study speculates that ISO could be a promising medication for the treatment of AGS.

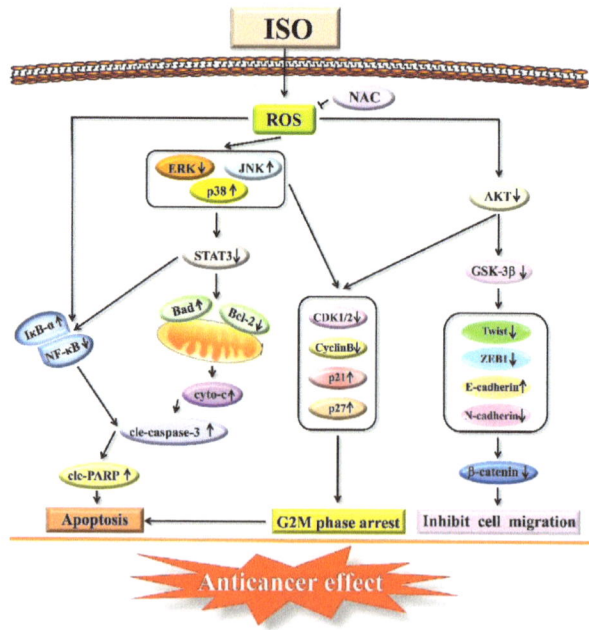

Figure 7. Schematic diagram of the signaling pathway of ISO in AGS cells to exert anti-cancer effects.

4. Materials and Methods

4.1. Cell Culture

Human gastric cancer cells and human normal lung cells were obtained from the American Type Culture Collection (ATCC, Manassas, VA, USA). Sage Biotechnology Co., Ltd. (Shanghai, China) provided the human normal gastric cells, liver cells, and renal cells. 10% FBS, 100 U/mL penicillin, and 100 µg/mL streptomycin in RPMI 1640 culture medium

(Gibco, Waltham, MA, USA) was used to culture a variety of cells, including gastric cancer cells (AGS, KATO–3, MKN–28, MKN–45, SNU–5, SNU–216, SNU–484, SNU–668), normal liver cells (L–02), and normal lung cells (IMR–90). Other gastric cancer cells, normal gastric cells (GES–1), and normal kidney cells (293T) were cultured in DMEM (Gibco) with the same contents. In sterile cell culture, all cells were cultured at 37 °C and 5% CO_2 in a SanYo incubator (Osaka, Japan).

4.2. Cell Viability Analyses

Four types of normal cells and twelve types of gastric cancer cells were seeded into 96–well plates (1×10^4 cells/well) and cultured overnight. They were treated with ISO and 5–FU (MedChem Express, Princeton, NJ, USA) at different concentrations for 24 h. The viability of the cells was determined using the Cell Counting Kit–8 (Solarbio, Beijing, China). Each cell was treated with 10 µL of a CCK-8 reagent for 3 h. Then, the results of the Microplate readers (BioTek Instruments Inc., Winooski, VT, USA) were used to calculate the half maximal inhibitory concentration (IC_{50}) value of the above-mentioned cells. Cell viability was determined by treating the cells with ISO and 5–FU IC_{50} values (0, 3, 6, 12, 24, and 36 h).

4.3. Cell Apoptosis Analysis

AGS cells were plated in 6–well dishes (1×10^5 cells/well) and cultured overnight. The cells were treated with 36.54 µM ISO and 36.54 µM 5–FU (the IC_{50} value of AGS cells) for 0, 3, 6, 12, and 24 h. Cell apoptosis was analyzed using the Apoptosis and Necrosis Assay Kit (Beyotime, Shanghai, China). A total of 200 µL of cell staining buffer, 3 µL of Hoechst, and 2 µL of PI were added. Cells were observed using the cell imaging system (Thermo Fisher Scientific, Shanghai, China). In addition, 100 µL of an Annexin V-binding buffer, 4 µL of Annexin V–FITC, and 3 µL PI were added to ISO–treated AGS cells, and flow cytometry (Beckman Coulter, Brea, CA, USA), and the cell imaging system was used.

4.4. Mitochondrial Membrane Potential Analysis

AGS cells were seeded in 3.5 cm Petri dishes (1×10^5 cells/dish) and cultured overnight. For 0, 3, 6, 12, and 24 h, the cells were exposed to 36.54 µM ISO. The JC–1 Assay Kit was used to assess the mitochondrial membrane potential of AGS cells (Solarbio). After centrifugation, AGS cells were collected and incubated with 1 mL JC–1 at 37 °C for 30 min. Then, AGS cells were suspended in a 1 mL binding solution two times and were detected by flow cytometry.

4.5. Extraction of Nucleoproteins

AGS cells were seeded into 3.5 cm Petri dishes and treated with 36.54 µM ISO for 0, 3, 6, 12, and 24 h. Samples were prepared with a Nuclear Protein Extraction Kit (Solarbio). Centrifugation was performed at 500 g for 2 min to separate the supernatant from the precipitation and was preserved for later use. A total of 100 mL of plasma protein extract was added to the precipitate and incubated with ice. After oscillation, they were centrifuged at 14,000 g at 4°C for 15 min, and 80 µL of nuclear protein extract was added to the precipitation. The supernatant was centrifuged again under the same conditions to prepare the sample.

4.6. Western Blot Analysis

AGS cells were seeded into 6 cm Petri dishes (6×10^5 cells/dish) and treated with 36.54 µM ISO for 0, 3, 6, 12, and 24 h. A 30 min centrifugation at 12,000 rpm and 4 °C was followed by mixing the supernatants with a 5× buffer and boiling them for five minutes. The OD value was measured at 595 nm with a spectrophotometer, and the protein concentrations were normalized. Proteins (20 µL per sample) were separated by 8–12% SDS–PAGE gel electrophoresis and were transferred to a nitrocellulose filtration membrane (NC membrane) and incubated with 5% skim milk for 2 h. The primary antibody was incubated overnight at 4 °C on the NC membrane. Santa Cruz Biotechnology (Dallas, TX, USA) provided all the primary antibodies. The primary antibodies used were Bad (1:1500; cat. no. sc–493), Bcl–2 (1:1500; cat. no. sc–7382), cyto–c (1:2000; cat. no. sc–13156), cle–caspase–3 (1:1500; cat. no. sc–373730), cle–PARP (1:1500; cat. no. sc–8007), α–tubulin (1:2500; cat. no. sc–47778), p–ERK (1:1500; cat. no. sc–7383), ERK (1:1000; cat. no. sc–154), p–JNK (1:1500; cat. no. sc–6254), JNK (1:1500; cat. no. sc–7345), p–p38 (1:1500; cat. no. sc–7973), p38 (1:1500; cat. no. sc–7149), p–STAT3 (1:1500; cat. no. sc–8059), STAT3 (1:1500; cat. no. sc–8019), NF–κB (1:1500; cat. no. sc–8008), IκBα (1:1500; cat. no. sc–1643), p–IκBα (1:1500; cat. no. sc–8404), Lamin B1 (1:2500; cat. no. sc–374015), p–AKT (1:1000; cat. no. sc–7985–R), AKT (1:1000; cat. no. sc–8312), CDK1/2 (1:1500; cat. no. sc–53219), Cyclin B (1:1500; cat. no. sc–245), p21 (1:1500; cat. no. sc–397), p27 (1:1500; cat. no. sc–528), p–GSK–3β (1:1000; cat. no. sc–373800), GSK–3β (1:1500; cat. no. sc–377213), Twist (1:1500; cat. no. sc–81417), ZEB1 (1:1000; cat. no. sc–515797), E–cadherin (1:1000; cat. no. sc–8426), N–cadherin (1:1000; cat. no. sc–59987), and β–catenin (1:1000; cat. no. sc–7963). Secondary antibodies (ZSGB–bio, Beijing, China) labeled with horseradish peroxidase were then added, and the NC blots were incubated at room temperature for 2 h before being combined with the enhanced chemiluminescence (ECL) substrate (Thermo Fisher Scientific). An Amersham Imager 600 (GE Healthcare, Beijing, China) was used to detect changes in protein expression. Protein relative densities were calculated using the Image J program. The endogenous controls were α-tubulin and Lamin B1. In addition, the protein content was determined by pretreatment with ERK inhibitors (FR180204, 10 μM), JNK inhibitors (SP600125, 10 μM), p38 inhibitors (SB203580, 10 μM) (MCE, Middlesex, NJ, USA), or reactive oxygen scavengers NAC (10 mM) (Beyotime) for 30 min prior to ISO treatment.

4.7. Measurement of ROS Generation

AGS cells and GES–1 cells were seeded in 3.5 cm Petri dishes and treated with 36.54 μM ISO for 0, 3, 6, 12, and 24 h, respectively. ROS levels in the AGS and GES–1 cells were measured using the ROS Assay Kit (Beyotime). The AGS cells were spun at 8000 rpm for 5 min before being treated with 10 μM of DCFH–DA fluorescent probe for 30 min. ROS accumulation in AGS and GES–1 cells was measured using flow cytometry. N–acetyl–L–cysteine (NAC, Beyotime) was given to AGS cells for 30 min before ISO treatment to assess the ROS accumulation in AGS cells.

4.8. Cell Cycle Analysis

AGS cells were plated in 3.5 cm dishes and treated with 36.54 μM ISO for 0, 3, 6, 12, and 24 h. The DNA Content Detection Kit (Solarbio) was used to examine the cell cycle. The AGS cells were collected and fixed in 70% alcohol overnight. The cell samples were incubated with 100 μL RNase for 30 min at 37 °C to eliminate RNA and were then stained with 400 μL of PI for 30 min at 4 °C and were detected by flow cytometry.

4.9. Cell Migration Analyses

AGS cells were plated in 6–well dishes and used a 10 μL pipette tip to perform a vertical swipe when the cells were confluent. After careful washing with PBS, 36.54 μM ISO was used to treat the AGS cells, and the cell migration at each moment was observed using an Auto Cell Imaging System (MSHOT, Guangzhou, China). Image J was used to calculate the migratory areas of the cells. In addition, AGS cells were plated in the upper chamber of the 6–well Transwell plate. A total of 36.54 μM ISO was used to treat the AGS cells; 0.1% crystal violet staining solution was added and washed with PBS. The number of cell migrations was observed and counted under a microscope.

4.10. Statistical Analysis

Three separate experiments were run, and the results are presented as the mean ± SD. GraphPad Prism 5.0 was used to determine the IC_{50} of ISO. Tukey's post hoc test was performed using SPSS version 21.0, and multiple comparisons across the groups were conducted using a one-way analysis of variance. Statistically significant differences are shown by the symbols * $p < 0.05$, ** $p < 0.01$, and *** $p < 0.001$.

Author Contributions: Conceptualization and writing—original draft preparation, T.Z.; writing—review and editing, Y.-H.X.; methodology, H.X. and Y.-N.L.; software, J.-L.C. and W.-S.H.; data analysis, J.L., Y.-H.C. and T.X.; supervision, Y.W. and C.-H.J. All authors have read and agreed to the published version of the manuscript.

Funding: This research was funded by the National Key Research and Development Project of China, grant number 2020YFD1001400, Program of HeiLongJiang BaYi Agricultural University, grant number XDB201818, the Central Government Supports Local College Reform, and Development Fund Talent Training Projects, grant number 2020GSP16, and Heilongjiang Touyan Innovation Team Program, grant number 2019HTY078.

Institutional Review Board Statement: Not applicable.

Informed Consent Statement: Not applicable.

Data Availability Statement: Data is contained within the article.

Conflicts of Interest: The authors declare no conflict of interest.

References

1. Shan, C.; Zhang, Y.; Hao, X.; Gao, J.; Chen, X.; Wang, K. Biogenesis, functions and clinical significance of circRNAs in gastric cancer. *Mol. Cancer* **2019**, *18*, 136. [CrossRef] [PubMed]
2. Wang, S.M.; Zheng, R.S.; Zhang, S.W.; Zeng, H.M.; Chen, R.; Sun, K.X.; Gu, X.Y.; Wei, W.W.; He, J. Epidemiological characteristics of gastric cancer in China, 2015. *Zhonghua Liu Xing Bing Xue Za Zhi* **2019**, *40*, 1517–1521. [PubMed]
3. Chen, W.Q.; Zheng, R.S.; Zhang, S.W.; Zeng, H.; Xia, C.; Zuo, T.; Yang, Z.; Zou, X.; He, J. Analysis of cancer incidence and mortality in elderly population in China, 2013. *Zhonghua Liu Xing Bing Xue Za Zhi* **2017**, *39*, 60–66.
4. Pilleron, S.; Sarfati, D.; Janssen-Heijnen, M.; Vignat, J.; Ferlay, J.; Bray, F.; Soerjomataram, I. Global cancer incidence in older adults, 2012 and 2035: A population-based study. *Int. J. Cancer* **2019**, *144*, 49–58. [CrossRef] [PubMed]
5. Wagner, A.D.; Syn, N.L.; Moehler, M.; Grothe, W.; Yong, W.P.; Tai, B.C.; Ho, J.; Unverzagt, S. Chemotherapy for advanced gastric cancer. *Cochrane Database Syst. Rev.* **2017**, *8*, CD004064. [CrossRef]
6. Créhange, G.; Huguet, F.; Quero, L.; N'Guyen, T.V.; Mirabel, X.; Lacornerie, T. Radiotherapy in cancers of the oesophagus, the gastric cardia and the stomach. *Cancer Radiothérapie* **2016**, *20*, S161–S168. [CrossRef]
7. Jiao, L.; Dong, C.; Liu, J.; Chen, Z.; Zhang, L.; Xu, J.; Shen, X.; Che, J.; Yang, Y.; Huang, H.; et al. Effects of Chinese Medicine as Adjunct Medication for Adjuvant Chemotherapy Treatments of Non-Small Cell Lung Cancer Patients. *Sci. Rep.* **2017**, *7*, 46524. [CrossRef]
8. Guo, H.; Liu, J.X.; Li, H.; Baak, J.P.A. In Metastatic Non-small cell Lung Cancer Platinum-Based Treated Patients, Herbal Treatment Improves the Quality of Life. A Prospective Randomized Controlled Clinical Trial. *Front. Pharmacol.* **2017**, *8*, 454. [CrossRef]
9. Li, A.; Qu, X.; Li, Z.; Qu, J.; Song, N.; Ma, Y.; Liu, Y. Secreted protein acidic and rich in cysteine antagonizes bufalin-induced apoptosis in gastric cancer cells. *Mol. Med. Rep.* **2015**, *12*, 2926–2932. [CrossRef]
10. Peng, J.; Fan, G.; Hong, Z.; Chai, Y.; Wu, Y. Preparative separation of isovitexin and isoorientin from Patrinia villosa Juss by high-speed counter-current chromatography. *J. Chromatogr. A* **2005**, *1074*, 111–115. [CrossRef]
11. Wedler, J.; Daubitz, T.; Schlotterbeck, G.; Butterweck, V. In vitro anti-inflammatory and wound-healing potential of a Phyllostachys edulis leaf extract–identification of isoorientin as an active compound. *Planta Med.* **2014**, *80*, 1678–1684. [CrossRef] [PubMed]
12. Da Silva, I.C.V.; Kaluđerović, G.N.; de Oliveira, P.F.; Guimarães, D.O.; Quaresma, C.H.; Porzel, A.; Muzitano, M.F.; Wessjohann, L.A.; Leal, I.C.R. Apoptosis Caused by Triterpenes and Phytosterols and Antioxidant Activity of an Enriched Flavonoid Extract from Passiflora mucronata. *Anticancer Agents Med. Chem.* **2018**, *18*, 1405–1416. [CrossRef] [PubMed]
13. Anilkumar, K.; Reddy, G.V.; Azad, R.; Yarla, N.S.; Dharmapuri, G.; Srivastava, A.; Kamal, M.A.; Pallu, R. Evaluation of Anti-Inflammatory Properties of Isoorientin Isolated from Tubers of Pueraria tuberosa. *Oxidative Med. Cell. Longev.* **2017**, *2017*, 5498054. [CrossRef] [PubMed]
14. Mykhailenko, O.; Petrikaite, V.; Korinek, M.; Chang, F.R.; El-Shazly, M.; Yen, C.H.; Bezruk, I.; Chen, B.H.; Hsieh, C.F.; Lytkin, D.; et al. Pharmacological Potential and Chemical Composition of Crocus sativus Leaf Extracts. *Molecules* **2021**, *27*, 10. [CrossRef]
15. Aljubiri, S.M.; Mahgoub, S.A.; Almansour, A.I.; Shaaban, M.; Shaker, K.H. Isolation of diverse bioactive compounds from Euphorbia balsamifera: Cytotoxicity and antibacterial activity studies. *Saudi J. Biol. Sci.* **2021**, *28*, 417–426. [CrossRef]
16. Bai, F.; Huang, Q.; Wei, J.; Lv, S.; Chen, Y.; Liang, C.; Wei, L.; Lu, Z.; Lin, X. Gypsophila elegans isoorientin-2″-O-α-l-arabinopyranosyl ameliorates porcine serum-induced immune liver fibrosis by inhibiting NF-κB signaling pathway and suppressing HSC activation. *Int. Immunopharmacol.* **2018**, *54*, 60–67. [CrossRef]
17. Czemplik, M.; Mierziak, J.; Szopa, J.; Kulma, A. Flavonoid C-glucosides Derived from Flax Straw Extracts Reduce Human Breast Cancer Cell Growth In vitro and Induce Apoptosis. *Front. Pharmacol.* **2016**, *7*, 282. [CrossRef]

18. Liu, S.C.; Huang, C.S.; Huang, C.M.; Hsieh, M.S.; Huang, M.S.; Fong, I.H.; Yeh, C.T.; Lin, C.C. Isoorientin inhibits epithelial-to-mesenchymal properties and cancer stem-cell-like features in oral squamous cell carcinoma by blocking Wnt/β-catenin/STAT3 axis. *Toxicol. Appl. Pharmacol.* **2021**, *424*, 115581. [CrossRef]
19. Lin, X.; Wei, J.; Chen, Y.; He, P.; Lin, J.; Tan, S.; Nie, J.; Lu, S.; He, M.; Lu, Z.; et al. Isoorientin from Gypsophila elegans induces apoptosis in liver cancer cells via mitochondrial-mediated pathway. *J. Ethnopharmacol.* **2016**, *187*, 187–194. [CrossRef]
20. Huang, D.; Jin, L.; Li, Z.; Wu, J.; Zhang, N.; Zhou, D.; Ni, X.; Hou, T. Isoorientin triggers apoptosis of hepatoblastoma by inducing DNA double-strand breaks and suppressing homologous recombination repair. *Biomed. Pharmacother.* **2018**, *101*, 719–728. [CrossRef]
21. Yuan, Z.F.; Tang, Y.M.; Xu, X.J.; Li, S.S.; Zhang, J.Y. 10-Hydroxycamptothecin induces apoptosis in human neuroblastoma SMS-KCNR cells through p53, cytochrome c and caspase 3 pathways. *Neoplasma* **2016**, *63*, 72–79. [CrossRef] [PubMed]
22. Sinha, K.; Das, J.; Pal, P.B.; Sil, P.C. Oxidative stress: The mitochondria-dependent and mitochondria-independent pathways of apoptosis. *Arch. Toxicol.* **2013**, *87*, 1157–1180. [CrossRef] [PubMed]
23. Nakagami, H.; Morishita, R.; Yamamoto, K.; Taniyama, Y.; Aoki, M.; Matsumoto, K.; Nakamura, T.; Kaneda, Y.; Horiuchi, M.; Ogihara, T. Mitogenic and antiapoptotic actions of hepatocyte growth factor through ERK, STAT3, and AKT in endothelial cells. *Hypertension* **2001**, *37*, 581–586. [CrossRef] [PubMed]
24. Xu, X.; Zou, L.; Yao, Q.; Zhang, Y.; Gan, L.; Tang, L. Silencing DEK downregulates cervical cancer tumorigenesis and metastasis via the DEK/p-Ser9-GSK-3β/p-Tyr216-GSK-3β/β-catenin axis. *Oncol. Rep.* **2017**, *38*, 1035–1042. [CrossRef]
25. Yan, Z.; Lai, Z.; Lin, J. Anticancer Properties of Traditional Chinese Medicine. *Comb. Chem. High Throughput Screen.* **2017**, *20*, 423–429. [CrossRef]
26. Wang, X.; Fang, G.; Pang, Y. Chinese Medicines in the Treatment of Prostate Cancer: From Formulas to Extracts and Compounds. *Nutrients* **2018**, *10*, 283. [CrossRef]
27. Wu, X.; Chung, V.C.H.; Lu, P.; Poon, S.K.; Hui, E.P.; Lau, A.Y.L.; Balneaves, L.G.; Wong, S.Y.S.; Wu, J.C.Y. Chinese Herbal Medicine for Improving Quality of Life Among Nonsmall Cell Lung Cancer Patients: Overview of Systematic Reviews and Network Meta-Analysis. *Medicine* **2016**, *95*, e2410. [CrossRef]
28. Ślefarska-Wolak, D.; Heinzle, C.; Leiherer, A.; Ager, C.; Muendlein, A.; Mezmale, L.; Leja, M.; Corvalan, A.H.; Drexel, H.; Krόlicka, A.; et al. Volatilomic Signatures of AGS and SNU-1 Gastric Cancer Cell Lines. *Molecules* **2022**, *27*, 4012. [CrossRef]
29. Xu, W.T.; Shen, G.N.; Li, T.Z.; Zhang, Y.; Zhang, T.; Xue, H.; Zuo, W.B.; Li, Y.N.; Zhang, D.J.; Jin, C.H. Isoorientin induces the apoptosis and cell cycle arrest of A549 human lung cancer cells via the ROS-regulated MAPK, STAT3 and NF-κB signaling pathways. *Int. J. Oncol.* **2020**, *57*, 550–561. [CrossRef]
30. Yuan, L.; Wang, J.; Xiao, H.; Xiao, C.; Wang, Y.; Liu, X. Isoorientin induces apoptosis through mitochondrial dysfunction and inhibition of PI3K/Akt signaling pathway in HepG2 cancer cells. *Toxicol. Appl. Pharmacol.* **2012**, *265*, 83–92. [CrossRef]
31. Blokhina, O.; Virolainen, E.; Fagerstedt, K.V. Antioxidants, oxidative damage and oxygen deprivation stress: A review. *Ann. Bot.* **2003**, *91*, 179–194. [CrossRef] [PubMed]
32. Wang, Y.; Qian, J.; Cao, J.; Wang, D.; Liu, C.; Yang, R.; Li, X.; Sun, C. Antioxidant Capacity, Anticancer Ability and Flavonoids Composition of 35 Citrus (Citrus reticulata Blanco) Varieties. *Molecules* **2017**, *22*, 1114. [CrossRef] [PubMed]
33. Yuan, L.; Wang, J.; Wu, W.; Liu, Q.; Liu, X. Effect of isoorientin on intracellular antioxidant defence mechanisms in hepatoma and liver cell lines. *Biomed. Pharmacother.* **2016**, *81*, 356–362. [CrossRef] [PubMed]
34. Wang, J.R.; Luo, Y.H.; Piao, X.J.; Zhang, Y.; Feng, Y.C.; Li, J.Q.; Xu, W.T.; Zhang, Y.; Zhang, T.; Wang, S.N.; et al. Mechanisms underlying isoliquiritigenin-induced apoptosis and cell cycle arrest via ROS-mediated MAPK/STAT3/NF-κB pathways in human hepatocellular carcinoma cells. *Drug Dev. Res.* **2019**, *80*, 461–470. [CrossRef]
35. Ye, T.; Su, J.; Huang, C.; Yu, D.; Dai, S.; Huang, X.; Chen, B.; Zhou, M. Isoorientin induces apoptosis, decreases invasiveness, and downregulates VEGF secretion by activating AMPK signaling in pancreatic cancer cells. *OncoTargets Ther.* **2016**, *9*, 7481–7492. [CrossRef]

Article

Antimicrobial Quantitative Relationship and Mechanism of Plant Flavonoids to Gram-Positive Bacteria

Ganjun Yuan [1,2,*], Xuexue Xia [1,2], Yingying Guan [2], Houqin Yi [2], Shan Lai [1,2], Yifei Sun [2] and Seng Cao [1,2]

[1] Biotechnological Engineering Center for Pharmaceutical Research and Development, Jiangxi Agricultural University, Nanchang 330045, China
[2] Laboratory of Natural Medicine and Microbiological Drug, College of Bioscience and Bioengineering, Jiangxi Agricultural University, Nanchang 330045, China
* Correspondence: gyuan@jxau.edu.cn; Tel.: +86-0791-83813459

Abstract: Antimicrobial resistance (AMR) poses a serious threat to human health, and new antimicrobial agents are desperately needed. Plant flavonoids are increasingly being paid attention to for their antibacterial activities, for the enhancing of the antibacterial activity of antimicrobials, and for the reversing of AMR. To obtain more scientific and reliable equations, another two regression equations, between the minimum inhibitory concentration (MIC) (y) and the lipophilicity parameter ACD/LogP or LogD$_{7.40}$ (x), were established once again, based on the reported data. Using statistical methods, the best one of the four regression equations, including the two previously reported, with regard to the antimicrobial quantitative relationship of plant flavonoids to Gram-positive bacteria, is $y = -0.1285\ x^6 + 0.7944\ x^5 + 51.785\ x^4 - 947.64\ x^3 + 6638.7\ x^2 - 21{,}273\ x + 26{,}087$; here, x is the LogP value. From this equation, the MICs of most plant flavonoids to Gram-positive bacteria can be calculated, and the minimum MIC was predicted as approximately 0.9644 µM and was probably from 0.24 to 0.96 µM. This more reliable equation further proved that the lipophilicity is a key factor of plant flavonoids against Gram-positive bacteria; this was further confirmed by the more intuitive evidence subsequently provided. Based on the antibacterial mechanism proposed in our previous work, these also confirmed the antibacterial mechanism: the cell membrane is the major site of plant flavonoids acting on the Gram-positive bacteria, and this involves the damage of the phospholipid bilayers. The above will greatly accelerate the discovery and application of plant flavonoids with remarkable antibacterial activity and the thorough research on their antimicrobial mechanism.

Keywords: flavonoid; lipophilicity; MIC; relationship; bacteria; cell membrane

1. Introduction

Antimicrobial resistance (AMR) has become a serious threat to the public health; meanwhile, the COVID-19 pandemic has further accelerated this global problem [1]. So, new antimicrobial agents are desperately needed [2,3]. After antibiotics have been used for the treatment of bacterial infection, most of them will also bring about some adverse reactions and eventually be resistant in the clinic [4]. However, some plant metabolites with moderate antimicrobial activities [5], being nontoxic to the human body, can enhance the antibacterial activity of some antibiotics, and even reverse the AMR [6,7]. Among them, plant flavonoids have received close attention [8–12]. Some of their structure–activity relationships against bacteria were summarized in various degrees [7,8,13,14], together with some sporadic ones [15,16]. In addition, the quantitative structure–activity relationship (QSAR) analyses for 30 prenylated (iso)flavonoids against *Listeria monocytogenes* and *Escherichia coli* were performed, respectively, with an accuracy of 71–88% [17]. However, a universal and systematic conclusion remains unclear due to the extensive structural diversity of plant flavonoids, and some of the conclusions are even contradictory [7,8,13,14].

In our previous work [18], two regression equations were established for calculating the antibacterial activities of plant flavonoids towards Gram-positive bacteria, based on the data pairs, consisting of the physicochemical parameter ACD/LogP or LogD$_{7.40}$ and the minimum inhibitory concentration (MIC, an indicator of antibacterial activity), of 66 reported flavonoids [19–24]. Subsequently, these two equations were further verified by the data pairs of another 68 reported flavonoids [6,25–30] and presented the accuracy of 85.3%. Combined with the literature analyses, it concluded that the lipophilicity is a key factor for flavonoids against Gram-positive bacteria and that the cell membrane is the major action site [18].

To obtain more scientific and reliable regression equations for the prediction of the MIC values of plant flavonoids, those data, as a greater sample, were reanalyzed, and two regression equations were reestablished. Using statistical methods, a regression equation with a larger correlation coefficient (r) of 0.9703 eventually proved to be the best one for fitting the correlation between the antibacterial activity (MIC) and the lipophilicity (LogP). This equation has shown to be more accurate and more reliable and can be practically considered as the quantitative relationship of plant flavonoids against Gram-positive bacteria. Moreover, the regression curves between the $\log_{10}$ (MIC) (y) and the LogP (or LogD$_{7.40}$) value (x) provide more intuitive evidence for the correlations between the antibacterial activity and the lipophilicity and for the antibacterial mechanism of the plant flavonoids acting on the cell membrane. The above are diagrammatically presented in Figure 1.

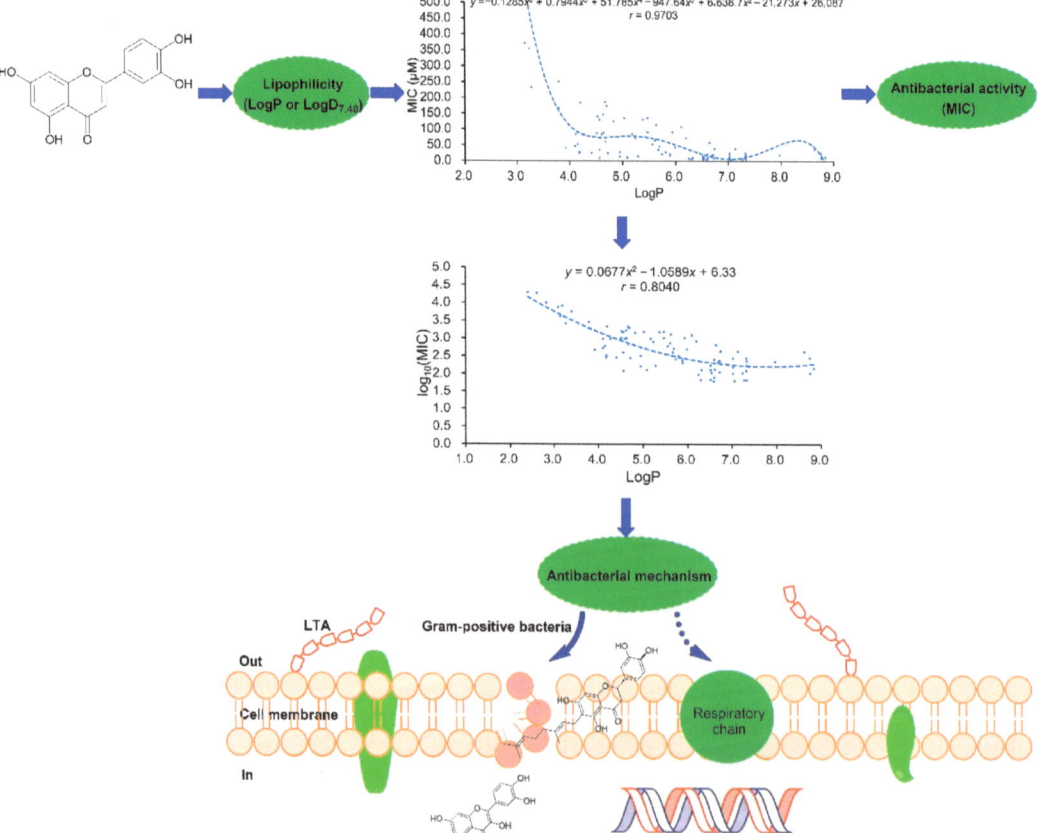

Figure 1. Diagrammatic presentation for the lipophilicity, the antibacterial activities, and the mechanisms of plant flavonoids. MIC, minimum inhibitory concentration; LTA, Lipoteichoic acid.

2. Results

2.1. Structure, Antibacterial Activity, and Physicochemical Parameters

The one hundred and thirty-four flavonoids published in the previous work [18], from twelve papers [19–30], were reorganized, and 92 compounds were screened out, according to the procedure in the methods section, for subsequent regression analyses. These flavonoids involve eleven subclasses, which mainly include flavones, dihydroflavones, flavonols, dihydroflavonols, isoflavones, dihydroisoflavones, dihydroisoflavane, and chalcones. The serial numbers of these compounds remain unchanged and correspond to those in the previous work [18]. Their physicochemical parameters (ACD/LogP and LogD$_{7.40}$) and antimicrobial activities (MICs) are listed in Table 1. If possible, the average MIC or MIC$_{90}$ of a certain flavonoid to different pathogenic bacteria was considered as its MIC. In other cases, the MIC of a certain flavonoid to pathogenic bacteria was processed according to the rules in the methods section.

Table 1. Plant flavonoids together with their structure types, physicochemical parameters, and antimicrobial activities, used for the regression analyses [18].

Compounds [a]	Structure Types	LogP [b]	LogD$_{7.40}$ [b]	MIC (μM) [c]	Log$_{10}$(MIC) [c]
2	Dihydroflavones	5.09	4.92	11.3	1.0531
3	Dihydroflavones	7.02	6.8	8.85	0.9469
4	Dihydroflavones	5.29	5.09	14.7	1.1673
6	Dihydroflavones	7.02	6.81	23.7	1.3747
7	Dihydroflavones	4.18	4.09	25.9	1.4133
8	Dihydroflavones	4.18	3.98	25.9	1.4133
9	Dihydroflavonols	5.74	5.5	22.7	1.3560
10	Dihydroflavones	6.52	6.33	5.9	0.7709
11	Dihydroflavones	6.30	6.08	5.7	0.7559
12	Dihydroflavones	7.05	6.83	5.5	0.7404
13	Dihydroflavones	7.27	7.09	5.7	0.7559
16	Dihydroflavones	7.24	7.06	9.15	0.9614
17	Dihydroflavones	4.56	4.37	10.5	1.0212
20	Dihydroflavones	5.56	5.34	52.8	1.7226
21	Dihydroflavones	6.54	6.32	9.15	0.9614
22	Dihydroflavones	6.61	6.39	11.35	1.0550
23	Dihydroflavones	5.18	4.96	85.05	1.9297
24	Dihydroflavonols	6.25	5.97	8.05	0.9058
25	Dihydroflavones	7.02	6.81	13.65	1.1351
26	Dihydroflavones	7.32	7.12	10.6	1.0253
27	Dihydroflavones	6.72	6.51	20.4	1.3096
28	Dihydroflavones	3.27	3.04	233.7	2.3687
29	Dihydroflavones	4.60	4.38	84.4	1.9263
30	Dihydroflavones	4.27	4.05	84.1	1.9248
31	Dihydroflavones	4.67	4.46	186.4	2.2704
32	Dihydroflavones	6.10	5.76	107.3	2.0306
33	Dihydroflavones	5.63	5.29	113.6	2.0554
34	Flavonols	4.52	3.84	140.2	2.1467
35	Flavonols	4.52	3.93	140.2	2.1467
36	Flavonols	6.20	5.53	73	1.8633
37	Dihydroflavones	6.72	6.51	9.5	0.9777
38	Dihydroflavones	7.32	7.12	14.75	1.1688
39	Dihydroflavones	8.75	8.54	24.45	1.3883
40	Dihydroflavones	7.32	7.13	24.6	1.3909
41	Dihydroflavones	5.94	5.75	90.8	1.9581
42	Dihydroflavones	7.97	7.78	19	1.2788
43	Dihydroflavones	6.74	6.50	37.9	1.5786
44	Dihydroflavones	8.84	8.64	12.25	1.0881
45	Dihydroflavonols	3.79	3.67	251.75	2.4010

Table 1. Cont.

Compounds [a]	Structure Types	LogP [b]	LogD$_{7.40}$ [b]	MIC (μM) [c]	Log$_{10}$(MIC) [c]
46	Dihydroflavonols	3.79	3.53	167.8	2.2248
47	Dihydroflavonols	3.92	3.59	42.1	1.6243
48	Dihydroflavonols	4.67	4.35	61	1.7853
49	Dihydroflavonols	4.11	3.67	84.5	1.9269
52	Dihydroflavonols	4.51	4.27	87.8	1.9435
53	Dihydroflavonols	2.42	2.11	1734.6	3.2392
54	Dihydroflavonols	4.64	4.34	88.3	1.9460
55	Dihydroflavones	6.52	6.33	11.05	1.0434
56	Dihydroflavones	8.76	8.70	9	0.9542
57	Dihydroflavones	4.72	4.51	24.25	1.3847
58	Dihydroflavones	6.52	6.33	14.7	1.1673
59	Dihydroflavones	5.89	5.67	17.75	1.2492
60	Dihydroflavones	5.89	5.68	21.3	1.3284
61	Dihydroflavones	6.60	6.35	22.05	1.3434
62	Dihydroflavones	5.81	5.62	28.4	1.4533
63	Dihydroflavones	5.81	5.62	28.4	1.4533
64	Dihydroflavones	4.56	4.37	35.1	1.5453
66	Dihydroflavones	3.19	2.96	734.6	2.8661
67	Flavones	4.20	3.77	184.7	2.2665
70	Flavonols	3.10	2.32	670.5	0.7597
72	Isoflavones	7.33	6.89	5.75	2.9485
73	Flavonols	2.83	2.16	888.1	1.5653
75	Dihydroflavonols	8.63	8.17	36.75	0.7284
76	Flavones	6.59	6.40	5.35	0.8325
77	Dihydroflavones	6.60	6.42	6.8	1.4518
81	Chalcones	4.95	4.82	28.3	1.1508
82	Chalcones	4.95	4.82	14.15	1.5502
86	Isoflavones	5.67	5.07	35.5	2.5715
87	Isoflavones	3.15	2.91	372.8	2.1166
88	Isoflavones	5.38	5.12	130.8	1.7239
89	Flavonols	4.15	3.48	52.95	1.0434
91	Dihydroisoflavane	6.32	6.32	11.05	1.4031
92	Dihydroisoflavane	4.41	4.4	25.3	1.4609
93	Dihydroisoflavane	4.18	4.18	28.9	1.7649
94	Other type	6.64	6.63	58.2	3.2186
97	Flavonols	2.62	1.95	1654.3	2.5505
113	Chalcones	3.23	3.10	355.2	2.6985
114	Chalcones	3.40	3.26	499.5	2.1318
115	Isoflavones	5.03	4.48	135.45	2.1649
116	Isoflavones	4.63	4.07	146.2	2.2399
118	Isoflavones	5.69	5.4	45.41	1.2940
119	Isoflavones	7.33	7.16	19.68	1.8510
120	Isoflavones	5.24	4.69	70.95	2.2398
121	Isoflavones	4.70	4.27	173.7	1.5786
122	Isoflavones	7.13	6.89	37.9	2.1149
123	Dihydroisoflavones	4.56	4.27	130.3	2.1318
124	Dihydroisoflavones	5.47	5.21	135.45	1.9557
125	Dihydroisoflavones	5.47	5.21	90.3	2.0964
126	Dihydroisoflavones	4.83	4.67	124.85	1.2765
127	Dihydroisoflavones	6.69	6.5	18.9	1.6375
128	Other type	5.99	5.98	43.4	2.5224
130	Other type	5.61	5.59	65.15	1.6721
133	Other type	4.10	4.10	47	0.7597

[a]: The chemical structures of flavonoids shown in previous work [18]. [b]: The LogP and LogD$_{7.40}$ values were calculated using software ACD/Labs 6.0. [c]: MIC, minimum inhibitory concentration; here, a processed MIC of a certain flavonoid to various Gram-positives, including *Staphylococcus aureus*, *S. epidermidis*, or/and *Bacillus subtilis*, etc., was presented; log$_{10}$(MIC) means log$_{10}$ of MIC.

2.2. Regression Equation between the MICs and the Physicochemical Parameters

The regression analyses for the MICs (y) to Gram-positive bacteria and the physicochemical parameters LogP or LogD$_{7.40}$ (x) of these flavonoids were achieved. Two regression curves are shown on Figure 2; their regression equations were established and are shown in Figure 2 and in Table 2, together with their correlation coefficients (r).

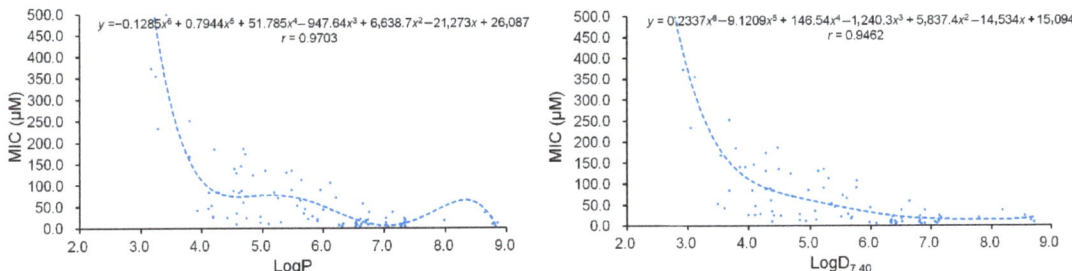

Figure 2. Polynomial regression analyses for the physicochemical parameter LogP or LogD$_{7.40}$ (x) and the MIC (y) to Gram-positive bacteria, mainly including *Staphylococcus aureus*, *S. epidermidis*, or/and *Bacillus subtilis* of 92 plant flavonoids.

Table 2. Regression equations for the correlation between the physicochemical parameter (x) and the antimicrobial activity (y) to Gram-positive bacteria of plant flavonoids [a].

Equation Number	Sample Numbers (n)	Parameters [b] (x)	Regression Equation (r [c])
(1)	92	LogP	$y = -0.1285 x^6 + 0.7944 x^5 + 51.785 x^4 - 947.64 x^3 + 6638.7 x^2 - 21{,}273 x + 26{,}087$ (0.9703)
(2)	92	LogD$_{7.40}$	$y = 0.2337 x^6 - 9.1209 x^5 + 146.54 x^4 - 1240.3 x^3 + 5837.4 x^2 - 14{,}534 x + 15{,}094$ (0.9462)
(3)	66 [d]	LogP	$y = -1.6745 x^5 + 56.143 x^4 - 741.93 x^3 + 4831.8 x^2 - 15{,}531 x + 19{,}805$ (0.9349)
(4)	66 [d]	LogD$_{7.40}$	$y = -1.1474 x^5 + 38.802 x^4 - 515.39 x^3 + 3361.9 x^2 - 10{,}789 x + 13{,}706$ (0.9309)

[a]: The antimicrobial activity (y) was the average MIC (or MIC$_{90}$) of a certain flavonoid to Gram-positive bacteria, mainly including *Staphylococcus aureus*, *S. epidermidis*, and *Bacillus subtilis*. [b]: The physicochemical parameter (x) was calculated using software ACD/Labs 6.0. [c]: r, correlation coefficient; the significant level α was set as 0.01, and the critical values of $r_{0.995}$ (90) and $r_{0.995}$ (64) were equal to 0.27 and 0.32, respectively. [d]: The regression equations were established in previous work [18].

From Figure 2, the characteristics of these two regression curves were similar to those established from the 66 flavonoids [18]. However, they presented larger r values (Table 2) and thereby indicated more significant correlations between the physicochemical parameter LogP or LogD$_{7.40}$ and the MIC of the plant flavonoids to Gram-positive bacteria, especially for that between the parameter LogP and the MIC, which presented the largest r value of 0.9703 (Table 2). Thereby, these two equations have a greater potency in proving that the antibacterial activities of plant flavonoids to Gram-positive bacteria are close related to their lipophilicities.

2.3. Antimicrobial Quantitative Relationship

Including the two regression equations reported [18], four regression equations were established for fitting the correlation between the antimicrobial activity (MIC) and the physicochemical parameter (LogP or Log D$_{7.40}$). To compare the goodness of fit, two statistical parameters, the coefficient of determination (R^2), and the residual standard deviation (s) were calculated, respectively, for these four equations and presented in Table 3. Generally, the closer the R^2 is to 1, the higher the goodness of fit and the closer the calculated value is, on the whole, to the actual one. The smaller s is, the smaller the mean deviation between the calculated value and the actual one. From Table 3, the largest value of the R^2 (0.9413) and the smallest value of s (68.1127) indicated that Equation (1) (Table 2) is the most reliable and the best one for fitting the quantitative relationship between the LogP and the MIC of the plant flavonoids to Gram-positive bacteria. Considering that the accuracy predicted from Equation (4) is approximately 85.3% [18], the above sufficiently indicated that that which is from Equation (1) has greater accuracy and is more than 85.3%, as it has a larger R^2 value and a far lower **s** value than Equation (4). Therefrom, the MICs (y) of most plant flavonoids to Gram-positive bacteria can be more accurately calculated from this equation by substituting their LogP values (x) (calculated by ACD/Labs 6.0).

Table 3. The goodness of fit of the regression equations [a].

Equation Number	Coefficient of Determination (R^2)	Residual Standard Deviation (s)	Goodness of Fit
(1)	0.9413	68.1127	The best one
(2)	0.8949	91.1187	The better one
(3)	0.8740	89.5452	—
(4)	0.8666	92.1391	—

[a]: Equations (3) and (4) were reported in previous work [18], and therefrom, the R^2 and s values were calculated from the 66 data pairs.

2.4. Regression Equation between the Log_{10}(MIC) and the Physicochemical Parameter

Based on the regression equations previously established and the literature analyses, the antibacterial mechanism of the plant flavonoids acting on the cell membranes of Gram-positive bacteria was proposed [18]. To more intuitively observe the correlation between the antibacterial activity and the lipophilic parameters, the regression analyses for the common logarithm (log_{10}) of the MIC (y) to Gram-positive bacteria and the LogP or LogD$_{7.40}$ (x) of these plant flavonoids were further performed. Their regression curves and regression equations, with the r values of 0.8040 and 0.8212, are shown, respectively, in Figure 3.

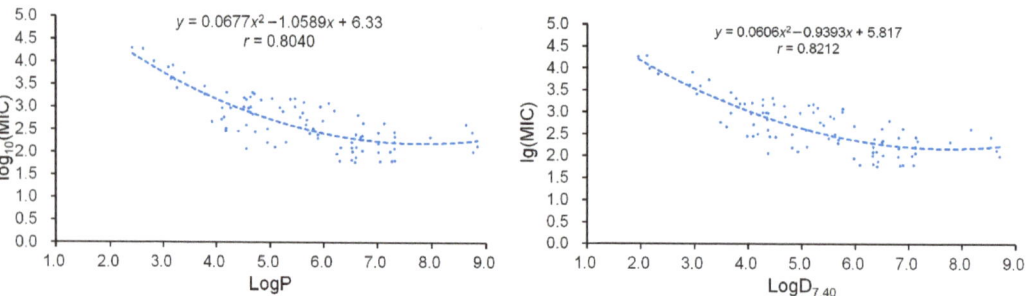

Figure 3. Regression analyses for the physicochemical parameter LogP or LogD$_{7.40}$ (x) and the log_{10}(MIC) (y) to Gram-positive bacteria of ninety-two plant flavonoids.

Both r values are greater than 0.27, which is the critical value when α is set at 0.01 and the sample number is ninety-two. This indicates that there is a very significant correlation between the log_{10}(MIC) and the LogP or LogD$_{7.40}$. Along with the increase of the LogP or LogD$_{7.40}$ value in an approximate range from 2.0 to 8.0, the log_{10}(MIC) value decreases, i.e., the antibacterial activity increases. These, more intuitively, demonstrated that the antibacterial activities of plant flavonoids to the Gram-positive bacteria are directly related to their lipophilicities.

3. Discussion

Flavonoids are an important class of secondary metabolites widely distributed in various parts of the plant, and so far, approximately 10,000 compounds have been discovered. These compounds have various bioactivities, such as antioxidation, antibiosis, an estrogen-like effect, and the prevention and treatment of cardiovascular diseases [6,31,32]. After some of them were discovered to have the potency to enhance the antibacterial effect of some antibiotics and/or even reverse the AMR [6,7], their antibacterial activities have been increasingly receiving close attention [8–12]. However, the antimicrobial activities of most flavonoids remain unknown after being discovered. Here, two equations between the lipophilicity (LogP or LogD$_{7.40}$) and the antimicrobial activity (MIC) were established and verified by r-test according to the statistical analyses. Comparing the goodness-of-fit of four equations, including the two reported ones [18], Equation (1) is the best one for calculating the MICs of plant flavonoids to Gram-positive bacteria, and the predicted accuracy is at least 85.3%. This equation can be widely used for many works related to the antimicrobial research of plant flavonoids: (1) the antimicrobial MICs of a larger amount of plant flavonoids already reported can be calculated and predicted, and therefrom, the plant flavonoids with the remarkable antimicrobial activity could be quickly screened from the flavonoids databases if one wanted; (2) based on the correlations between the lipophilicity and the antimicrobial activity and between the chemical structure and the lipophilicity, the antimicrobial activity can be quickly narrowed into a range after a compound is identified; (3) furthermore, the MIC values of the plant flavonoids to Gram-positive bacteria can be quickly predicted after they are isolated and identified, which would help to quickly target the desired one and simplify the MIC test; (4) as a good reference and guide, it will help to modify and optimize the chemical structure of plant flavonoids for potent antimicrobial agents; and (5) it can also provide a good reference for the structural modification and optimization of the plant flavonoids and reduce trial and error. All these will save a large amount of workload and human and material resources for the discovery of potent antimicrobial agents.

Based on the previous report [18], here the correlation between the ACD/LogP or LogD$_{7.40}$ values and the MICs to Gram-positive bacteria of the plant flavonoids was further proved by a larger sample (n = 92), and both r values of the two regression equations were, respectively, 0.9703 and 0.9462, larger than those previously published. Thereby, these more powerfully proved that there is a direct correlation between the lipophilicity and the antibacterial activity of plant flavonoids. The statistical analyses, including the calculation and comparison of R^2 and s (Table 3), concluded that equation (1), as $y = -0.1285\, x^6 + 0.7944\, x^5 + 51.785\, x^4 - 947.64\, x^3 + 6638.7\, x^2 - 21{,}273\, x + 26{,}087$, is the most scientific and reliable and is the best one. Specifically, the predicted value is more accurate and closer to the actual one, and/or the acceptable probability of the predicted MIC value is higher, at more than 85.3%, according to the same rule stating that the predicted MICs ranging from $1/4\times$ to $4\times$ the determined ones were acceptable [18]. More importantly, this equation was established from the data of eleven flavonoid subclasses, including seven main ones, while the equations previously reported were from those of three flavonoid subclasses. Thereby, the above together indicated that Equation (1) is more widely applicable and can be considered as the antimicrobial quantitative relationship of plant flavonoids to Gram-positive bacteria. Simultaneously, it can present an accuracy of approximate 94% (Table 3) according to the statistic principle, which is higher than the accuracy of 71–88% predicted from the QSAR of prenylated (iso)flavonoids against test bacterial isolates [17]. Moreover, Equation (1) can be at least used for the MIC calculation of eleven flavonoid subclasses against most Gram-positive bacteria, while the QSAR can only be used for that of prenylated (iso)flavonoids against two bacterial isolates.

In addition, here the correlations between the ACD/LogP or LogD$_{7.40}$ values and the MICs to Gram-positive bacteria of plant flavonoids were further proved by a lager sample (n = 92), and both r values (0.9703 and 0.9462) of the two regression equations were larger than those previously published. Thereby, both of the two equations were better and more scientific in proving that there is a direct correlation between the lipophilicity and the antibacterial activity of plant flavonoids. The statistical evaluation procedure, including the calculation and comparison of R^2 and s (Table 3), concluded that Equation (1), as $y = -0.1285\, x^6 + 0.7944\, x^5 + 51.785\, x^4 - 947.64\, x^3 + 6638.7\, x^2 - 21{,}273\, x + 26{,}087$, between the LogP value (x) and the MICs (y), is the most reliable and the best one. More importantly, this equation was established on the data of eleven subclasses of flavonoids, including seven main subclasses, while those previously published were generated from the data of three subclasses of flavonoids. Thereby, the above together indicated that Equation (1) is more scientific, reliable, and universal and can be considered as the antimicrobial quantitative relationship of plant flavonoids to Gram-positive bacteria.

As many factors involving the methods and details of the MIC test may have an influence on the experimental MIC value, the antibacterial activities of a compound to different pathogens are usually varied [18]. Therefore, the tested MICs would fluctuate within a reasonable range, especially from $1/2\times$ to $2\times$ the actual values [18], since the MICs were generally tested by the double dilution method. Simultaneously, the LogP value calculated by soft ACD/Labs 6.0 generally presents as a range. Thereby, the determined MICs would probably range from $1/2\times$ to $2\times$ the predicted one or more probably from $1/4\times$ to $4\times$ the predicted one. Based on these, the MIC (more accurately, MIC_{90}) for a certain compound of flavonoids to Gram-positive bacteria can be calculated by substituting its ACD/LogP value (x) into Equation (1). Furthermore, the minimum MIC of plant flavonoids to Gram-positive bacteria can be predicted as approximately 0.9644 μM, and at this time, the LogP value is equal to about 7.055. Considering that the experimental MICs would fluctuate, the minimum MIC tested would more probably range from 0.24 to 0.96 μM.

The MICs of most plant flavonoids to Gram-positive bacteria can be correctly calculated from this equation, even if those flavonoid subclasses were not included when Equation (1) was established. For example, the MIC of α-mangostin, a xanthone from mangosteen, against Gram-positive bacteria was calculated as 8.16 μM (3.35 μg/mL), and so, it is deduced that the MICs tested would fall into the range from 0.84 to 13.4 μg/mL. This is, by and large, consistent with the determined MIC value of 1 or 0.5 μg/mL (0.5 μg/mL for MIC_{90}) [33] and is also approved by the antibacterial tests repeated by two students at different times on S. aureus ATCC 25923 in our laboratory (0.5, 1 or 2 μg/mL for the MICs). Of course, a few of the plant flavonoids, such as baicalein, a rare 5,6,7-trihydroxyl flavonoid from *Scutellaria baicalensis*, probably present incorrect predictions [34]. However, the structural modification of baicalein for increasing the lipophilicity of molecules will increase the antibacterial activity [35]. This indicated that the correlation between the antibacterial activity and the lipophilicity is also suitable for baicalein, an ortho-trihydroxyl flavonoid.

As there were few data pairs in the LogP value range from 7.4 to 8.9 (Figure 2), the reliability of the calculation is possibly lower at this moment. It was already confirmed that the lipophilicity is a key factor of plant flavonoids against Gram-positive bacteria [18], while the influence of the dissociative state of plant flavonoids on their lipophilicities would gradually increase, along with the increase in the lipophilicity of plant flavonoids. Thereby, the $LogD_{7.40}$, as the LogP at pH 7.40, is better to reflect the actual state of a compound in the medium of MIC determination, especially when the LogP value is large enough. Considering this, the parameter $LogD_{7.40}$ should be more scientific and reliable than the LogP for fitting the correlation between the lipophilicity and the MIC, when the LogP value is more than 7.4. This was also supported by the change tendency of the two regression curves and the data pairs of the LogP values from 7.4 to 8.9 (Figure 2), as it is less possible for the regression curve to appear to drop twice according to the antimicrobial mechanism of plant flavonoids, especially when there is already a concave curve with a similar goodness of fit between the $LogD_{7.40}$ and the MIC. Thereby, it should be more accurate to calculate the MIC values from the $LogD_{7.40}$ values using Equation (2), when the LogP values range from 7.4 to 8.9. It is probable that when the LogP values of the plant flavonoids are more than 8.9, this equation can be still used for the crude calculation for their MIC values against the Gram-positive pathogenic bacteria.

Similar to previous analyses [18], according to a similar procedure, the more reliable regression equations for a certain subclass of flavonoids, with a larger r value, can also established for the more accurate calculations for the MICs and for the structural modification and optimization of the plant flavonoids. It is worth noting that this equation is not necessarily suitable for the antibacterial calculation of all structural derivatives from plant flavonoids, especially those introducing heteroatoms, such as nitrogen and halogen.

In addition, there are some differences among the LogP or LogD$_{7.40}$ values calculated by various software. As the LogP or LogD$_{7.40}$ values in the equations were calculated by software ACD/Labs 6.0, both the lipophilic parameters must be calculated by the software ACD/Labs 6.0 (or updated edition) when the equations are applied. As previously reported [18], the correlations between the MIC and the LogP were not so significant and reliable if the LogP was calculated by ChemBioDraw Ultra 12.0 (CambridgeSoft Corporation, USA). Although the calculations of the lipophilic parameters are relatively mature, it is worth noting that some factors were still not considered, such as the stereochemistries of the chiral centers. Fortunately, plant flavonoids have few chiral centers, except for their pyran or furan rings, if they have even them, on which the chiral centers generally present identical stereochemistries. Thereby, the influence from some factors not considered will be reduced.

To better apply the antimicrobial quantitative relationship in practice, the main relationships between the lipophilicity (LogP) and the structure of the plant flavonoids, together with their consistency with some of the structure–activity relationships of the reported plant flavonoids [7,8,13–17], are presented in Table 4, in which some novel structure–activity relationships are also proposed. As everyone knows, the lipophilicity is influenced by many factors, such as the molecular structure and the pH environment, and the former also includes various substituent groups and their positions, etc. Some main factors contributed to the lipophilicity of the plant flavonoids, including the structural skeleton ring C, the hydroxyl groups, and the isopentenyl chains, and are presented in Table 4. Among them, the introduction of isopentenyl groups into rings A or B is the most important one, and it can remarkably enhance the LogP value and lead to the increase in the antimicrobial activity. Usually, this would mask the influences from other factors. However, the LogP value would sharply reduce when the hydroxylation occurred for the double bond of the isopentenyl groups, and thereby, it is deduced that the antimicrobial activity would remarkably reduce. These are completely consistent with the experimental MICs reported [8,18] and can be considered as novel structure–activity relationships of plant flavonoids against Gram-positive bacteria (Table 4). It is likely that the above are responsible for the confused, unsystematic, and even contradictory structure–activity relationships (SARs) of the plant flavonoids [7,8,13–15], especially for the effect of hydroxyls at the structural skeletons and their methylations on the antibacterial activities of the plant flavonoids. Moreover, the numbers and subclasses of plant flavonoids used for the establishments of most reported SARs are different and limited, which might be another reason for the confused and even contradictory SARs. Conversely, this further confirmed that the correlation between the lipophilicity and the antimicrobial activity of plant flavonoids, being established from 92 flavonoids including eleven subclasses, is scientific and reliable.

It is worth noting that the lipophilicity reflects the comprehensive characteristics of the whole molecular structure, while the traditional structure–activity relationships usually describe the contribution of a certain group and its position in the molecular structure to the antibacterial activity. As plant flavonoids include many structural subclasses, it is very difficult to conclude the universal structure–activity relationships, and different subclasses generally present different structure–activity relationships. Thereby, the simple summary of the structure–activity relationship of plant flavonoids against pathogenic bacteria easily leads to confused or inappropriate conclusions and even some contradictory results. This was also confirmed by the structure–activity relationships summarized from different laboratories [7,8,13,14]. As concluded above, the lipophilicity is the key factor responsible for the antimicrobial activity of plant flavonoids, including various subclasses, and therefrom, a universal quantitative relationship can be established. Thereby, these differences from different laboratories would be likely eliminated, especially that stating that the predicted MICs ranging from 1/4× to 4× the determined ones were acceptable [18]. Furthermore, the more accurate MIC values can be predicted from the calculated ones, with the help of some of the structure–activity relationships reported in [7,8,13,14] and proposed in Table 4.

Table 4. The relationship between the structure and the lipophilicity (LogP) and some novel structure–activity relationships of plant flavonoids.

Structural Segment	Contribution for the Lipophilicity Parameter LogP Value	The Antimicrobial Structure–Activity Relationship of Plant Flavonoids
Structural skeleton (Ring C)	(1) The LogP value for Chalcones > dihydrochalcones, flavonols > flavones, dihydroisoflavones, dihydroflavones > isoflavones, dihydroflavonols. (2) When ring C is open, the LogP values remarkably increase, such as chalcones and dihydrochalcones.	Overall consistency with that reported [7,8,13,14].
Hydroxyl group	(1) The hydroxyl group substituting on ring A rather than ring B has greater contribution for the LogP value of flavonoids. (2) Generally, the contribution of hydroxyl groups substituting on ring A for the LogP value of flavonoids as: for flavones: 7-OH > 5-OH > 5,7-di-OH; for flavonols: 5-OH ≈ 7-OH > 5,7-di-OH; for chalcone, dihydrochalcones, dihydroisoflavones, dihydroflavones, isoflavones and dihydroflavonols: 5-OH > 5,7-di-OH > 7-OH. (3) Generally, the contribution of hydroxyl groups substituting on ring B for the LogP value of flavonoids as: 2′-OH ≥ 4′-OH (≈ 2′,4′-di-OH) > 3′,4′-di-OH (≈ 3′,4′,5′-tri-OH) > 2′,4′,5′-tri-OH > 2′,4′,6′-tri-OH. (4) The LogP values will be increased a little or remain unchanged when the hydroxyl groups are methylated.	(1) Uncertain. (2) and (3) Overall, the contributions of hydroxyl groups for antimicrobial activity were consistent with that reported [7,8,13,14], while the contributed sequence was not presented. A new SAR was proposed as follows: The hydroxyls will increase the antimicrobial activity, while the molecules must have enough lipophilicity. Otherwise, the increase in hydroxyl would reduce the antimicrobial activity. Namely, the molecular lipophilicity would likely mask the influences on antimicrobial activity from the hydroxyls. (4) Antimicrobial activity increases or not depending on the position of methylated hydroxyls and the structural subclass [7,13,14].
Isopentenyl chains	(1) The introductions of isopentenyl groups into the skeleton would remarkably increase the LogP values, while their substituted positions present no obvious influence on the LogP values. In addition, the number increase of isopentenyl units on structural skeleton will remarkably increase the LogP values. However, the dissociations of hydroxyls on structural skeleton will decrease along with the increase of isopentenyl units. (2) The introductions of the hydroxyl group into the isopentenyl side chain would sharply reduce the LogP values.	(1) Antimicrobial activity will remarkably increase, which is consistent with that reported [7,8,13,14]. However, a new SAR was proposed as follows: (1) the substituted positions of isopentenyl chains into the skeleton likely present no obvious influence on the antimicrobial activity; (2) the number increase of isopentenyl units on structural skeleton would increase the antimicrobial activity. However, too many isopentenyl units (usually, above 4) would lead to the slight decrease in antimicrobial activity. Both the above SARs were mainly summarized from the data of previous reports [18]. (2) Antimicrobial activity would sharply reduce, which was first summarized from the data of previous reports [18].

As a previous work suggested [18], the cell-membrane is the major site of plant flavonoids acting on Gram-positive bacteria and likely involves the disruption or damage of the phospholipid bilayers. This was further supported by recent reports [15,17,33]. Here, more reliable regression equations further proved that the lipophilicity is a key factor responsible for the antibacterial activity of plant flavonoids to Gram-positive bacteria. Combined with previous work [18], the regression analyses for the correlation between the $\log_{10}(MIC)$ and the LogP or $LogD_{7.40}$ more intuitively confirmed the antibacterial mechanism of plant flavonoids acting on the cell membrane of Gram-positive bacteria. As previously pointed out [18], many other antibacterial mechanisms were mentioned in recent reviews [6,8,10], while most experiments were performed for the influence on the in vitro determination of enzyme activities [36,37], the molecular docking of plant flavonoids with various synthases [36,38], and the proteomic change without the intracellular verification and the consideration of whether the chicken or the egg came first [39]. In addition, the authors concluded that some mechanisms other than DNA gyrase inhibition may play a role in the antibacterial activity of flavonoids [29]. Therefore, together with many previous works [15,17,18,33], it is undoubted that the cell membrane is the main region of plant flavonoids acting on Gram-positive bacteria and likely involves the disruption or damage of phospholipid bilayers or some others. Therefrom, the prior direction for clarifying the mechanism of flavonoids against Gram-positive bacteria is ascertained.

Recently, many antimicrobial mechanisms and SARs of plant flavonoids against Gram-negative bacteria have been reported [17,40,41]. As this research focused on the antimicrobial quantitative relationships and mechanisms of the plant flavonoids against Gram-positive bacteria, those of the plant flavonoids against Gram-negative bacteria were not discussed here. In addition, it can be deduced that there are likely to be different antimicrobial mechanisms for plant flavonoids against Gram-positive and Gram-negative bacteria.

Furthermore, as plant flavonoids belong to phenols, our laboratory tried to explore whether similar equations could be established for phenols and found that there are also similar correlations between their lipophilicities and their inhibitory activities towards Gram-positive bacteria. However, there is no extensive applicability for phenols as their structural diversity is too great. For some specific structural types of phenols, which one is the larger or the largest compound against Gram-positive bacteria can also be roughly deduced from their lipophilicities, such as abietane diterpenoids [42,43]. In addition, the anti-MRSA activities of trimethylhydroquinone and vitamin K_3 were successfully predicted and verified by our laboratory [44], referring to the initial assumptions of the above conclusions.

Based on the above, the antibacterial activity and mechanism of plant flavonoids against Gram-positive bacteria were diagrammatically presented in Figure 1, and some errors in Figure 9 of the published paper were incidentally corrected [8].

4. Materials and Methods
4.1. Data and Processing

Based on all the data on the plant flavonoids in the previous work [18], the data processing was reperformed. As no clear MIC value was presented for the many flavonoids used for the verification of the two regression equations in that paper [18], such as the MIC of compound **84** expressed as more than one hundred (>100 μM), these data were processed according to the following rules: (1) discard all the ambiguous data which the MICs expressed as more than a certain value; (2) for the MICs expressed as more than or equal to a certain value, the boundary value is considered as the MIC, such as the MIC for compound **69** as 636.4 μM; (3) for the MICs expressed as more than a range, the latter is considered as the MIC because it is a clear MIC value, such as the MIC for compound **73** as 888.1 μM; and (4) for the MIC expressed as a range, the average of the two boundary values is considered as the MIC because these two boundary values are the MICs of a certain flavonoid to different pathogenic strains, such as the MIC for compound **71** as 520.3 μM. Finally, based on the variation tendency of MIC, along with the lipophilicity parameters of LogP or LogD previously reported, and in view of the probable fluctuation at the determination of the MICs, the probable outliers were discarded using a scatter diagram. All the rest of the data were used as the data of this article for the subsequent analyses. The physicochemical parameter LogP or $LogD_{7.40}$ (the log_{10} of oil/water distribution coefficient at pH 7.40) was calculated using the software ACD/Labs 6.0 (Advanced Chemistry Development, Inc., Toronto, ON, Canada).

4.2. Regression Analyses

For establishing the antimicrobial quantitative relationship of plant flavonoids to Gram-positive bacteria, the regression analysis between the MICs (y) and the physicochemical parameter LogP or $LogD_{7.40}$ (x) was performed using Microsoft Excel software (Microsoft Corporation, USA), and the r value was also calculated. To discover more powerful evidence for supporting the antibacterial mechanism of plant flavonoids acting on the cell membrane of Gram-positive bacteria, the MIC was further transformed to the log_{10}(MIC), and subsequently, the regression analysis between the log_{10}(MIC) (y) and the physicochemical parameter LogP or $LogD_{7.40}$ (x) was further achieved.

4.3. Statistical Analyses

To ensure that one is the most reliable, further statistical analyses were performed for all the regression equations, including those reported in the previous paper [18]. In the process, two statistical parameters, the coefficient of determination (R^2), and the residual standard deviation (s) were calculated, respectively, according to Equations (5) and (6).

$$R^2 = 1 - \frac{\sum(y_i - \hat{y}_i)^2}{\sum(y_i - \overline{y})^2} \quad (5)$$

$$s = \sqrt{\frac{\sum(y_i - \hat{y}_i)^2}{n-2}} \quad (6)$$

where y_i is the MIC of a certain flavonoid i. Correspondingly, $\hat{y}_i$ is the predicted MIC of flavonoid i, $\overline{y}$ is the average MIC of all flavonoids in Table 1, and n (n = 92) is the number of all flavonoids.

When comparing the goodness of fit of these regression curves, the closer the R^2 is to 1, the higher the goodness of fit and the closer the predicted value is to the actual one, on the whole. The smaller s is, the smaller the mean deviation between the predicted value and the actual one. Generally, a consistent result will be presented from these two statistical parameters.

5. Conclusions

In conclusion, the MICs (y) of most plant flavonoids to Gram-positive bacteria can be calculated by substituting their physicochemical parameter ACD/LogP (x) into the equation $y = -0.1285\ x^6 + 0.7944\ x^5 + 51.785\ x^4 - 947.64\ x^3 + 6638.7\ x^2 - 21{,}273\ x + 26{,}087$. More reliable equations than before further proved that the lipophilicity is a key factor of plant flavonoids against Gram-positive bacteria, and more intuitive evidence powerfully confirmed the antibacterial mechanism, which is that the cell membrane is the major site of plant flavonoids acting on the Gram-positive bacteria and likely involves the damage of phospholipid bilayers. The above will greatly accelerate the discovery and application of plant flavonoids with remarkable antibacterial activity and accelerate the screening for the leading antibacterial compounds from the reported plant flavonoids. In addition, it can also provide a good reference for the structural modification and optimization of plant flavonoids if no heteroatom is introduced into their structures and can reduce trial and error. Simultaneously, all of the above provide good references for exploring the antibacterial activity and mechanisms of plant flavonoids against Gram-negative bacteria.

Author Contributions: Conceptualization, G.Y.; methodology, G.Y.; software, G.Y.; validation, G.Y.; formal analysis, G.Y.; investigation, G.Y., X.X., and Y.G.; resources, G.Y.; data curation, G.Y.; writing—original draft preparation, G.Y., X.X., Y.G., H.Y., S.L., Y.S., and S.C.; writing—review and editing, G.Y., H.Y., S.L., Y.S., and S.C.; visualization, G.Y.; supervision, G.Y.; project administration, G.Y.; funding acquisition, G.Y. All authors have read and agreed to the published version of the manuscript.

Funding: This work was financially supported by grants from the National Natural Science Foundation of China (No. 82073745 and 81960636) and the Natural Science Foundation of Jiangxi Province, China (Grant No. 20202BABL206156).

Institutional Review Board Statement: Not applicable.

Informed Consent Statement: Not applicable.

Data Availability Statement: The raw data of all compounds, which generated the data of Table 1 in this study, were reported by us in Springer Nature and are available from the link at https://www.nature.com/articles/s41598-021-90035-7 (accessed on 18 May 2021). All other data generated or analyzed during this study are included in this published article.

Conflicts of Interest: The authors declare no conflict of interest.

References

1. Murray, C.J.L.; Ikuta, K.S.; Sharara, F.; Swetschinski, L.; Aguilar, G.R.; Gray, A.; Han, C.; Bisignano, C.; Rao, P.; Wool, E.; et al. Global burden of bacterial antimicrobial resistance in 2019: A systematic analysis. *Lancet* **2022**, *399*, 629–655. [CrossRef]
2. Laxminarayan, R.; Sridhar, D.; Blaser, M.; Wang, M.; Woolhouse, M. Achieving global targets for antimicrobial resistance. *Science* **2016**, *353*, 874–875. [CrossRef]
3. Kurosu, M.; Siricilla, S.; Mitachi, K. Advances in MRSA drug discovery: Where are we and where do we need to be? *Exp. Opin. Drug Discov.* **2013**, *8*, 1095–1116. [CrossRef] [PubMed]
4. Xu, X.; Xu, L.; Yuan, G.; Wang, Y.; Qu, Y.; Zhou, M. Synergistic combination of two antimicrobial agents closing each other's mutant selection windows to prevent antimicrobial resistance. *Sci. Rep.* **2018**, *8*, 7237. [CrossRef] [PubMed]
5. Liang, M.; Ge, X.; Xua, H.; Ma, K.; Zhang, W.; Zan, Y.; Efferth, T.; Xue, Z.; Hua, X. Phytochemicals with activity against methicillin-resistant *Staphylococcus aureus*. *Phytomedicine* **2022**, *100*, 154073. [CrossRef] [PubMed]
6. Górniak, I.; Bartoszewski, R.; Króliczewski, J. Comprehensive review of antimicrobial activities of plant flavonoids. *Phytochem. Rev.* **2019**, *18*, 241–272. [CrossRef]
7. Farhadi, F.; Khameneh, B.; Iranshahi, M.; Iranshahy, M. Antibacterial activity of flavonoids and their structure-activity relationship: An update review. *Phytother. Res.* **2019**, *33*, 13–40. [CrossRef] [PubMed]
8. Xie, Y.; Yang, W.; Tang, F.; Chen, X.; Ren, L. Antibacterial activities of flavonoids: Structure-activity relationship and mechanism. *Curr. Med. Chem.* **2015**, *22*, 132–149. [CrossRef] [PubMed]
9. Tan, Z.; Deng, J.; Ye, Q.; Zhang, Z. The antibacterial activity of natural-derived flavonoids. *Curr. Top. Med. Chem.* **2022**, *22*, 1009–1019. [CrossRef]
10. Song, L.; Hu, X.; Ren, X.; Liu, J.; Liu, X. Antibacterial modes of herbal flavonoids combat resistant bacteria. *Front. Pharmacol.* **2022**, *13*, 873374. [CrossRef] [PubMed]
11. Wu, S.C.; Yang, Z.Q.; Liu, F.; Peng, W.J.; Qu, S.Q.; Li, Q.; Song, X.B.; Zhu, K.; Shen, J.Z. Antibacterial effect and mode of action of flavonoids from licorice against methicillin-resistant *Staphylococcus aureus*. *Front. Microbiol.* **2019**, *10*, 2489. [CrossRef] [PubMed]
12. Zhou, K.; Yang, S.; Li, S.M. Naturally occurring prenylated chalcones from plants: Structural diversity, distribution, activities and biosynthesis. *Nat. Prod. Rep.* **2021**, *38*, 2236–2260. [CrossRef]
13. Panda, L.; Duarte-Sierra, A. Recent advancements in enhancing antimicrobial activity of plant-derived polyphenols by biochemical means. *Horticulturae* **2022**, *8*, 401. [CrossRef]
14. Shamsudin, N.F.; Ahmed, Q.U.; Mahmood, S.; Ali Shah, S.A.; Khatib, A.; Mukhtar, S.; Alsharif, M.A.; Parveen, H.; Zakaria, Z.A. Antibacterial effects of flavonoids and their structure-activity relationship study: A comparative interpretation. *Molecules* **2022**, *27*, 1149. [CrossRef]
15. Echeverría, J.; Opazo, J.; Mendoza, L.; Urzúa, A.; Wilkens, M. Structure-activity and lipophilicity relationships of selected antibacterial natural flavones and flavanones of *Chilean flora*. *Molecules* **2017**, *22*, 608. [CrossRef]
16. Magozwi, D.K.; Dinala, M.; Mokwana, N.; Siwe-Noundou, X.; Krause, R.W.M.; Sonopo, M.; McGaw, L.J.; Augustyn, W.A.; Tembu, V.J. Flavonoids from the *Genus Euphorbia*: Isolation, structure, pharmacological activities and structure-activity relationships. *Pharmaceuticals* **2021**, *14*, 428. [CrossRef] [PubMed]
17. Araya-Cloutier, C.; Vincken, J.P.; van de Schans, M.G.; Hageman, J.; Schaftenaar, G.; den Besten, H.M.; Gruppen, H. QSAR-based molecular signatures of prenylated (iso)flavonoids underlying antimicrobial potency against and membrane-disruption in Gram positive and Gram negative bacteria. *Sci. Rep.* **2018**, *8*, 9267. [CrossRef] [PubMed]
18. Yuan, G.; Guan, Y.; Yi, H.; Lai, S.; Sun, Y.; Cao, S. Antibacterial activity and mechanism of plant flavonoids to gram-positive bacteria predicted from their lipophilicities. *Sci. Rep.* **2021**, *11*, 10471. [CrossRef]
19. Kuroyanagi, M.; Arakawa, T.; Hirayama, Y.; Hayashi, T. Antibacterial and antiandrogen flavonoids from *Sophora flavescens*. *J. Nat. Prod.* **1999**, *62*, 1595–1599. [CrossRef] [PubMed]
20. Šmejkal, K.; Chudík, S.; Klouček, P.; Marek, R.; Cvačka, J.; Urbanová, M.; Julínek, O.; Kokoška, L.; Šlapetová, T.; Holubová, P.; et al. Antibacterial C-geranylflavonoids from *Paulownia tomentosa* fruits. *J. Nat. Prod.* **2008**, *71*, 706–709. [CrossRef] [PubMed]
21. Navrátilová, A.; Schneiderová, K.; Veselá, D.; Hanáková, Z.; Fontana, A.; Dall'Acqua, S.; Cvačka, J.; Innocenti, G.; Novotná, J.; Urbanová, M.; et al. Minor C-geranylated flavanones from Paulownia tomentosa fruits with MRSA antibacterial activity. *Phytochemistry* **2013**, *89*, 104–113. [CrossRef] [PubMed]
22. Inui, S.; Hosoya, T.; Shimamura, Y.; Masuda, S.; Ogawa, T.; Kobayashi, H.; Shirafuji, K.; Moli, R.T.; Kozone, I.; Shin-ya, K.; et al. Solophenols B–D and solomonin: New prenylated polyphenols isolated from propolis collected from the solomon islands and their antibacterial activity. *J. Agric. Food Chem.* **2012**, *60*, 11765–11770. [CrossRef]
23. Sasaki, H.; Kashiwada, Y.; Shibata, H.; Takaishi, Y. Prenylated flavonoids from Desmodium caudatum and evaluation of their anti-MRSA activity. *Phytochemistry* **2012**, *82*, 136–142. [CrossRef] [PubMed]
24. Tsuchiya, H.; Sato, M.; Miyazaki, T.; Fujiwara, S.; Tanigaki, S.; Ohyama, M.; Tanaka, T.; Iinuma, M. Comparative study on the antibacterial activity of phytochemical flavanones against methicillin-resistant *Staphylococcus aureus*. *J. Ethnopharmacol.* **1996**, *50*, 27–34. [CrossRef]
25. Edziri, H.; Mastouri, M.; Mahjoub, M.A.; Mighri, Z.; Mahjoub, A.; Verschaeve, L. Antibacterial, antifungal and cytotoxic activities of two flavonoids from *Retama raetam* flowers. *Molecules* **2012**, *17*, 7284–7293. [CrossRef] [PubMed]
26. Sufian, A.S.; Ramasamy, K.; Ahmat, N.; Zakaria, Z.A.; Yusof, M.I.M. Isolation and identification of antibacterial and cytotoxic compounds from the leaves of *Muntingia calabura* L. *J. Ethnopharmacol.* **2013**, *146*, 198–204. [CrossRef]

27. Fukai, T.; Marumo, A.; Kaitou, K.; Kanda, T.; Terada, S.; Nomura, T. Antimicrobial activity of licorice flavonoids against methicillin-resistant *Staphylococcus aureus*. *Fitoterapia* **2002**, *73*, 536–539. [CrossRef]
28. Fukai, T.; Marumo, A.; Kaitou, K.; Kanda, T.; Terada, S.; Nomura, T. Anti-*Helicobacter pylori* flavonoids from licorice extract. *Life Sci.* **2002**, *71*, 1449–1463. [CrossRef]
29. Ohemeng, K.A.; Schwender, C.F.; Fu, K.P.; Barrett, J.F. DNA gyrase inhibitory and antibacterial activity of some flavones (l). *Bioorg. Med. Chem. Lett.* **1993**, *3*, 225–230. [CrossRef]
30. Hatano, T.; Shintani, Y.; Aga, Y.; Shiota, S.; Tsuchiya, T.; Yoshida, T. Phenolic constituents of Licorice. VIII. Structures of glicophenone and glicoisoflavanone, and effects of licorice phenolics on methicillin-resistant *Staphylococcus aureus*. *Chem. Pharm. Bull.* **2000**, *48*, 1286–1292. [CrossRef] [PubMed]
31. Chen, X.; Mukwaya, E.; Wong, M.S.; Zhang, Y. A systematic review on biological activities of prenylated flavonoids. *Pharm. Biol.* **2014**, *52*, 655–660. [CrossRef]
32. Veitch, N.C.; Grayer, R.J. Flavonoids and their glycosides, including anthocyanins. *Nat. Prod. Rep.* **2011**, *28*, 1626–1695. [CrossRef]
33. Song, M.; Liu, Y.; Li, T.; Liu, X.; Hao, Z.; Ding, S.; Panichayupakaranant, P.; Zhu, K.; Shen, J. Plant natural flavonoids against multidrug resistant pathogens. *Adv. Sci.* **2021**, *8*, 2100749. [CrossRef] [PubMed]
34. Qiu, F.; Meng, L.; Chen, J.; Jin, H.; Jiang, L. In vitro activity of five flavones from *Scutellaria baicalensis*in combination with Cefazolin against methicillin resistant *Staphylococcus aureus* (MRSA). *Med. Chem. Res.* **2016**, *25*, 2214–2219. [CrossRef]
35. Wang, S.; Chen, C.; Lo, C.; Feng, J.; Lin, H.; Chang, P.; Yang, L.; Chen, L.; Liu, Y.; Kuo, C.; et al. Synthesis and biological evaluation of novel 7-O-lipophilic substituted baicalein derivatives as potential anticancer agents. *Med. Chem. Commun.* **2015**, *6*, 1864–1873. [CrossRef]
36. Donadio, G.; Mensitieri, F.; Santoro, V.; Parisi, V.; Bellone, M.L.; de Tommaso, N.; Izzo, V.; Dal Piaz, F. Interactions with microbial proteins driving the antibacterial activity of flavonoids. *Pharmaceutics* **2021**, *13*, 660. [CrossRef] [PubMed]
37. Jeong, K.; Lee, J.; Kang, D.; Lee, J.; Shin, S.Y.; Kim, Y. Screening of flavonoids as candidate antibiotics against *Enterococcus faecalis*. *J. Nat. Prod.* **2009**, *72*, 719–724. [CrossRef] [PubMed]
38. Rammohan, A.; Bhaskar, B.V.; Venkateswarlu, N.; Rao, V.L.; Gunasekar, D.; Zyryanov, G.V. Isolation of flavonoids from the flowers of *Rhynchosia beddomei* Baker as prominent antimicrobial agents and molecular docking. *Microb. Pathog.* **2019**, *136*, 103667. [CrossRef]
39. Elmasri, W.A.; Zhu, R.; Peng, W.; Al-Hariri, M.; Kobeissy, F.; Tran, P.; Hamood, A.N.; Hegazy, M.F.; Paré, P.W.; Mechref, Y. Multitargeted flavonoid inhibition of the pathogenic bacterium *Staphylococcus aureus*: A proteomic characterization. *J. Proteome Res.* **2017**, *16*, 2579–2586. [CrossRef] [PubMed]
40. Mohamed, M.S.; Abdelkader, K.; Gomaa, H.A.M.; Batubara, A.S.; Gamal, M.; Sayed, A.M. Mechanistic study of the antibacterial potential of the prenylated flavonoid auriculasin against *Escherichia coli*. *Arch. Pharm.* **2022**, *27*, e2200360. [CrossRef] [PubMed]
41. Fang, Y.; Lu, Y.; Zang, X.; Wu, T.; Qi, X.; Pan, S.; Xu, X. 3D-QSAR and docking studies of flavonoids as potent *Escherichia coli* inhibitors. *Sci. Rep.* **2016**, *6*, 23634. [CrossRef] [PubMed]
42. Machumi, F.; Samoylenko, V.; Yenesew, A.; Derese, S.; Midiwo, J.O.; Wiggers, F.T.; Jacob, M.R.; Tekwani, B.L.; Khan, S.I.; Walker, L.A.; et al. Antimicrobial and antiparasitic abietane diterpenoids from the roots of *Clerodendrum eriophyllum*. *Nat. Prod. Commun.* **2010**, *5*, 841–992. [CrossRef]
43. Abdissa, N.; Frese, M.; Sewald, N. Antimicrobial abietane-type diterpenoids from *Plectranthus punctatus*. *Molecules* **2017**, *22*, 1919. [CrossRef] [PubMed]
44. Yuan, G.; Zhu, X.; Li, P.; Zhang, Q.; Cao, J. New activity for old drug: In vitro activities of vitamin K_3 and menadione sodium bisulfite against methicillin-resistant *Staphylococcus aureus*. *Afr. J. Pharm. Pharmacol.* **2014**, *8*, 364–371.

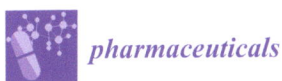

Review

Quercetin in the Prevention and Treatment of Coronavirus Infections: A Focus on SARS-CoV-2

Amin Gasmi [1], Pavan Kumar Mujawdiya [2], Roman Lysiuk [3,4], Mariia Shanaida [5], Massimiliano Peana [6], Asma Gasmi Benahmed [7], Nataliya Beley [5], Nadiia Kovalska [8] and Geir Bjørklund [9,*]

1 Société Francophone de Nutrithérapie et de Nutrigénétique Appliquée, 69100 Villeurbanne, France
2 Birla Institute of Technology and Science-Pilani, Hyderabad 500078, India
3 Department of Pharmacognosy and Botany, Danylo Halytsky Lviv National Medical University, 79010 Lviv, Ukraine
4 CONEM Ukraine Life Science Research Group, Danylo Halytsky Lviv National Medical University, 79010 Lviv, Ukraine
5 I. Horbachevsky Ternopil National Medical University, 46001 Ternopil, Ukraine
6 Department of Chemical, Physics, Mathematics and Natural Sciences, University of Sassari, 07100 Sassari, Italy
7 Académie Internationale de Médecine Dentaire Intégrative, 75000 Paris, France
8 Bogomolets National Medical University, 01601 Kyiv, Ukraine
9 Council for Nutritional and Environmental Medicine (CONEM), Toften 24, 8610 Mo i Rana, Norway
* Correspondence: bjorklund@conem.org

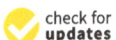

Citation: Gasmi, A.; Mujawdiya, P.K.; Lysiuk, R.; Shanaida, M.; Peana, M.; Gasmi Benahmed, A.; Beley, N.; Kovalska, N.; Bjørklund, G. Quercetin in the Prevention and Treatment of Coronavirus Infections: A Focus on SARS-CoV-2. *Pharmaceuticals* **2022**, *15*, 1049. https://doi.org/10.3390/ph15091049

Academic Editors: Fernando Calzada and Miguel Valdes

Received: 29 July 2022
Accepted: 20 August 2022
Published: 25 August 2022

Publisher's Note: MDPI stays neutral with regard to jurisdictional claims in published maps and institutional affiliations.

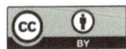

Copyright: © 2022 by the authors. Licensee MDPI, Basel, Switzerland. This article is an open access article distributed under the terms and conditions of the Creative Commons Attribution (CC BY) license (https://creativecommons.org/licenses/by/4.0/).

Abstract: The COVID-19 outbreak seems to be the most dangerous challenge of the third millennium due to its highly contagious nature. Amongst natural molecules for COVID-19 treatment, the flavonoid molecule quercetin (QR) is currently considered one of the most promising. QR is an active agent against SARS and MERS due to its antimicrobial, antiviral, anti-inflammatory, antioxidant, and some other beneficial effects. QR may hold therapeutic potential against SARS-CoV-2 due to its inhibitory effects on several stages of the viral life cycle. In fact, QR inhibits viral entry, absorption, and penetration in the SARS-CoV virus, which might be at least partly explained by the ability of QR and its derivatives to inhibit 3-chymotrypsin-like protease (3CLpro) and papain-like protease (PLpro). QR is a potent immunomodulatory molecule due to its direct modulatory effects on several immune cells, cytokines, and other immune molecules. QR-based nanopreparations possess enhanced bioavailability and solubility in water. In this review, we discuss the prospects for the application of QR as a preventive and treatment agent for COVID-19. Given the multifactorial beneficial action of QR, it can be considered a very valid drug as a preventative, mitigating, and therapeutic agent of COVID-19 infection, especially in synergism with zinc, vitamins C, D, and E, and other polyphenols.

Keywords: quercetin; coronavirus; COVID-19; infection; SARS-CoV-2; nanopreparations; prevention; treatment

1. Introduction

Coronaviruses are positive-sense RNA viruses belonging to the family Coronaviridae and fall under the Nidovirales order. Since the beginning of the 21st century, coronaviruses have caused some of the most lethal outbreaks across the globe. For example, the SARS outbreak of 2002–2003 and Middle East respiratory syndrome coronavirus (MERS-CoV) outbreaks were caused by coronaviruses with a lethality rate of 10% and 37%, respectively [1]. A new member of the coronavirus family, SARS-CoV-2, is responsible for COVID-19, a highly contagious disorder that affects the respiratory system and leads to death in severe cases. Although the death rate of COVID-19 is much lower (~3.4%) than those of SARS and MERS, the highly contagious global outbreak has made COVID-19 one of the most lethal infections. The disease was first reported in Wuhan, China, in December 2019 and spread rapidly worldwide within months. COVID-19 has been declared a global pandemic by the WHO, and the number of coronavirus cases and the number of deaths continue to rise inexorably with a series of contagion waves [2–4]. Individuals infected with SARS-CoV-2 show pneumonia-like symptoms and develop a dry cough, intense fever, lung damage and inflammation, and breathing difficulty. In severe cases, lung damage is extensive and irreversible, leading to death. SARS-CoV-2 is a member of the β-coronavirus family and shares 79.5% sequence homology with the SARS-CoV virus (responsible for the SARS outbreak). SARS-CoV-2 also shares 96% sequence homology with bat SARS coronavirus, indicating that the novel coronavirus may have originated in bats. Once SARS-CoV-2 enters the body, the spike proteins of the virus interact with angiotensin-converting enzyme 2 (ACE2) receptors of the human alveolar epithelial cells. This interaction facilitates the entry of the virus into the host cells [5]. Studies have shown that SARS-CoV-2 is more lethal in patients with previous chronic disorders, such as diabetes, cardiovascular disorders, and lung diseases [5]. The current median incubation period of SARS-CoV-2 is 5.2 days (range: 0–24 days), and the median time between the symptoms and death is 14 days [5]. Despite the severity of the disease, no cure for COVID-19 is available. Some coronavirus proteins are essential to viral entry and replication; among them, the most attractive targets for drug development are papain-like protease (PLpro), 3C-like protease (3CLpro), and spike protein (S) [6].

Several scientific groups across the globe have started exploring various natural molecules for COVID-19 treatment. One such small molecule is quercetin (QR), a flavonoid molecule found in many natural products, such as vegetables, fruits, herbs, and bee products. QR, an antiviral agent, has been found effective in both SARS and MERS treatments. The present review is an attempt to understand various biological, pharmacological, and immunomodulatory properties of QR, which may be beneficial in the prevention and treatment of COVID-19. In addition, will be discussed the synergic effect of QR in combination with micronutrients, vitamins, trace elements, or other polyphenols.

2. Quercetin Sources and Properties

The increasing interest in recent years in naturally occurring plant phytochemicals for the healing of various diseases is because they are generally less expensive and have fewer side effects than synthetic drugs. QR and several other natural polyphenols act as antioxidants, scavengers of ROS and other free radicals, and induce phase II detoxification enzymes [7,8]. QR is a hydrophobic citron-yellow crystal and plant-derived substance that has been subject to experimental validation to evaluate its characteristics and biological properties [9]. QR is one of the most ubiquitous flavonoid molecules. The characteristic feature of QR is the presence of five hydroxyl groups at positions 3, 5, 7, 3′, and 4′ with the electron-donating activity (Figure 1).

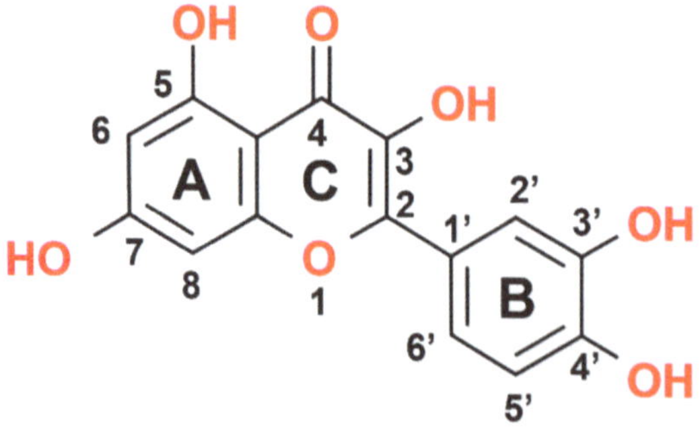

Figure 1. The structural formula of quercetin.

QR possesses several biological effects, including antioxidant, anti-inflammatory, antiviral, anticarcinogenic, cardioprotective, psychostimulant, and neuroprotective properties [9].

atherosclerosis in rabbits. One-month administration of QR decreased atherosclerotic lesion areas in the aorta [29]. In the same animal model, the QR derivative corvitin suppressed lipid peroxidation [30]. QR exhibited an antioxidant effect and a positive impact on endothelial function in patients with acute coronary syndrome with ST-segment elevation [31]. Treatment with QR-containing medicines positively affected hemodynamics and decreased about threefold the cardiac fibrosis area [32]. The anti-ischemic activity of intravenous QR in patients with ST-segment elevation myocardial infarction has been demonstrated [33].

4. Quercetin in Immunomodulation

QR is a potent immunomodulatory molecule due to its direct modulatory effects on several immune cells, cytokines, and other immune molecules. For instance, QR treatment reduces the expression of major histocompatibility complex (MHC) class II and other molecules that stimulate dendritic cells (DCs). DCs isolated from mouse bone marrow display reduced activation when administered with LPS. QR also decreases the LPS-induced migration of DCs. The reduction of DC activation reduces the antigen-specific activation of T-cells in the body [34,35]. The action of QR on immunity and inflammation is carried out by acting primarily on leukocytes and targeting different intracellular signaling kinases and phosphatases, enzymes, and membrane proteins [36].

Flavonoids exhibit numerous biological effects. In addition to antioxidant, anti-inflammatory, and antiviral properties, hepatoprotective and antiallergic properties have also been demonstrated [37]. The "cytokine storm", an increased release of tumor necrosis factor (TNF), interferon-gamma (IFN-γ), interleukins, and other cytokines, is one of the main characteristics of severe viral infections, including SARS and COVID-19 disease [1]. Flavonoids are considered promising anti-inflammatory therapeutic agents due to several studies on their in vitro inhibitory activity towards various inflammatory mediators, including cytokines [36]. QR shows potent immunomodulatory properties by inhibiting the expression of several proinflammatory cytokines and signaling pathways. Rogerio et al. demonstrated that treatment with QR-loaded microemulsion (QR-ME) (3 or 10 mg/kg) during a 22-day study reduced airway inflammation by decreasing the expression of IL-5 and IL-4. QR-ME also reduced the activation of the NF-κB inflammatory pathway and the expression levels of P-selectins [38]. QR (20 mg/kg/day, intraperitoneally) decreased hyperoxic lung injury in neonatal mice by reducing inflammation and enhancing alveolarization with an impaired degree of neutrophil and macrophage infiltration [39]. Another study by Stemberg et al. showed that QR modulates the activity of peripheral blood mononuclear cells (PBMCs) isolated from multiple sclerosis patients. QR treatment significantly reduced the PBMC proliferation dose-dependently and consequently reduced the expression levels of TNF-α and IL-1β. The modulating effect was more pronounced when QR was given in combination with IFN-β [40]. QR treatment also modulates the activity of cytokines, such as IL-4 and IL-5 secreted by Th2 cells.

Moreover, a reduction in specific immunoglobulin E (sIgE) levels was observed, leading to a reduced anaphylactic reaction. These immunomodulatory properties of QR are useful in alleviating asthma symptoms [41]. QR treatment in immunized mice increased B-cell proliferation under ex vivo conditions and enhanced the numbers of IgM-producing lymphocytes [42]. The immunomodulatory properties of QR were also evident in inflammatory responses induced by the influenza A virus. In such cases, QR treatment increased the secretion of IL-27 and reduced TNF-α expression [43]. A study by Zhang et al. demonstrated that QR possesses antifatigue properties, which is attributed to reduced TNFα expression and increased the expression of IL-10 in a strenuous exercise mice model [44]. The intake of QR is also beneficial in treating food allergy induced by peanuts by reducing the expression of immunoglobulin E responses [45]. QR also modulates the immune system by decreasing the expression of IL-4, inhibiting the activity of eosinophils, improving Th1/Th2 balance, and reducing the levels of leukotrienes and prostaglandins [45].

Its ability to inhibit free radicals, the cause of oxidative stress, can decrease the risk of metabolic disorders, cardiovascular diseases, and certain types of cancer [8,10].

Some common food ingredients rich in QR are apples, berries, grapes, citrus fruits, tea, many seeds, nuts, honey, propolis, and medicinal plants [11–14]. High QR content was evaluated in some commonly eaten vegetables in Japan. During the acquisition period in the summer of 2013, it was found that the content of QR was 30.6 mg/100 g in red leaf lettuce (*Lactuca sativa* L. var. *crispa*), 23.6 mg/100 g in asparagus (*Asparagus officinalis* L.), 12.0 mg/100 g in romaine lettuce (*Lactuca sativa* L. var. *longifolia*), 11.0 mg/100 g in onion (*Allium cepa* L.), and 9.9 mg/100 g in green pepper (*Capsicum annuum* L.), and 2.1 mg/100 mL of QR in green tea infusion [15]. QR was the most abundant phenolic compound in acacia honey samples, ranging from 123.5 to 240.2 µg/100 g of honey [16].

This flavonol is widely distributed in plants, primarily as water-soluble QR glycosides [12]. The QR and derivatives are stable in the stomach of the human body under the gastric acid influence; glucosides are hydrolyzed in the small intestine by brush border enzymes, such as lactase phlorizin hydrolase, beta-glucosidase enzyme to the aglycone form, and then absorbed [17,18]. Thus, before absorption into the enterocyte, sugars must be removed from the molecule [18].

3. Antioxidant, Anti-Inflammatory, and Antitumor Activities of Quercetin

Various research groups have reported the pharmacological properties of QR, such as antioxidant, anti-inflammatory, and antitumor properties. Due to these properties, QR is recommended for managing various disorders where oxidative stress, inflammation, and abnormal cell proliferation are major underlying causes. Zhang et al. observed that QR has a higher reduction potential than curcumin, comparable to the standard antioxidant Trolox. Moreover, QR reduced lipopolysaccharide (LPS)-induced production of reactive oxygen species and nitric oxide levels. The data indicated that QR is a powerful antioxidant and anti-inflammatory agent [14,19]. QR also increased the oxidative stress-fighting ability of the cells by stimulating the synthesis and expression of antioxidant enzymes, such as catalase, glutathione peroxidase, and superoxide dismutase. These enzymes' QR-induced expression protects the tissues from oxidative damage and injury [20]. Oxidative stress and inflammation are interlinked in the way that the presence of one of these phenomena induces the appearance of the other, and both are commonly observed in several chronic disorders, such as obesity, type 2 diabetes mellitus (T2DM), and cardiovascular disorders (CVDs) [21]. This indicates that reducing oxidative stress/inflammation profoundly alleviates the symptoms of chronic diseases, and consequently, QR can be used as a powerful therapeutic strategy to treat these chronic disorders [21]. QR inhibits inflammation by reducing the expression of the cyclooxygenase (COX) and lipoxygenase (LOX) enzymes. The inhibition of these enzymes by QR reduces the synthesis of leukotrienes and prostaglandins, critical mediators of inflammation in the body [22,23]. Another key marker of inflammation in the body is C-reactive protein (CRP), and elevated levels of CRP have been implicated in several disorders, such as obesity, T2DM, and CVDs. QR inhibits the levels of several proinflammatory molecules, such as nitric oxide, COX, and CRP in hepatocyte cell lines [24].

Moreover, in [25], a dose of 80 mg significantly reduced chronic inflammation and helped in cases of adjuvant-induced arthritis. QR is also a potent anticancer agent by promoting apoptosis in cancer cells (CT-26, LNCaP, MOLT-4, and Raji cell lines) and reducing the volume of tumors [26]. QR inhibits cancer cell proliferation, reduces neovascularization of tumors, induces apoptosis, and prevents tumor metastasis [27]. QR (100 µM) causes cell growth inhibition and halts the proliferation of human T leukemic lymphoblasts (Jurkat) [28].

Considering its potent antioxidant properties, QR is actively investigated as a promising substance for the prevention and treatment of CVDs [29]. QR contributes to a decreased incidence of stroke due to radioprotective characteristics mediated by its impact on proteasomal proteolysis, as demonstrated in an experimental model of cholesterol-induced polyphenols and vitamins shows a synergistic effect and helps the speedy clearance of the virus. The combination of QR and other polyphenols is a strategy to control the viral infection by attacking several targets simultaneously [77]. This combination also helps reduce the doses of flavonoids and polyphenols, thus diminishing the development of viruses resistant to drugs/natural compounds [77]. For example, a recent study by Aslam et al. demonstrated that a combination of various herbal extracts rich in flavonoids and polyphenols showed synergism and displayed improved antioxidant capacity and free radical scavenging potential [78].

Moreover, a combination of plants has been reported to treat viral infections causing respiratory tract, throat, skin, and nasal cavity [79]. Taken together, using QR in combination with other polyphenols and vitamins can be a better therapeutic choice than using them individually [75,80]. Using a specific and well-designed combination of polyphenols has the advantage of a high safety profile without causing significant side effects [81].

9. Quercetin in Combination with Other Polyphenols

Since SARS-CoV-2 is a novel coronavirus, no study reports a synergistic effect of QR with other polyphenols. However, the synergistic antiviral properties of QR are well documented in previous studies on other viruses. For example, QR synergistically affected herpes simplex virus type 1. In this study, a combination of QR (0.4 mM) and apigenin (0.4 mM) showed synergistic behavior in clearing the virus in the cell culture. It is important to highlight that synergistic action is observed only when both molecules act on different targets to inhibit virus growth. This leads to the inhibition of multiple molecular pathways or concurrent inhibition of targets leading to synergistic behavior [82]. In another study, a combination of QR, naringenin, and pinocembrin showed a synergistic effect in inhibiting canine distemper virus. The study reported that combining QR, naringenin, and pinocembrin before viral infection enhanced cell survival and inhibited CDV-NP gene expression [83]. Chiow et al. reported that a combination of QR and quercitrin at a 1:1 ratio displayed increased inhibition of the virus and lower cell cytotoxicity than using them individually. The study reported the synergistic antiviral behavior of QR in the DENV-2 virus [84]. A recent report on COVID-19 recommended several traditional Chinese medicinal plants/formulations where QR is one of the major constituents of the proposed formulation. As per the report, 26 herbs cataloged for treating respiratory infections (caused by viruses) may contain QR in combination with other flavonoids and polyphenols. For example, Shufeng Jiedu Capsule (SFJDC), a well-known formulation in traditional Chinese medicine (TCM), contains QR in combination with other polyphenols and flavonoids, such as rutin, kaempferol, liquiritigenin, liquiritin, resveratrol, emodin, and rhein. SFJDC is one of the recommended TCM formulations for the treatment of influenza in China [85].

Zhang et al. [6] conducted in silico screening of 125 species of TCM and found that several phenolics (QR, kaempferol, and lignin) may inhibit COVID-19 reproduction. Among the investigated constituents of 121 herbs in a study, luteolin and tetra-O-galloyl-β-d-glucose inhibited SARS-CoV entry into a host cell [66].

After the screening of thousands of potential antiviral phytoconstituents in a medicinal plant database, the following were found to be the most promising polyphenols for inhibiting SARS-CoV-2 3CL virus replication [86]: myricitrin, myricetin 3-O-beta-D-glucopyranoside, methyl rosmarinate, flavanone-3-O-beta-D-glucopyranoside, 5,7,3′,4′-tetrahydroxy-2′-(3,3-dimethylallyl) isoflavone, (2S)-eriodictyol 7-O-(6″-O-galloyl)-beta-D-glucopyranoside, and calceolarioside B. A phenolic aloe-emodin compound, isolated from *Isatis indigotica* root, dose-dependently inhibited the 3CLpro cleavage activity (IC_{50} = 366 mM) [87]. Yu et al. found in vitro that the flavonoids myricetin and scutellarein can inhibit the SARS-CoV helicase protein [88]. Glycosides of the flavonol kaempferol may be good antiviral agents for 3a channel proteins of coronaviruses [89].

The geranylated flavonoids tomentins (A, B, C, D, and E), isolated from the *Paulownia tomentosa* fruit extract, inhibited the papain-like protease of SARS-CoV [90]. Isobavachalcone and psoralidin in *Psoralea corylifolia* seeds also decrease the SARS-CoV papain-like protease activity [91]. Papyriflavonol from *Broussonetia papyrifera* extract was, in a study the most potent inhibitor of papain-like coronavirus cysteine proteases (IC_{50} = 3.7 µM) [92].

Cinnamomi cortex butanol extract demonstrated anti-SARS-CoV activities through several mechanisms due to the yield of different compounds or mixtures. Still, procyanidins were evaluated as the main constituents with such properties [93]. Unique compounds found among the green tea polyphenols were epigallocatechin-3-gallate and its lipophilic derivatives [94]. Fatty acid monoesters of epigallocatechin-3-O-gallate showed an antiviral effect against several viruses, probably due to their affinity for viruses and cellular membranes [95]. Investigation of the 3CL(Pro) inhibitory effect of extracts from seven different teas revealed that the polyphenol theaflavin-3,3′-digallate possesses this activity [96]. Besides QR, such flavonoids as luteolin, apigenin, kaempferol, amentoflavone, epigallocatechin, gallocatechin gallate, and epigallocatechin gallate were found as efficient blockers of the SARS-CoV 3CLpro enzymatic activity [97]. Ellagic acid proved to be the most potent 3CLpro inhibitor among numerous polyphenols tested by in silico molecular docking and molecular dynamics supported by in vitro assays [98]. According to Ryu et al. [99], after the fractionation of the *Torreya nucifera* leaf extract, a good SARS-CoV 3CL inhibitory activity was revealed by the biflavone amentoflavone (IC_{50} = 8.3 µM).

It has been observed that seriously ill patients with COVID-19 show pulmonary inflammation, and the pulmonary inflammation load score is higher in patients with an advanced stage of COVID-19 than in patients with a mild condition. Thus, reducing inflammation is a critical target for reducing the severity of COVID-19 [100]. A study by Heeba et al. demonstrated that a combination of QR and curcumin (both 50 mg/kg) showed synergistic behavior in reducing inflammation and oxidative stress in a rat model. The mixture was more effective in reducing inflammatory cytokine TNF-α, MDA (an indication of lipid peroxidation), and nitric oxide levels. Moreover, the combination increased heme oxygenase-1 levels and restored the levels of GSH, indicating reduced oxidative stress [101].

10. Quercetin in Combination with Vitamins and Trace Elements

Vitamins are essential for several physiological processes in the system and boost immunity. Using vitamins in combination with QR can alleviate the symptoms of COVID-19. Vitamin C is a potent antioxidant molecule and could be beneficial in reducing the symptoms of coronavirus. Several recent clinical trials on COVID-19 used vitamin C to treat infected patients. The RTC NCT04468139 is based on an approach of quadruple therapy including QR, vitamin C, zinc, and bromelain (https://clinicaltrials.gov/ct2/show/NCT04468139, accessed on 29 July 2022).

It has been reported that a higher level of intracellular zinc increases intracellular pH inhibiting SARS-CoV-2's RNA-dependent RNA polymerase, leading to damage to the virus replication mechanism [102]. QR as zinc ionophore helps increase intracellular zinc influx. The dietary supplement bromelain (a proteolytic enzyme from the pineapple plant) has been shown to diminish the expression of ACE2 and TMPRSS2 and to inhibit SARS-CoV-2 infection in Vero E6 cells [103]. In COVID-19, SARS-CoV-2-induced sepsis leads to a surge in the levels of proinflammatory cytokines, leading to increased accumulation of neutrophils in the lungs and further destruction of alveolar capillaries. Vitamin C cannot only prevent this accumulation, but it also does alveolar fluid.

Moreover, vitamin C prevents vascular injury by inhibiting the formation of neutrophil extracellular traps. Vitamin C also averts the common cold and protects against influenza [104]. Since COVID-19 patients show fever, cough, inflammation, and respiratory distress, a combination of vitamin C and QR can be useful in treating the disorder because both are potent antioxidant and anti-inflammatory molecules. Although QR is a ubiquitous flavonoid, and its dietary intake can be easily enhanced by changing nutritional habits, its lower absorption rate in the gastrointestinal tract limits its therapeutic effects. Normally, the absorption rate of QR in the intestine is between 30% and 50%, but a higher half-life of 25 h can help maintain the plasma levels of QR. It has been observed that vitamin C increases the absorption rate of QR in the intestine and elevates plasma QR levels [105].

Vitamin C also reduces flavonol's oxidative degradation, thus helping maintain higher plasma levels of flavonoids, such as QR [105]. Vitamin D is a major immunomodulatory vitamin and controls the immune system. Studies have established that vitamin D prevents respiratory distress by regulating the activity of the immune system and eliminating viral pathogens. It downregulates excessive cytokine secretion during viral infection and helps clear the pathogen [106]. These properties of vitamin D can be beneficial in combination with QR. In addition, QR shows synergistic behavior with vitamin E and protects against oxidative damage. The combination of QR and vitamin E reduces free radical damage and augments cellular defense against ROS [107]. In another observation, QR and vitamin E combination significantly reduced metal intoxication, particularly towards the nonessential cadmium [108,109]. Several studies have shown that combining QR and vitamins can synergistically increase the antioxidant capacity, reduce inflammation, and eliminate viral pathogens. These properties are beneficial in treating COVID-19, where oxidative stress, respiratory distress, and inflammation are important symptoms. However, further research in this direction is needed to explore the appropriate combinations and ratios of QR and vitamins.

11. Quercetin-Based Nanopreparations

Nanotechnology is a modern and promising area of science and technology that allows solving several problems in many fields, including medicine. The reduction of the particle sizes in the nanometer scale enhances their solubility, activity, and bioavailability [110,111]. Nanomaterials improve active principles' physical, chemical, and biological characteristics [112].

Due to poor bioavailability (low aqueous solubility and permeability) and instability in physiological media of QR, high doses of this substance are required for administration, which is the main limitation of its clinical application.

QR-based nanosystems, reducing hydrophobicity and increasing the bioavailability of the active ingredient, can have promising proficiency as antiviral agents. Several scientific studies apply various techniques to obtain QR formulations with enhanced bioavailability and water solubility [113–119]. A chemically and photostable QR nanosuspension with a significantly increased dissolution level was obtained by Gao and colleagues [113]. Poly(lactic-co-glycolic acid) nanoparticles loaded with QR were successfully tested on the human triple-negative breast (MDA-MB-231) and larynx epidermoid carcinoma (HEp-2) cell lines, revealing potent antiproliferative and cytotoxic effects on cancer cell lines [115]. Encapsulated in solid–liquid, QR exhibited a sustained QR release until 48 h and higher efficacy in inhibiting MCF-7 human breast cancer cells [118]. QR nanoparticles revealed activity towards mechanisms involved in amyloid-related diseases [116]. A more soluble and safe food-grade formulation of QR based on lecithin (quercetin phytosome) was recently developed. In comparison with QR alone, quercetin phytosome showed improved oral absorption with the detection of 20-fold exceeded QR in the plasma [119]. Several studies have reported that patients treated with QR phytosome supplementation have better clinical outcomes than those treated with standard therapy [120].

12. Conclusions

COVID-19 is a severe respiratory disorder caused by SARS-CoV-2. The disease is highly contagious and spreads quickly in the community through contagion waves. Since no cure for COVID-19 is available, several scientific groups worldwide have shifted their focus to finding treatment from natural sources. Natural substances have been found effective in treating SARS and MERS due to their inhibitory effects on virus entry, absorption, penetration, and replication. Quercetin, a flavonoid naturally occurring in fruits, vegetables, tea, medicinal plants, and bee products, is a potent antiviral drug molecule against SARS and MERS.

Consequently, it has been proposed as possibly useful for the COVID-19 cure. The potential beneficial effect of quercetin in the treatment of COVID-19 has been evaluated in recent case-control clinical studies that found its efficacy in inhibiting SARS-CoV-2. Quercetin shows multifactor beneficial action against SARS-CoV-2 to counterbalance the COVID-19 infection (Figure 2).

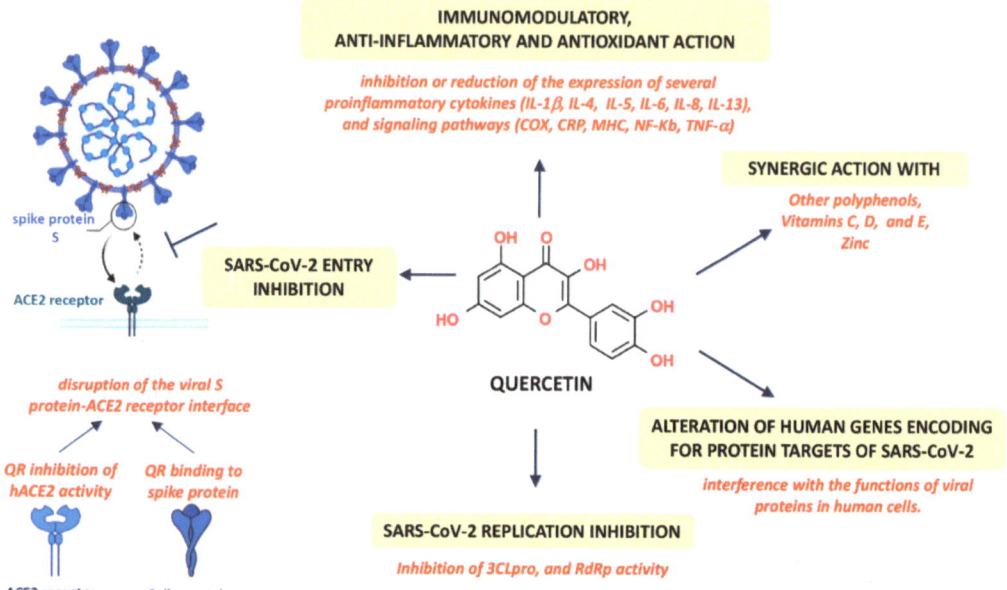

Figure 2. Beneficial multifactorial action of quercetin as a preventive, mitigative, and therapeutic agent of COVID-19 infection.

Quercetin showed inhibitory effects on several stages of the viral life cycle, from entry to replication. In particular, quercetin could directly bind the glycoprotein spike and inhibit the activity of ACE2, thus disrupting the viral–host recognition interface and preventing the SARS-CoV-2 entry. Quercetin can alter the expression of several human genes encoding protein targets of SARS-CoV-2, thus potentially interfering with the functions of the viral proteins in human cells. Quercetin inhibits viral replication by interfering with the activity of 3-chymotrypsin-like protease (3CLpro), papain-like protease (PLpro), and RNA-dependent RNA polymerase (RdRp). Moreover, quercetin possesses a wide spectrum of antioxidant, anti-inflammatory, and immunomodulation actions contributing to mitigating the disease consequences.

Besides quercetin, several phenolic compounds are prospective for treating COVID-19 infection. The efficacy of quercetin can be amplified with the synergism with these polyphenols and with the beneficial action of vitamins C, D, and E and zinc. Several clinical trials related to the monotherapy of quercetin and their compositions, including zinc, vitamin C, curcumin, vitamin D3, and drugs such as hydroxychloroquine, azithromycin, masitinib, and ivermectin, have been launched. Among the available results, the confirmation of the efficacy of some combinations tested for the prevention of COVID-19 is evident [121].

However, large well-designed RCTs of quercetin-based compositions are still needed to identify an effective COVID-19 treatment, considering the emerging SARS-CoV-2 variants. Further research will need to improve the bioavailability and solubility of quercetin and its drug combinations to improve the absorption rate.

Nanopreparations appear to be among the most promising solutions.

Author Contributions: Conceptualization, A.G., P.K.M., R.L., M.S., M.P., A.G.B., N.B., N.K. and G.B.; writing—original draft preparation, A.G., P.K.M., R.L., M.S., A.G.B., N.B. and N.K.; writing—review and editing, M.P. and G.B.; visualization, M.P.; supervision, G.B. All authors have read and agreed to the published version of the manuscript.

Funding: This research received no external funding.

Institutional Review Board Statement: Not applicable.

Informed Consent Statement: Not applicable.

Data Availability Statement: Data sharing not applicable.

Conflicts of Interest: The authors declare no conflict of interest.

References

1. Huang, C.; Wang, Y.; Li, X.; Ren, L.; Zhao, J.; Hu, Y.; Zhang, L.; Fan, G.; Xu, J.; Gu, X.; et al. Clinical features of patients infected with 2019 novel coronavirus in Wuhan, China. *Lancet* **2020**, *395*, 497–506. [CrossRef]
2. Zhou, Y.; Hou, Y.; Shen, J.; Huang, Y.; Martin, W.; Cheng, F. Network-based drug repurposing for novel coronavirus 2019-nCoV/SARS-CoV-2. *Cell Discov.* **2020**, *6*, 14. [CrossRef] [PubMed]
3. Worldmeters. COVID-19 Coronavirus Pandemic. Available online: https://www.worldometers.info/coronavirus/ (accessed on 22 July 2022).
4. Contreras, S.; Priesemann, V. Risking further COVID-19 waves despite vaccination. *Lancet Infect. Dis.* **2021**, *21*, 745–746. [CrossRef]
5. Wang, L.; Wang, Y.; Ye, D.; Liu, Q. Review of the 2019 novel coronavirus (SARS-CoV-2) based on current evidence. *Int. J. Antimicrob. Agents* **2020**, *55*, 105948. [CrossRef]
6. Zhang, D.H.; Wu, K.L.; Zhang, X.; Deng, S.Q.; Peng, B. In silico screening of Chinese herbal medicines with the potential to directly inhibit 2019 novel coronavirus. *J. Integr. Med.* **2020**, *18*, 152–158. [CrossRef]
7. Bjørklund, G.; Dadar, M.; Chirumbolo, S.; Lysiuk, R. Flavonoids as detoxifying and pro-survival agents: What's new? *Food Chem. Toxicol.* **2017**, *110*, 240–250. [CrossRef]
8. Chirumbolo, S.; Bjorklund, G.; Lysiuk, R.; Vella, A.; Lenchyk, L.; Upyr, T. Targeting Cancer with Phytochemicals via Their Fine Tuning of the Cell Survival Signaling Pathways. *Int. J. Mol. Sci.* **2018**, *19*, 3568. [CrossRef]
9. Davis, J.M.; Murphy, E.A.; Carmichael, M.D. Effects of the dietary flavonoid quercetin upon performance and health. *Curr. Sports Med. Rep.* **2009**, *8*, 206–213. [CrossRef]
10. Anand David, A.V.; Arulmoli, R.; Parasuraman, S. Overviews of Biological Importance of Quercetin: A Bioactive Flavonoid. *Pharm. Rev.* **2016**, *10*, 84–89. [CrossRef]
11. Zheng, Y.Z.; Deng, G.; Liang, Q.; Chen, D.F.; Guo, R.; Lai, R.C. Antioxidant Activity of Quercetin and Its Glucosides from Propolis: A Theoretical Study. *Sci. Rep.* **2017**, *7*, 7543. [CrossRef]
12. Li, Y.; Yao, J.; Han, C.; Yang, J.; Chaudhry, M.T.; Wang, S.; Liu, H.; Yin, Y. Quercetin, Inflammation and Immunity. *Nutrients* **2016**, *8*, 167. [CrossRef]
13. Jaganathan, S.K.; Mandal, M. Antiproliferative effects of honey and of its polyphenols: A review. *J. Biomed. Biotechnol.* **2009**, *2009*, 830616. [CrossRef]
14. Ozarowski, M.; Karpinski, T.M. Extracts and Flavonoids of Passiflora Species as Promising Anti-inflammatory and Antioxidant Substances. *Curr. Pharm. Des.* **2021**, *27*, 2582–2604. [CrossRef]
15. Nishimuro, H.; Ohnishi, H.; Sato, M.; Ohnishi-Kameyama, M.; Matsunaga, I.; Naito, S.; Ippoushi, K.; Oike, H.; Nagata, T.; Akasaka, H.; et al. Estimated daily intake and seasonal food sources of quercetin in Japan. *Nutrients* **2015**, *7*, 2345–2358. [CrossRef]
16. Stanek, N.; Kafarski, P.; Jasicka-Misiak, I. Development of a high performance thin layer chromatography method for the rapid qualification and quantification of phenolic compounds and abscisic acid in honeys. *J. Chromatogr. A* **2019**, *1598*, 209–215. [CrossRef]
17. Almeida, A.F.; Borge, G.I.A.; Piskula, M.; Tudose, A.; Tudoreanu, L.; Valentová, K.; Williamson, G.; Santos, C.N. Bioavailability of Quercetin in Humans with a Focus on Interindividual Variation. *Compr. Rev. Food Sci. Food Saf.* **2018**, *17*, 714–731. [CrossRef]
18. Day, A.J.; Canada, F.J.; Diaz, J.C.; Kroon, P.A.; McLauchlan, R.; Faulds, C.B.; Plumb, G.W.; Morgan, M.R.; Williamson, G. Dietary flavonoid and isoflavone glycosides are hydrolysed by the lactase site of lactase phlorizin hydrolase. *FEBS Lett.* **2000**, *468*, 166–170. [CrossRef]
19. Zhang, M.; Swarts, S.G.; Yin, L.; Liu, C.; Tian, Y.; Cao, Y.; Swarts, M.; Yang, S.; Zhang, S.B.; Zhang, K.; et al. Antioxidant properties of quercetin. *Adv. Exp. Med. Biol.* **2011**, *701*, 283–289. [CrossRef]
20. Xu, D.; Hu, M.J.; Wang, Y.Q.; Cui, Y.L. Antioxidant Activities of Quercetin and Its Complexes for Medicinal Application. *Molecules* **2019**, *24*, 1123. [CrossRef]
21. Biswas, S.K. Does the Interdependence between Oxidative Stress and Inflammation Explain the Antioxidant Paradox? *Oxid. Med. Cell Longev.* **2016**, *2016*, 5698931. [CrossRef]
22. Xiao, X.; Shi, D.; Liu, L.; Wang, J.; Xie, X.; Kang, T.; Deng, W. Quercetin suppresses cyclooxygenase-2 expression and angiogenesis through inactivation of P300 signaling. *PLoS ONE* **2011**, *6*, e22934. [CrossRef] [PubMed]

23. Warren, C.A.; Paulhill, K.J.; Davidson, L.A.; Lupton, J.R.; Taddeo, S.S.; Hong, M.Y.; Carroll, R.J.; Chapkin, R.S.; Turner, N.D. Quercetin may suppress rat aberrant crypt foci formation by suppressing inflammatory mediators that influence proliferation and apoptosis. *J. Nutr.* **2009**, *139*, 101–105. [CrossRef]
24. Yahfoufi, N.; Alsadi, N.; Jambi, M.; Matar, C. The Immunomodulatory and Anti-Inflammatory Role of Polyphenols. *Nutrients* **2018**, *10*, 1618. [CrossRef]
25. Garcia-Mediavilla, V.; Crespo, I.; Collado, P.S.; Esteller, A.; Sanchez-Campos, S.; Tunon, M.J.; Gonzalez-Gallego, J. The anti-inflammatory flavones quercetin and kaempferol cause inhibition of inducible nitric oxide synthase, cyclooxygenase-2 and reactive C-protein, and down-regulation of the nuclear factor kappaB pathway in Chang Liver cells. *Eur. J. Pharmacol.* **2007**, *557*, 221–229. [CrossRef]
26. Hashemzaei, M.; Delarami Far, A.; Yari, A.; Heravi, R.E.; Tabrizian, K.; Taghdisi, S.M.; Sadegh, S.E.; Tsarouhas, K.; Kouretas, D.; Tzanakakis, G.; et al. Anticancer and apoptosis-inducing effects of quercetin in vitro and in vivo. *Oncol. Rep.* **2017**, *38*, 819–828. [CrossRef]
27. Tang, S.M.; Deng, X.T.; Zhou, J.; Li, Q.P.; Ge, X.X.; Miao, L. Pharmacological basis and new insights of quercetin action in respect to its anti-cancer effects. *Biomed. Pharm.* **2020**, *121*, 109604. [CrossRef]
28. Seremet, T.; Dumitrescu, M.; Radesi, S.; Katona, G.; DoagĂ, I.; Radu, E.; HorvÁTh, J.; Tanos, E.; Katona, L.; Katona, E. Photobiomodulation of quercetin antiproliferative effects seen in human acute T leukemic Jurkat cells. *Rom. J. Biophys.* **2007**, *17*, 33–43.
29. Pashevin, D.A.; Tumanovska, L.V.; Dosenko, V.E.; Nagibin, V.S.; Gurianova, V.L.; Moibenko, A.A. Antiatherogenic effect of quercetin is mediated by proteasome inhibition in the aorta and circulating leukocytes. *Pharmacol. Rep.* **2011**, *63*, 1009–1018. [CrossRef]
30. Shysh, A.; Pashevin, D.O.; Dosenko, V.; Moibenko, O.O. Correction of lipid peroxidation and antioxidant system disorders by bioflavonoids during modeling of cholesterol atherosclerosis in rabbits. *Fiziol. Zh.* **2011**, *57*, 19–26. [CrossRef]
31. Lutai, Y.M.; Parkhomeko, O.; Ryzhkova, N.; Havrylenko, T.; Irkin, O.; Kozhukhov, S.; Stepura, A.; Bilyi, D. Effects of Intravenous 5-Lipoxygenase Inhibitor Quercetin Therapy on Endothelial Function, Severity of Systemic Inflammation and Oxidative Stress in Acute ST Elevation Myocardial Infarction. *Emerg. Med.* **2016**, *72*, 111–119. [CrossRef]
32. Kuzmenko, M.A.; Pavlyuchenko, V.B.; Tumanovskaya, I.V.; Dosenko, V.E.; Moybenko, A.A. Experimental therapy of cardiac remodeling with quercetin-containing drugs. *Patol. Fiziol. Eksp. Ter.* **2013**, *2*, 17–22.
33. Parkhomenko, A.; Kozhukhov, S.; Lutay, Y. Multicenter randomized clinical trial of the efficacy and safety of intravenous quercetin in patients with ST-elevation acute myocardial infarction. *Eur. Heart J.* **2018**, *39*, 10–1093. [CrossRef]
34. Verna, G.; Liso, M.; Cavalcanti, E.; Bianco, G.; Di Sarno, V.; Santino, A.; Campiglia, P.; Chieppa, M. Quercetin Administration Suppresses the Cytokine Storm in Myeloid and Plasmacytoid Dendritic Cells. *Int. J. Mol. Sci.* **2021**, *22*, 8349. [CrossRef] [PubMed]
35. Delvecchio, F.R.; Vadrucci, E.; Cavalcanti, E.; De Santis, S.; Kunde, D.; Vacca, M.; Myers, J.; Allen, F.; Bianco, G.; Huang, A.Y.; et al. Polyphenol administration impairs T-cell proliferation by imprinting a distinct dendritic cell maturational profile. *Eur. J. Immunol.* **2015**, *45*, 2638–2649. [CrossRef]
36. Chirumbolo, S. The role of quercetin, flavonols and flavones in modulating inflammatory cell function. *Inflamm. Allergy Drug Targets* **2010**, *9*, 263–285. [CrossRef]
37. Lysiuk, R.; Hudz, N. Differential spectrophotometry: Application for quantification of flavonoids in herbal drugs and nutraceuticals. *Int. J. Trends Food Nutr.* **2017**, *1*, e102.
38. Rogerio, A.P.; Dora, C.L.; Andrade, E.L.; Chaves, J.S.; Silva, L.F.; Lemos-Senna, E.; Calixto, J.B. Anti-inflammatory effect of quercetin-loaded microemulsion in the airways allergic inflammatory model in mice. *Pharmacol. Res.* **2010**, *61*, 288–297. [CrossRef]
39. Maturu, P.; Wei-Liang, Y.; Androutsopoulos, V.P.; Jiang, W.; Wang, L.; Tsatsakis, A.M.; Couroucli, X.I. Quercetin attenuates the hyperoxic lung injury in neonatal mice: Implications for Bronchopulmonary dysplasia (BPD). *Food Chem. Toxicol.* **2018**, *114*, 23–33. [CrossRef]
40. Sternberg, Z.; Chadha, K.; Lieberman, A.; Hojnacki, D.; Drake, A.; Zamboni, P.; Rocco, P.; Grazioli, E.; Weinstock-Guttman, B.; Munschauer, F. Quercetin and interferon-β modulate immune response(s) in peripheral blood mononuclear cells isolated from multiple sclerosis patients. *J. Neuroimmunol.* **2008**, *205*, 142–147. [CrossRef]
41. Gupta, K.; Kumar, S.; Gupta, R.K.; Sharma, A.; Verma, A.K.; Stalin, K.; Chaudhari, B.P.; Das, M.; Singh, S.P.; Dwivedi, P.D. Reversion of Asthmatic Complications and Mast Cell Signalling Pathways in BALB/c Mice Model Using Quercetin Nanocrystals. *J. Biomed. Nanotechnol.* **2016**, *12*, 717–731. [CrossRef]
42. Valentova, K.; Sima, P.; Rybkova, Z.; Krizan, J.; Malachova, K.; Kren, V. (Anti)mutagenic and immunomodulatory properties of quercetin glycosides. *J. Sci. Food Agric.* **2016**, *96*, 1492–1499. [CrossRef]
43. Mehrbod, P.; Abdalla, M.A.; Fotouhi, F.; Heidarzadeh, M.; Aro, A.O.; Eloff, J.N.; McGaw, L.J.; Fasina, F.O. Immunomodulatory properties of quercetin-3-O-alpha-L-rhamnopyranoside from Rapanea melanophloeos against influenza a virus. *BMC Complement Altern. Med.* **2018**, *18*, 184. [CrossRef]
44. Zhang, W.-q. Evaluation of anti-fatigue and immunomodulating effects of quercetin in strenuous exercise mice. *IOP Conf. Ser. Earth Environ. Sci.* **2017**, *61*, 012046. [CrossRef]
45. Mlcek, J.; Jurikova, T.; Skrovankova, S.; Sochor, J. Quercetin and Its Anti-Allergic Immune Response. *Molecules* **2016**, *21*, 623. [CrossRef]
46. Jaisinghani, R.N. Antibacterial properties of quercetin. *Microbiol. Res.* **2017**, *8*, 6877. [CrossRef]

47. Wang, S.; Yao, J.; Zhou, B.; Yang, J.; Chaudry, M.T.; Wang, M.; Xiao, F.; Li, Y.; Yin, W. Bacteriostatic Effect of Quercetin as an Antibiotic Alternative In Vivo and Its Antibacterial Mechanism In Vitro. *J. Food Prot.* **2017**, *81*, 68–78. [CrossRef]
48. Geoghegan, F.; Tsui, V.W.; Wong, R.W.; Rabie, A.B. Inhibitory effect of quercetin on periodontal pathogens. *Ann. R. Australas. Coll. Dent. Surg.* **2008**, *19*, 157–158.
49. Siriwong, S.; Teethaisong, Y.; Thumanu, K.; Dunkhunthod, B.; Eumkeb, G. The synergy and mode of action of quercetin plus amoxicillin against amoxicillin-resistant Staphylococcus epidermidis. *BMC Pharmacol. Toxicol.* **2016**, *17*, 39. [CrossRef]
50. Hirai, I.; Okuno, M.; Katsuma, R.; Arita, N.; Tachibana, M.; Yamamoto, Y. Characterisation of anti-Staphylococcus aureus activity of quercetin. *Int. J. Food Sci. Technol.* **2010**, *45*, 1250–1254. [CrossRef]
51. Wu, W.; Li, R.; Li, X.; He, J.; Jiang, S.; Liu, S.; Yang, J. Quercetin as an Antiviral Agent Inhibits Influenza A Virus (IAV) Entry. *Viruses* **2015**, *8*, 6. [CrossRef]
52. Nayak, D.P.; Hui, E.K.; Barman, S. Assembly and budding of influenza virus. *Virus Res.* **2004**, *106*, 147–165. [CrossRef] [PubMed]
53. Yao, C.; Xi, C.; Hu, K.; Gao, W.; Cai, X.; Qin, J.; Lv, S.; Du, C.; Wei, Y. Inhibition of enterovirus 71 replication and viral 3C protease by quercetin. *Virol. J.* **2018**, *15*, 116. [CrossRef] [PubMed]
54. Ganesan, S.; Faris, A.N.; Comstock, A.T.; Wang, Q.; Nanua, S.; Hershenson, M.B.; Sajjan, U.S. Quercetin inhibits rhinovirus replication in vitro and in vivo. *Antiviral. Res.* **2012**, *94*, 258–271. [CrossRef] [PubMed]
55. Qiu, X.; Kroeker, A.; He, S.; Kozak, R.; Audet, J.; Mbikay, M.; Chrétien, M. Prophylactic Efficacy of Quercetin 3-β-O-d-Glucoside against Ebola Virus Infection. *Antimicrob. Agents Chemother.* **2016**, *60*, 5182–5188. [CrossRef]
56. Wong, G.; He, S.; Siragam, V.; Bi, Y.; Mbikay, M.; Chretien, M.; Qiu, X. Antiviral activity of quercetin-3-β-O-D-glucoside against Zika virus infection. *Virol. Sin.* **2017**, *32*, 545–547. [CrossRef]
57. Derosa, G.; Maffioli, P.; D'Angelo, A.; Di Pierro, F. A role for quercetin in coronavirus disease 2019 (COVID-19). *Phytother. Res.* **2020**, *35*, 1230–1236. [CrossRef]
58. Pawar, A.; Pal, A. Molecular and functional resemblance of dexamethasone and quercetin: A paradigm worth exploring in dexamethasone-nonresponsive COVID-19 patients. *Phytother. Res.* **2020**, *34*, 3085–3088. [CrossRef]
59. Bastaminejad, S.; Bakhtiyari, S. Quercetin and its relative therapeutic potential against COVID-19: A retrospective review and prospective overview. *Curr. Mol. Med.* **2020**, *21*, 385–391. [CrossRef]
60. Aucoin, M.; Cooley, K.; Saunders, P.R.; Cardozo, V.; Remy, D.; Cramer, H.; Neyre Abad, C.; Hannan, N. The effect of quercetin on the prevention or treatment of COVID-19 and other respiratory tract infections in humans: A rapid review. *Adv. Integr. Med.* **2020**, *7*, 247–251. [CrossRef]
61. Colunga Biancatelli, R.M.L.; Berrill, M.; Catravas, J.D.; Marik, P.E. Quercetin and Vitamin C: An Experimental, Synergistic Therapy for the Prevention and Treatment of SARS-CoV-2 Related Disease (COVID-19). *Front. Immunol.* **2020**, *11*, 1451. [CrossRef]
62. Glinsky, G.V. Tripartite Combination of Candidate Pandemic Mitigation Agents: Vitamin D, Quercetin, and Estradiol Manifest Properties of Medicinal Agents for Targeted Mitigation of the COVID-19 Pandemic Defined by Genomics-Guided Tracing of SARS-CoV-2 Targets in Human Cells. *Biomedicines* **2020**, *8*, 129. [CrossRef]
63. Yang, Y.; Islam, M.S.; Wang, J.; Li, Y.; Chen, X. Traditional Chinese Medicine in the Treatment of Patients Infected with 2019-New Coronavirus (SARS-CoV-2): A Review and Perspective. *Int. J. Biol. Sci.* **2020**, *16*, 1708–1717. [CrossRef]
64. Liu, C.; Zhou, Q.; Li, Y.; Garner, L.V.; Watkins, S.P.; Carter, L.J.; Smoot, J.; Gregg, A.C.; Daniels, A.D.; Jervey, S.; et al. Research and Development on Therapeutic Agents and Vaccines for COVID-19 and Related Human Coronavirus Diseases. *ACS Cent. Sci.* **2020**, *6*, 315–331. [CrossRef]
65. Liu, X.; Raghuvanshi, R.; Ceylan, F.D.; Bolling, B.W. Quercetin and Its Metabolites Inhibit Recombinant Human Angiotensin-Converting Enzyme 2 (ACE2) Activity. *J. Agric. Food Chem.* **2020**, *68*, 13982–13989. [CrossRef]
66. Yi, L.; Li, Z.; Yuan, K.; Qu, X.; Chen, J.; Wang, G.; Zhang, H.; Luo, H.; Zhu, L.; Jiang, P.; et al. Small molecules blocking the entry of severe acute respiratory syndrome coronavirus into host cells. *J. Virol.* **2004**, *78*, 11334–11339. [CrossRef]
67. Chen, L.; Li, J.; Luo, C.; Liu, H.; Xu, W.; Chen, G.; Liew, O.W.; Zhu, W.; Puah, C.M.; Shen, X.; et al. Binding interaction of quercetin-3-beta-galactoside and its synthetic derivatives with SARS-CoV 3CL(pro): Structure-activity relationship studies reveal salient pharmacophore features. *Bioorg. Med. Chem.* **2006**, *14*, 8295–8306. [CrossRef]
68. Nguyen, T.T.; Woo, H.J.; Kang, H.K.; Nguyen, V.D.; Kim, Y.M.; Kim, D.W.; Ahn, S.A.; Xia, Y.; Kim, D. Flavonoid-mediated inhibition of SARS coronavirus 3C-like protease expressed in Pichia pastoris. *Biotechnol. Lett.* **2012**, *34*, 831–838. [CrossRef]
69. Zhang, L.; Lin, D.; Sun, X.; Curth, U.; Drosten, C.; Sauerhering, L.; Becker, S.; Rox, K.; Hilgenfeld, R. Crystal structure of SARS-CoV-2 main protease provides a basis for design of improved alpha-ketoamide inhibitors. *Science* **2020**, *368*, 409–412. [CrossRef]
70. Khaerunnisa, S.; Kurniawan, H.; Awaluddin, R.; Suhartati, S.; Soetjipto, S. Potential inhibitor of COVID-19 main protease (Mpro) from several medicinal plant compounds by molecular docking study. *Preprints* **2020**, 2020030226. [CrossRef]
71. Adem, S.; Eyupoglu, V.; Sarfraz, I.; Rasul, A.; Ali, M. Identification of potent COVID-19 main protease (Mpro) inhibitors from natural polyphenols: An in silico strategy unveils a hope against CORONA. *Preprints* **2020**, *6*, 664–672. [CrossRef]
72. Jo, S.; Kim, H.; Kim, S.; Shin, D.H.; Kim, M.-S. Characteristics of flavonoids as potent MERS-CoV 3C-like protease inhibitors. *Chem. Biol. Drug Des.* **2019**, *94*, 2023–2030. [CrossRef] [PubMed]
73. Ubani, A.; Agwom, F.; Shehu, N.Y.; Luka, P.; Umera, A.; Umar, U.; Omale, S.; Nnadi, N.E.; Aguiyi, J.C. Molecular Docking Analysis of Some Phytochemicals on Two Sars-CoV-2 Targets. *BioRxiv* **2020**. [CrossRef]

74. Munafo, F.; Donati, E.; Brindani, N.; Ottonello, G.; Armirotti, A.; De Vivo, M. Quercetin and luteolin are single-digit micromolar inhibitors of the SARS-CoV-2 RNA-dependent RNA polymerase. *Sci. Rep.* **2022**, *12*, 10571. [CrossRef] [PubMed]
75. Gasmi, A.; Tippairote, T.; Mujawdiya, P.K.; Peana, M.; Menzel, A.; Dadar, M.; Gasmi Benahmed, A.; Bjorklund, G. Micronutrients as immunomodulatory tools for COVID-19 management. *Clin. Immunol.* **2020**, *220*, 108545. [CrossRef]
76. Mora, J.R.; Iwata, M.; von Andrian, U.H. Vitamin effects on the immune system: Vitamins A and D take centre stage. *Nat. Rev. Immunol.* **2008**, *8*, 685–698. [CrossRef]
77. Moran-Santibanez, K.; Pena-Hernandez, M.A.; Cruz-Suarez, L.E.; Ricque-Marie, D.; Skouta, R.; Vasquez, A.H.; Rodriguez-Padilla, C.; Trejo-Avila, L.M. Virucidal and Synergistic Activity of Polyphenol-Rich Extracts of Seaweeds against Measles Virus. *Viruses* **2018**, *10*, 465. [CrossRef]
78. Aslam, S.; Jahan, N.; Rahman, K.-U.; Zafar, F.; Ashraf, M.Y. Synergistic interactions of polyphenols and their effect on antiradical potential. *Pak. J. Pharm. Sci.* **2017**, *30*, 1297–1304.
79. Shrivastava, R.; Shrivastava, C. Synergistic Compositions for the Treatment of Topical Viral Infections. U.S. Patent No. 8,709,506, 29 April 2014.
80. Gasmi, A.; Noor, S.; Tippairote, T.; Dadar, M.; Menzel, A.; Bjorklund, G. Individual risk management strategy and potential therapeutic options for the COVID-19 pandemic. *Clin. Immunol.* **2020**, *215*, 108409. [CrossRef]
81. Mehany, T.; Khalifa, I.; Barakat, H.; Althwab, S.A.; Alharbi, Y.M.; El-Sohaimy, S. Polyphenols as promising biologically active substances for preventing SARS-CoV-2: A review with research evidence and underlying mechanisms. *Food Biosci.* **2021**, *40*, 100891. [CrossRef]
82. Amoros, M.; Simoes, C.M.; Girre, L.; Sauvager, F.; Cormier, M. Synergistic effect of flavones and flavonols against herpes simplex virus type 1 in cell culture. Comparison with the antiviral activity of propolis. *J. Nat. Prod.* **1992**, *55*, 1732–1740. [CrossRef]
83. Gonzalez-Burquez, M.J.; Gonzalez-Diaz, F.R.; Garcia-Tovar, C.G.; Carrillo-Miranda, L.; Soto-Zarate, C.I.; Canales-Martinez, M.M.; Penieres-Carrillo, J.G.; Cruz-Sanchez, T.A.; Fonseca-Coronado, S. Comparison between In Vitro Antiviral Effect of Mexican Propolis and Three Commercial Flavonoids against Canine Distemper Virus. *Evid. Based Complement Alternat Med.* **2018**, *2018*, 7092416. [CrossRef]
84. Chiow, K.H.; Phoon, M.C.; Putti, T.; Tan, B.K.; Chow, V.T. Evaluation of antiviral activities of Houttuynia cordata Thunb. extract, quercetin, quercetrin and cinanserin on murine coronavirus and dengue virus infection. *Asian Pac. J. Trop. Med.* **2016**, *9*, 1–7. [CrossRef] [PubMed]
85. Tao, Z.; Yang, Y.; Shi, W.; Xue, M.; Yang, W.; Song, Z.; Yao, C.; Yin, J.; Shi, D.; Zhang, Y. Complementary and alternative medicine is expected to make greater contribution in controlling the prevalence of influenza. *Biosci. Trends* **2013**, *7*, 253–256. [CrossRef]
86. Ul Qamar, M.T.; Alqahtani, S.M.; Alamri, M.A.; Chen, L.L. Structural basis of SARS-CoV-2 3CL(pro) and anti-COVID-19 drug discovery from medicinal plants. *J. Pharm. Anal.* **2020**, *10*, 313–319. [CrossRef]
87. Lin, C.W.; Tsai, F.J.; Tsai, C.H.; Lai, C.C.; Wan, L.; Ho, T.Y.; Hsieh, C.C.; Chao, P.D. Anti-SARS coronavirus 3C-like protease effects of Isatis indigotica root and plant-derived phenolic compounds. *Antiviral. Res.* **2005**, *68*, 36–42. [CrossRef]
88. Yu, M.-S.; Lee, J.; Lee, J.M.; Kim, Y.; Chin, Y.-W.; Jee, J.-G.; Keum, Y.-S.; Jeong, Y.-J. Identification of myricetin and scutellarein as novel chemical inhibitors of the SARS coronavirus helicase, nsP13. *Bioorg. Med. Chem. Lett.* **2012**, *22*, 4049–4054. [CrossRef]
89. Schwarz, S.; Sauter, D.; Wang, K.; Zhang, R.; Sun, B.; Karioti, A.; Bilia, A.R.; Efferth, T.; Schwarz, W. Kaempferol derivatives as antiviral drugs against the 3a channel protein of coronavirus. *Planta. Med.* **2014**, *80*, 177–182. [CrossRef]
90. Cho, J.K.; Curtis-Long, M.J.; Lee, K.H.; Kim, D.W.; Ryu, H.W.; Yuk, H.J.; Park, K.H. Geranylated flavonoids displaying SARS-CoV papain-like protease inhibition from the fruits of Paulownia tomentosa. *Bioorg. Med. Chem.* **2013**, *21*, 3051–3057. [CrossRef]
91. Kim, D.W.; Seo, K.H.; Curtis-Long, M.J.; Oh, K.Y.; Oh, J.W.; Cho, J.K.; Lee, K.H.; Park, K.H. Phenolic phytochemical displaying SARS-CoV papain-like protease inhibition from the seeds of Psoralea corylifolia. *J. Enzyme. Inhib. Med. Chem.* **2014**, *29*, 59–63. [CrossRef]
92. Park, J.-Y.; Yuk, H.J.; Ryu, H.W.; Lim, S.H.; Kim, K.S.; Park, K.H.; Ryu, Y.B.; Lee, W.S. Evaluation of polyphenols from Broussonetia papyrifera as coronavirus protease inhibitors. *J. Enzyme. Inhib. Med. Chem.* **2017**, *32*, 504–512. [CrossRef]
93. Zhuang, M.; Jiang, H.; Suzuki, Y.; Li, X.; Xiao, P.; Tanaka, T.; Ling, H.; Yang, B.; Saitoh, H.; Zhang, L.; et al. Procyanidins and butanol extract of Cinnamomi Cortex inhibit SARS-CoV infection. *Antiviral. Res.* **2009**, *82*, 73–81. [CrossRef] [PubMed]
94. Hsu, S. Compounds Derived from Epigallocatechin-3-Gallate (EGCG) as a Novel Approach to the Prevention of Viral Infections. *Inflamm. Allergy Drug Targets* **2015**, *14*, 13–18. [CrossRef] [PubMed]
95. Kaihatsu, K.; Yamabe, M.; Ebara, Y. Antiviral Mechanism of Action of Epigallocatechin-3-O-gallate and Its Fatty Acid Esters. *Molecules* **2018**, *23*, 2475. [CrossRef]
96. Chen, C.N.; Lin, C.P.; Huang, K.K.; Chen, W.C.; Hsieh, H.P.; Liang, P.H.; Hsu, J.T. Inhibition of SARS-CoV 3C-like Protease Activity by Theaflavin-3,3'-digallate (TF3). *Evid. Based Complement Alternat Med.* **2005**, *2*, 209–215. [CrossRef]
97. Jo, S.; Kim, S.; Shin, D.H.; Kim, M.S. Inhibition of SARS-CoV 3CL protease by flavonoids. *J. Enzyme. Inhib. Med. Chem.* **2020**, *35*, 145–151. [CrossRef]
98. Bahun, M.; Jukic, M.; Oblak, D.; Kranjc, L.; Bajc, G.; Butala, M.; Bozovicar, K.; Bratkovic, T.; Podlipnik, C.; Poklar Ulrih, N. Inhibition of the SARS-CoV-2 3CL(pro) main protease by plant polyphenols. *Food Chem.* **2022**, *373*, 131594. [CrossRef]
99. Ryu, Y.B.; Jeong, H.J.; Kim, J.H.; Kim, Y.M.; Park, J.Y.; Kim, D.; Nguyen, T.T.; Park, S.J.; Chang, J.S.; Park, K.H.; et al. Biflavonoids from Torreya nucifera displaying SARS-CoV 3CL(pro) inhibition. *Bioorg. Med. Chem.* **2010**, *18*, 7940–7947. [CrossRef]

100. Yang, R.; Li, X.; Liu, H.; Zhen, Y.; Zhang, X.; Xiong, Q.; Luo, Y.; Gao, C.; Zeng, W. Chest CT Severity Score: An Imaging Tool for Assessing Severe COVID-19. *Radiol. Cardiothorac. Imaging* **2020**, *2*, e200047. [CrossRef]
101. Heeba, G.H.; Mahmoud, M.E.; El Hanafy, A.A. Anti-inflammatory potential of curcumin and quercetin in rats: Role of oxidative stress, heme oxygenase-1 and TNF-alpha. *Toxicol. Ind. Health* **2014**, *30*, 551–560. [CrossRef]
102. Hecel, A.; Ostrowska, M.; Stokowa-Soltys, K.; Watly, J.; Dudek, D.; Miller, A.; Potocki, S.; Matera-Witkiewicz, A.; Dominguez-Martin, A.; Kozlowski, H.; et al. Zinc(II)-The Overlooked Eminence Grise of Chloroquine's Fight against COVID-19? *Pharmaceuticals* **2020**, *13*, 228. [CrossRef]
103. Sagar, S.; Rathinavel, A.K.; Lutz, W.E.; Struble, L.R.; Khurana, S.; Schnaubelt, A.T.; Mishra, N.K.; Guda, C.; Broadhurst, M.J.; Reid, S.P.M.; et al. Bromelain Inhibits SARS-CoV-2 Infection in VeroE6 Cells. *Biorxiv Prepr. Serv. Biol.* **2020**. [CrossRef]
104. Peng, Z. Vitamin C Infusion for the Treatment of Severe 2019-nCoV Infected Pneumonia. ClinicalTrials.Gov. 2020. Available online: https://clinicaltrials.gov/ct2/show/NCT04264533 (accessed on 22 July 2022).
105. Kinker, B.; Comstock, A.T.; Sajjan, U.S. Quercetin: A promising treatment for the common cold. *J. Anc. Dis. Prev. Remedies* **2014**, *2*, 1–3. [CrossRef]
106. Yamshchikov, A.V.; Desai, N.S.; Blumberg, H.M.; Ziegler, T.R.; Tangpricha, V. Vitamin D for treatment and prevention of infectious diseases: A systematic review of randomized controlled trials. *Endocr. Pract.* **2009**, *15*, 438–449. [CrossRef]
107. Mostafavi-Pour, Z.; Zal, F.; Monabati, A.; Vessal, M. Protective effects of a combination of quercetin and vitamin E against cyclosporine A-induced oxidative stress and hepatotoxicity in rats. *Hepatol. Res.* **2008**, *38*, 385–392. [CrossRef] [PubMed]
108. Milton Prabu, S.; Shagirtha, K.; Renugadevi, J. Quercetin in combination with vitamins (C and E) improves oxidative stress and renal injury in cadmium intoxicated rats. *Eur. Rev. Med. Pharmacol. Sci.* **2010**, *14*, 903–914. [PubMed]
109. Zoroddu, M.A.; Aaseth, J.; Crisponi, G.; Medici, S.; Peana, M.; Nurchi, V.M. The essential metals for humans: A brief overview. *J. Inorg. Biochem.* **2019**, *195*, 120–129. [CrossRef] [PubMed]
110. Zoroddu, M.A.; Medici, S.; Ledda, A.; Nurchi, V.M.; Lachowicz, J.I.; Peana, M. Toxicity of nanoparticles. *Curr. Med. Chem.* **2014**, *21*, 3837–3853. [CrossRef]
111. Crisponi, G.; Nurchi, V.M.; Lachowicz, J.I.; Peana, M.; Medici, S.; Zoroddu, M.A. Chapter 18-Toxicity of Nanoparticles: Etiology and Mechanisms. In *Antimicrobial Nanoarchitectonics*; Grumezescu, A.M., Ed.; Elsevier: Amsterdam, The Netherlands, 2017; pp. 511–546. [CrossRef]
112. Jeevanandam, J.; Barhoum, A.; Chan, Y.S.; Dufresne, A.; Danquah, M.K. Review on nanoparticles and nanostructured materials: History, sources, toxicity and regulations. *Beilstein. J. Nanotechnol.* **2018**, *9*, 1050–1074. [CrossRef]
113. Gao, L.; Liu, G.; Wang, X.; Liu, F.; Xu, Y.; Ma, J. Preparation of a chemically stable quercetin formulation using nanosuspension technology. *Int. J. Pharm.* **2011**, *404*, 231–237. [CrossRef]
114. El-Rahmanand, S.N.A.; Suhailah, S. Quercetin nanoparticles: Preparation and characterization. *Indian J. Drugs* **2014**, *2*, 96–103.
115. Halder, A.; Mukherjee, P.; Ghosh, S.; Mandal, S.; Chatterji, U.; Mukherjee, A. Smart PLGA nanoparticles loaded with Quercetin: Cellular uptake and in-vitro anticancer study. *Mater. Today* **2018**, *5*, 9698–9705. [CrossRef]
116. Han, Q.; Wang, X.; Cai, S.; Liu, X.; Zhang, Y.; Yang, L.; Wang, C.; Yang, R. Quercetin nanoparticles with enhanced bioavailability as multifunctional agents toward amyloid induced neurotoxicity. *J. Mater. Chem. B* **2018**, *6*, 1387–1393. [CrossRef] [PubMed]
117. Nam, J.S.; Sharma, A.R.; Nguyen, L.T.; Chakraborty, C.; Sharma, G.; Lee, S.S. Application of Bioactive Quercetin in Oncotherapy: From Nutrition to Nanomedicine. *Molecules* **2016**, *21*, 108. [CrossRef] [PubMed]
118. Niazvand, F.; Orazizadeh, M.; Khorsandi, L.; Abbaspour, M.; Mansouri, E.; Khodadadi, A. Effects of Quercetin-Loaded Nanoparticles on MCF-7 Human Breast Cancer Cells. *Medicina* **2019**, *55*, 114. [CrossRef]
119. Riva, A.; Ronchi, M.; Petrangolini, G.; Bosisio, S.; Allegrini, P. Improved Oral Absorption of Quercetin from Quercetin Phytosome(R), a New Delivery System Based on Food Grade Lecithin. *Eur. J. Drug Metab. Pharmacokinet.* **2019**, *44*, 169–177. [CrossRef]
120. Rondanelli, M.; Perna, S.; Gasparri, C.; Petrangolini, G.; Allegrini, P.; Cavioni, A.; Faliva, M.A.; Mansueto, F.; Patelli, Z.; Peroni, G.; et al. Promising Effects of 3-Month Period of Quercetin Phytosome((R)) Supplementation in the Prevention of Symptomatic COVID-19 Disease in Healthcare Workers: A Pilot Study. *Life* **2022**, *12*, 66. [CrossRef]
121. Imran, M.; Thabet, H.K.; Alaqel, S.I.; Alzahrani, A.R.; Abida, A.; Alshammari, M.K.; Kamal, M.; Diwan, A.; Asdaq, S.M.B.; Alshehri, S. The Therapeutic and Prophylactic Potential of Quercetin against COVID-19: An Outlook on the Clinical Studies, Inventive Compositions, and Patent Literature. *Antioxidants* **2022**, *11*, 876. [CrossRef]

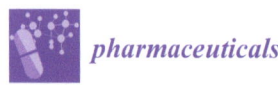

Article

Molecular Targets of Pinocembrin Underlying Its Regenerative Activities in Human Keratinocytes

Jirapak Ruttanapattanakul [1,2], Nitwara Wikan [1], Saranyapin Potikanond [1] and Wutigri Nimlamool [1,*]

[1] Department of Pharmacology, Faculty of Medicine, Chiang Mai University, Chiang Mai 50200, Thailand; jirapak.ken@gmail.com (J.R.); nitwara.wik@cmu.ac.th (N.W.); saranyapin.p@cmu.ac.th (S.P.)
[2] Graduate School, Chiang Mai University, Chiang Mai 50200, Thailand
[*] Correspondence: wutigri.nimlamool@cmu.ac.th; Tel.: +66-53-93-4597

Abstract: Pinocembrin is one of the well-known compounds in the group of flavonoids. The pharmacological activities of pinocembrin in association with wound-healing activities have been reported. However, its effects on the aspect of cellular interaction underlying growth and survival are still unidentified in human keratinocytes. Our previous study reported that *Boesenbergia rotunda* potently stimulated survival and proliferation of a human keratinocyte cell line (HaCaT). On the basis that pinocembrin is revealed to be one of the major constituents of this plant, we aimed to define the survival- and proliferation-enhancing effects of this compound at the cellular level. Results from the current study confirmed that pinocembrin induced an increase in HaCaT cell number. At the signaling perspective, we identified that pinocembrin significantly triggered ERK1/2 and Akt activation. The stimulating effects of pinocembrin were clearly inhibited by MEK and PI3K inhibitors authenticating that proliferation- and survival-promoting activities of pinocembrin were mainly acted on these two signaling cascades. Altogether, we successfully identified that pinocembrin functions to induce keratinocyte proliferation and survival, at least by provoking MAPK and PI3K pathways. Our study encourages the fact that pinocembrin is one of the interesting natural flavonoid compounds to be developed as a wound closure-promoting agent.

Keywords: flavonoids; pinocembrin; wound healing; keratinocyte; regenerative medicine

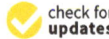

Citation: Ruttanapattanakul, J.; Wikan, N.; Potikanond, S.; Nimlamool, W. Molecular Targets of Pinocembrin Underlying Its Regenerative Activities in Human Keratinocytes. *Pharmaceuticals* **2022**, *15*, 954. https://doi.org/10.3390/ph15080954

Academic Editors: Fernando Calzada and Miguel Valdes

Received: 24 June 2022
Accepted: 27 July 2022
Published: 31 July 2022

Publisher's Note: MDPI stays neutral with regard to jurisdictional claims in published maps and institutional affiliations.

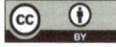

Copyright: © 2022 by the authors. Licensee MDPI, Basel, Switzerland. This article is an open access article distributed under the terms and conditions of the Creative Commons Attribution (CC BY) license (https://creativecommons.org/licenses/by/4.0/).

1. Introduction

Wound healing is an indispensable protective mechanism for both humans and animals. It consists of different crucial steps controlled by different stages composed of coagulation/hemostasis stage, inflammation stage, proliferation stage, and wound remodeling stage [1,2]. These phases are not individual but partly overlap on a sequence by hemostasis, inflammation, proliferation, and remodeling phase, respectively [3]. After a wound has occurred, coagulation cascade and platelet are activated by injured endothelial cells, and the next event is the generation of acute inflammation of the surrounding tissues for eliminating the pathogen [4]. Importantly, the proliferation step truly requires proliferation of surrounding cells which are activated by many growth factors including vascular endothelial growth factor (VEGF), platelet-derived growth factor (PDGF), and epidermal growth factor (EGF). The final phase called "wound remodeling period" is the longest phase which focuses on organization, degradation, and synthesis of the extracellular matrix in the dermis layer of the skin [5–7]. Natural delays in healing processes may occur in older individuals [8]. All phases of the healing process are affected, making cell proliferation, remodeling, and collagen synthesis to occur at a lesser degree. Moreover, in comparison with children and young adults, the elderly may have complications from certain diseases that greatly hamper the healing process [9]. Therefore, besides recently available healing therapies, discovery of novel active agents and special treatments that can effectively accelerate wound healing to the maximal level would be beneficial for the elderly to prevent possible complications such as septicemia. Considering this fact, natural compounds including flavonoids have emerged as interesting agents for enhancing wound healing.

Pinocembrin (PC) is one of the primary flavonoid compounds that is found in many plants belonging to different families, as *Boesenbergia rotunda* (Zingiberaceae) [10,11], and it has been previously reported that pinocembrin has many pharmacological effects including anti-inflammatory and anti-microbial effects, anti-aging activities, and wound-healing properties [12–16]. Regarding the wound-healing properties, our previous research found that *Boesenbergia rotunda* (BR), which is a plant in Zingiberaceae family [17], can promote keratinocyte cell proliferation via activating MAPK and PI3K pathways [18]. Additionally, it was found that *Boesenbergia rotunda* ethanolic extract contains pinocembrin as one of its major compounds [19]. Possibly, pinocembrin may be the responsible constituent of BR that stimulates proliferation of human keratinocytes. However, the wound healing-promoting activities of pinocembrin in keratinocytes has not been fully elucidated; especially in the view of specific activation of growth and survival pathways. On this basis, the major aims of this research are to determine the function of PC on keratinocyte proliferation and to monitor the expression and activation status of important kinase markers in the MAPK signal transduction pathway (ERK 1/2, pERK1/2) and PI3K/Akt signal transduction pathway (pAkt and Akt) in response to PC treatment.

Our study provided an insight into how an active compound, pinocembrin, functions at the cellular level for enhancing proliferation and survival which are crucial events for wound healing. This new understanding may guide for the possibility to develop this compound as an alternative wound healing-accelerating drug, especially for patients who have complications of diseases and are irresponsive to currently available standard treatments.

2. Results

2.1. Pinocembrin Affects the Viability of Human Keratinocytes

To investigate proliferation-enhancing effects of pinocembrin, we first performed cytotoxicity of pinocembrin in HaCaT cells which are immortalized human keratinocytes. Results demonstrated that 500 µM was the only concentration of pinocembrin which significantly reduced the viability of HaCaT cells. Interestingly, pinocembrin at the range be-tween 15.6 and 125 µM presented a dramatic increase in cell viability/cell proliferation, with a maximal peak at 62.5 µM where the cell viability of HaCaT cells was approximately 140% in comparison to that of the untreated cells (100%) (Figure 1). Human keratinocytes treated with DMSO (as a vehicle control) at all concentrations did not show any change in cell viability.

2.2. Effects of Pinocembrin on Accelerating Scratch Wound Closure of Human Keratinocyte Monolayer

From the MTT results demonstrating that pinocembrin from 15.6 to 62.5 µM could increase the viability of human keratinocytes, it is reasonable that this increased cell viability may also promote healing of keratinocyte monolayer. Therefore, we evaluated wound closure-accelerating effects of pinocembrin on human keratinocyte monolayer by choosing the highest concentration at 62.5 µM. Phase-contrast micrographs demonstrated that pinocembrin significantly accelerated the cellular wound healing over time (0, 3, 6, 24, and 48 h), compared to the DMSO vehicle control group (Figure 2).

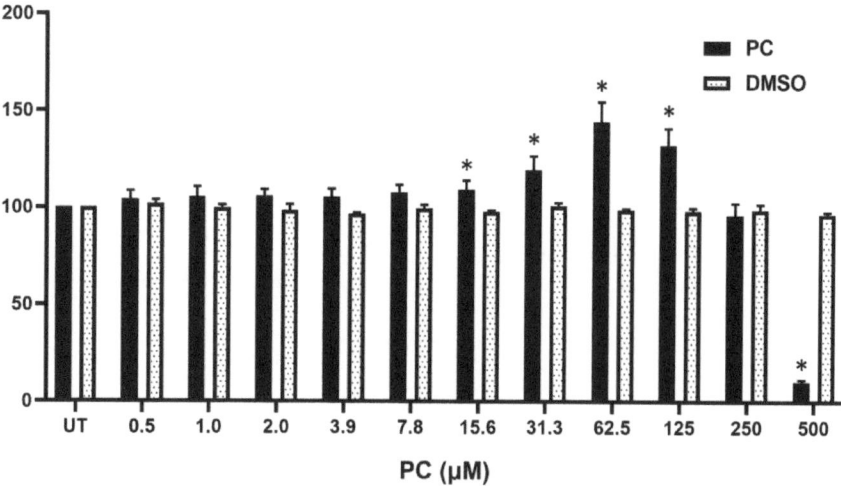

Figure 1. Cytotoxicity effects of pinocembrin on HaCaT cells determined by MTT assay. Human keratinocytes treated with different doses of pinocembrin for 48 h in serum-free media. Data were shown as percent cell viability/proliferation with mean ± SD. * $p < 0.05$ as compared with the un-treated group (UT).

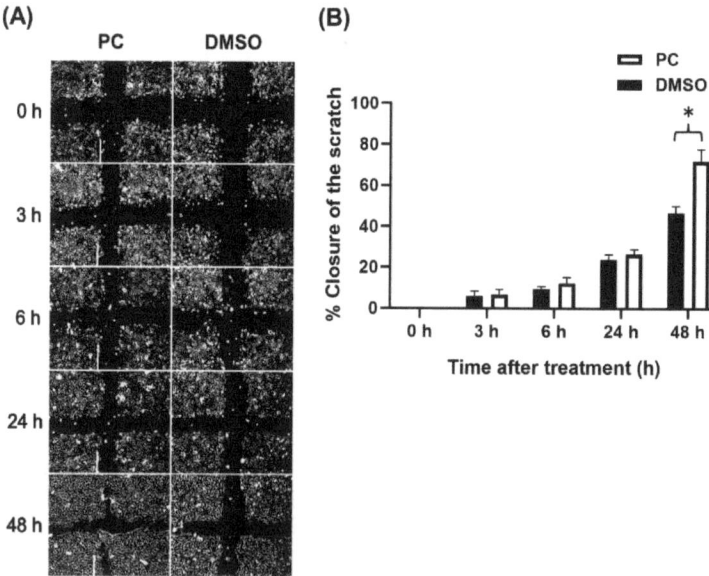

Figure 2. Effects of pinocembrin on accelerating closure of scratch wound of human keratinocyte monolayers. (**A**) Phase-contrast microscopy (10× magnification) of scratch wound-healing assay at various captured times (0 h, 3 h, 6 h, 24 h, and 48 h) in HaCaT treated with 62.5 µM pinocembrin; (**B**) Percent closure of the scratch wounded areas of human keratinocyte monolayer over the course of 48 h. Data were analyzed from three individual replicates and presented as mean ± SD. * $p < 0.05$ as compared with the DMSO control.

2.3. Pinocembrin Induces Proliferation and Increases the Size of HaCaT Colonies

To explore the role of pinocembrin in activating human keratinocyte proliferation, we seeded HaCaT cells at low density, treated the cells with 62.5 µM pinocembrin, and visualized the changes in colony size over 48 h. As presented in Figure 3A, pinocembrin clearly stimulated an increase in colony size of HaCaT cells over the course of 48 h while the growing colony pattern of the DMSO control group was similar to that of the untreated group. To test the hypothesis that pinocembrin may stimulate keratinocyte proliferation, we directly counted the number of cells. Results demonstrated that at the 0 h time point, the number and distribution of the keratinocytes were seen to be similar to those of the control group and pinocembrin group. Obviously, pinocembrin at 62.5 µM significantly induced an increase in cell number of keratinocytes at 24 h and 48 h when compared with the untreated group and DMSO-treated group (Figure 3B).

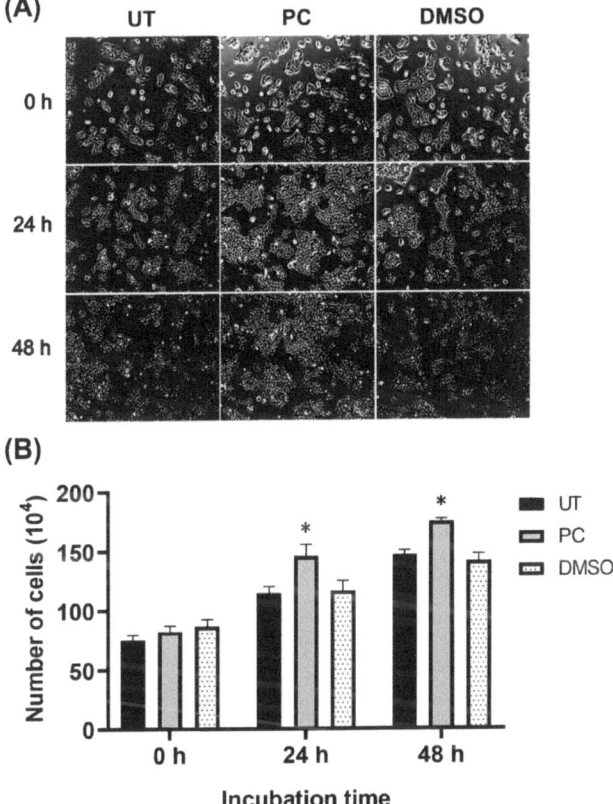

Figure 3. Effects of pinocembrin on human keratinocyte proliferation. (**A**) Phase-contrast observation of HaCaT cells treated with pinocembrin at 62.5 µM at 0, 24, and 48 h (10× magnification) compared with the untreated group and the DMSO control group; (**B**) Direct cell counting for number of human keratinocytes treated with pinocembrin at 62.5 µM and at 0, 24, and 48 h. Data from three experiments were analyzed and presented as mean ± SD. * $p < 0.05$ (compared to the untreated group, UT).

2.4. Effects of Pinocembrin on the Signaling Pathways Regulating Keratinocyte Proliferation

The MAPK and PI3K/Akt cascades are one of the most important cellular pathways for growth and survival of all type of cells including human keratinocytes. To inspect the effects of pinocembrin on these signaling cascades in human keratinocytes, the phosphorylation status of crucial cellular kinases (ERK1/2 and Akt) was monitored and measured upon treatment with pinocembrin at various time points (0–24 h). Results demonstrated that pinocembrin could rapidly activate phosphorylation of ERK1/2 protein within 2 min after pinocembrin addition. The signal intensity rapidly increased over time before it declined after 15 min (Figure 4A,B). The phosphorylation status of Akt was slightly delayed since a clear phosphorylation signal started to be seen 5 min post pinocembrin treatment, increased over time, and was stable for 1 h before it declined (Figure 4A,C). Noticeably, pinocembrin did not affect the expression of both ERK1/2 and Akt kinases.

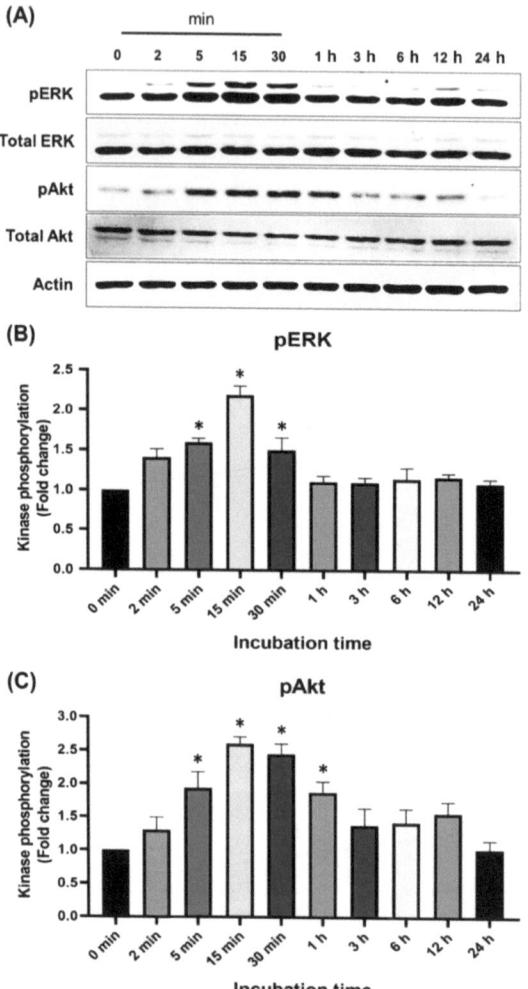

Figure 4. Effects of pinocembrin on MAPK and PI3K/Akt signaling pathways. (**A**) The activation status evaluated by the level of phosphorylation of ERK1/2 and Akt in the lysates of cells treated with 62.5 µM of pinocembrin at various time points; (**B**) Densitometric analysis of phosphorylated ERK1/2 in cells treated with pinocembrin at each time point; (**C**) Densitometric analysis of phosphorylated Akt in cells treated with pinocembrin at each time point. The total protein expression of each kinase was detected and used for normalization. Data from three experiments were analyzed and presented as mean ± SD. * $p < 0.05$ (compared to the 0 min group).

Moreover, we performed Western blotting to confirm the kinase-activating effects of pinocembrin at varied concentrations (15.6, 31.3, and 62.5 µM), and data clearly demonstrated that the phosphorylation form of the two kinases was significantly elevated when the dose of pinocembrin was increased without affecting the total protein level (Figure 5A). Quantification of immunoreactive signals demonstrated that after 15 min of pinocembrin treatment, phosphorylation of ERK1/2 and Akt was approximately 2-fold, 2.5- fold, and 3-fold for cells treated with pinocembrin at 15.6, 31.3, and 62.5 µM, respectively (Figure 5B,C).

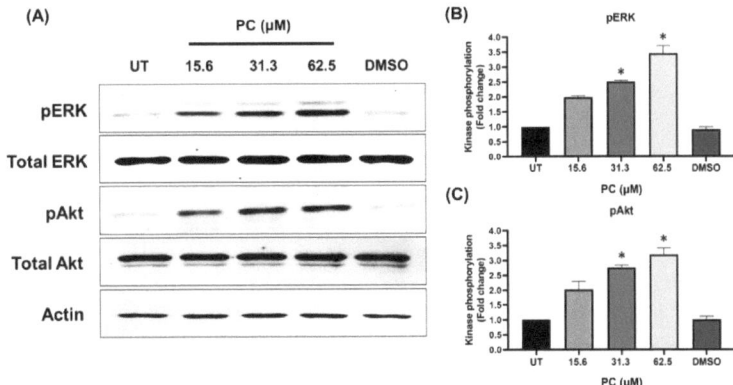

Figure 5. Concentration-dependent effects of pinocembrin on ERK1/2 and Akt activation. (**A**) Western blotting for ERK1/2 and Akt phosphorylation in HaCaT cells incubated with pinocembrin at 15.6, 31.3, or 62.5 µM for 15 min; (**B**) Densitometric analysis of phosphorylated ERK1/2 in lysates of cells treated with varied concentrations of pinocembrin; (**C**) Densitometric analysis of phosphorylated Akt in lysates of cells treated with varied concentrations of pinocembrin. Data from three experiments were analyzed and presented as mean ± SD. * $p < 0.05$ (compared to the control group, UT).

Concomitantly, immunofluorescence analysis for the phosphorylation form of ERK1/2 (Figure 6A(d–f)) and Akt (Figure 6B(d–f)) definitively verified that pinocembrin rapidly induced the activation of these two kinases in individual cells compared to those cells treated with DMSO (Figure 6A(a–c),B(a–c)).

2.5. Inhibitors That Specifically Inhibit MEK and PI3K Completely Block ERK1/2 and Akt Activation and HaCaT Cell Proliferation Induced by Pinocembrin

Specific inhibitors which included U0126 (MEK inhibitor) and LY294002 (a PI3K inhibitor) were used to confirm whether pinocembrin specifically activates MAPK and PI3K transduction pathways. Western blot results confirmed that when U0126 was used, complete inhibition of ERK1/2 but not Akt was seen in keratinocytes treated with pinocembrin alone. Likewise, when LY294002 was applied, the phosphorylation of Akt but not ERK1/2 was blocked (Figure 7). Apparently, when both U0126 and LY294002 were applied to keratinocytes, no phosphorylation signal of ERK1/2 and Akt was detected (Figure 7).

Scratch wound healing was performed as a functional test to verify the results obtained from the experiments where the inhibitors were included. As anticipated, U0126 could suppress keratinocyte monolayer closure accelerating effects of PC over the course of 48 h. In addition, LY294002-treated group demonstrated a similar pattern of scratch healing inhibition. Doubtlessly, keratinocyte monolayer treated with pinocembrin with the presence of both U0126 and LY294002 exhibited the slowest rate of wound closure (Figure 8). These results show that pinocembrin induces keratinocyte proliferation mainly through activating MAPK and PI3K/Akt kinases.

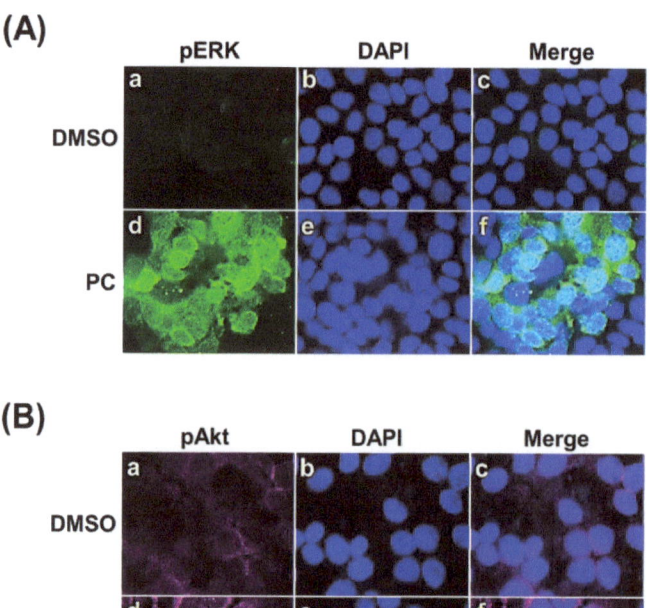

Figure 6. Immunofluorescence study determining ERK1/2 and Akt activation in cells treated with pinocembrin (62.5 µM). (**A**) Phosphorylated ERK1/2 (pERK1/2) (green); (**B**) Phosphorylated Akt (pAkt) (green). HaCaT cells were counterstained with DAPI to detect the nuclei (blue). Pictures were captured by a fluorescent microscope at 100× magnification.

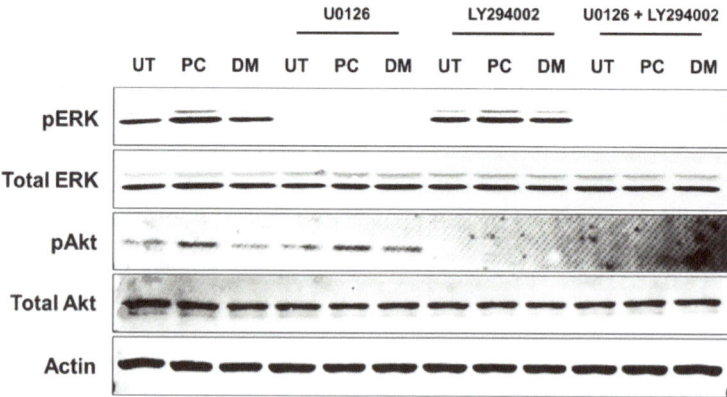

Figure 7. Western blot analysis detecting pERK1/2 and pAkt after incubation with pinocembrin at various concentrations (15.6, 31.3, and 62.5 µM) for 15 min in combination with U0126 and LY294002 which are specific inhibitors of MAPK and PI3K signaling. Data are obtained from three individual experiments.

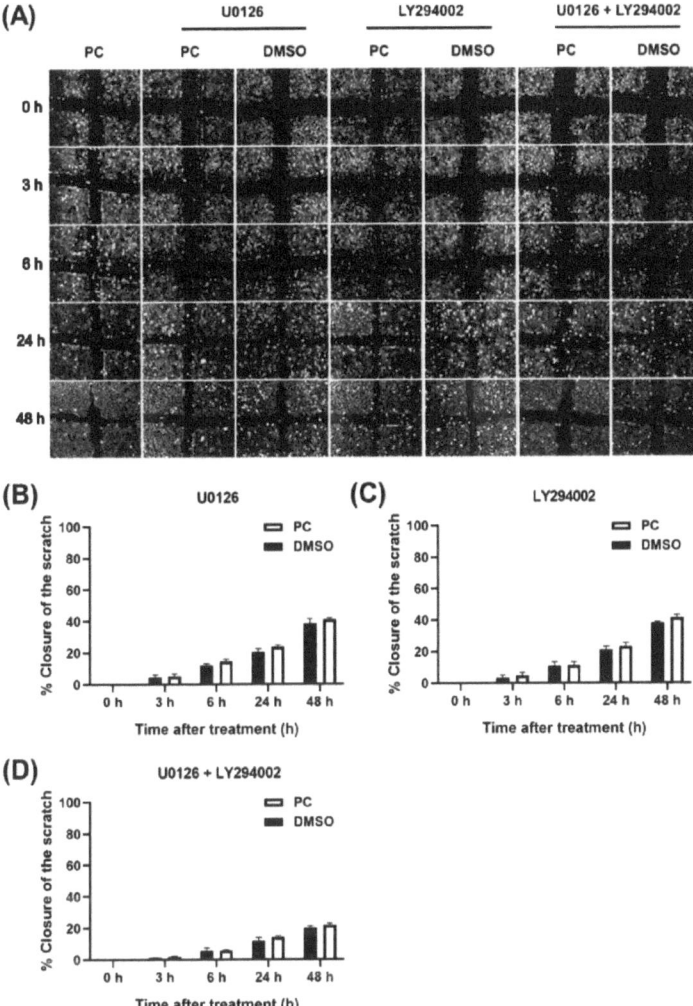

Figure 8. Scratch wound healing assay for investigating the monolayer wound closure accelerating effects of pinocembrin (62.5 μM) in the presence of U0126, LY294002, or combination of both U0126 and LY294002. (**A**) Phase-contrast microscopy (10× magnification) of scratch wound-healing assay with U0126, LY294002, or combination of U0126 and LY294002 over the course of 48 h. Percent closure of the scratch-wounded areas of human keratinocyte monolayer over the course of 48 h in the presence of (**B**) U0126, (**C**) LY294002, or (**D**) combination of both U0126 and LY294002. Data from three experiments were analyzed and presented as mean ± standard deviation.

3. Discussion

It is well known that the skin is an important organ that protects the internal viscera, prevents water loss, and protects against microorganisms and UV radiation. When an individual experiences open wound or skin damage, the sequential healing phases must occur for a specific duration at an optimal intensity to properly heal the wound [20]. In particular, wound healing is a complex process that requires the orchestration of different types of cells, cytokines, and growth factors in order to effectively close the wound [21]. Although the human body responds rapidly to reverse the functional integrity of skin, many negative factors may interfere with certain wound-healing phases causing delayed or improper tissue repair. One obvious factor is skin aging characterized by drying, roughness, atrophy, changes in pigmentation, wrinkling, and sagging which are caused by both intrinsic and extrinsic aging factors including exposure to ultraviolet irradiation [22]. Specifically, age-related delayed wound healing is linked to the aberration in the inflammation phase, and that includes slow infiltration of T-cell into the affected regions, changes in chemokine production, and reduced phagocytic activity of macrophages [23]. Additionally, angiogenesis, collagen synthesis, and re-epithelialization have been reported to be delayed in aged mice [24]. Besides an aspect of aging, other factors have been identified to be important factors that negatively influence wound healing. Those include oxygenation, infections, sex hormones, stress, diabetes, medications, obesity, alcohol consumption, smoking, and nutrition [25]. Improper or impaired wound healing caused by these factors may influence medical management and overall economy in every country. The United States has reported that the unmanaged skin trauma costs around 50 billion dollars, wound scarring from surgical treatments and trauma costs nearly 12 billion dollars, and burns cost 7.5 billion dollars per year [26]. Patients with complications, which are not responsive to currently available therapeutic agents, may experience delayed wound closure, and this enhances an increased risk of infections or development of certain new complications [27]. Therefore, the discovery of new wound healing-stimulating compounds would be clinically beneficial for the treatment of individuals who have a persistent skin wound with severe problems.

Since ancient times, humans have relied on traditional herbal medicine for curing and preventing many diseases and conditions. Those medicinal plants have been revealed to exhibit strong biological activities which include anti-microbial, anti-inflammatory, and wound healing properties [28,29]. Currently, many studies have reported specific pharmacological effects of certain medicinal plants [30,31]. For these reasons, interest in medicinal plants and their active compounds is currently increasing. Pinocembrin is a type of flavonoid which is found in certain plants in the family of Piperaceae, Lauraceae, and Asteraceae which are mainly distributed in tropical and subtropical regions [13]. Besides, it is prevalent in different dietary sources such as Calabrian honey [32], licorice (Glycyrrhiza glabra) [33], and fingerroot (*Boesenbergia rotunda*) [19]. Many studies have reported about the anti-bacterial effects of pinocembrin [34,35]. About the wound healing-promoting properties, it was shown that *Boesenbergia rotunda* which contains pinocembrin [11] demonstrated cell proliferation-activating effects on human keratinocytes by promoting MAPK and PI3K/Akt signal transduction pathways [18].

Our current study focused on investigating the specific cellular signaling pathways at which pinocembrin acts on to promote proliferation and survival of human keratinocytes. Cell viability testing demonstrated that pinocembrin at a specific non-toxic range could drastically increase human keratinocyte viability. These results suggest that pinocembrin may elevate the rate of keratinocyte division. We further examined this hypothesis by focusing mainly on the influence of pinocembrin on cell proliferation and con-firmed that this compound truly stimulated an increase in cell number and enhanced the rate of monolayer wound healing. Moreover, Western blot analysis and immunofluorescence study clearly verified that MAPK/ERK and PI3K/Akt signal transduction pathway were rapidly stimulated in response to pinocembrin. When specific inhibitors of these two pathways were used, the kinase-stimulating effects of pinocembrin completely disappeared. Data from our findings indicate that pinocembrin rapidly stimulates functional kinases responsible for stimulating the growth (MAPK) and survival (PI3K/Akt) of human keratinocytes. Similar effects at the level of signal transduction pathway have been reported previously by our group where the ethanolic extract of *Boesenbergia rotunda* was examined [18], and pinocembrin has been identified by many studies as one of the major constituents of this plant [11,36]. It is well characterized that major mitogen-activated protein (MAP) kinases are key molecular players that stimulate the proliferation and differentiation of many cells, including keratinocytes where the effect is stimulated by growth factors, the level of intracellular calcium, and cytokines [37]. Furthermore, this signaling conveyed by the upstream kinase (MEKK1) induces the expression of responsible genes involved in wound re-epithelialization [38]. The PI3K/Akt signaling cascade also regulates cell proliferation, cell migration, and cell survival [39,40]. Interestingly, a previous study demonstrated that pinocembrin and its linolenoyl ester derivatives can promote wound healing in human keratinocytes through a GPR120/FFA4 mediated pathway [12]. Specifically, this study showed that pinocembrin was hybridized with fatty acids by using pancreatic porcine lipase, and its wound healing activity was mediated by GPR120/β-arrestin complexation. GPR120 is a G-protein-coupled receptor 120 that has been reported to crosstalk with the PI3K/Akt–NF-kB pathway [41]. Similarly, it has been explored that ERK1/2 is a functional kinase working downstream of GPR120 to modulate a series of biologic processes [42,43]. Nevertheless, how pinocembrin exactly interacts with certain molecular players remains to be identified. One way to obtain such information is through conducting a structural interaction assay as well as rational redesign of a functional protein kinase-substrate interaction [44] to probe the functional consequences of specific phosphorylation events in keratinocytes upon pinocembrin stimulation.

On the basis that keratinocytes in the epidermis play a crucial role on re-epithelialization which is a process for the restoration of the epidermis after injury, and on our recent discovery that pinocembrin is an active compound that rapidly targets certain cellular molecules resulting in the activation of the MAPK and PI3K/Akt (as illustrated in Figure 9), this sheds light on this natural compound for the possible development as an alternative agent required for the full regenerative function of keratinocytes, especially in patients who are less responsive to other treatments or patients with delayed wound healing.

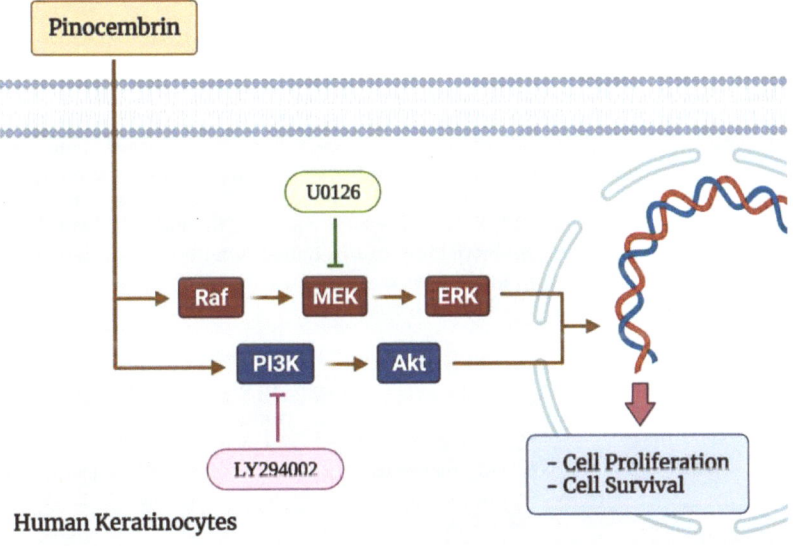

Figure 9. Schematic figure illustrating that pinocembrin regulates human keratinocyte proliferation and survival. Pinocembrin increases the proliferation and survival of keratinocytes through both MAPK signal transduction pathway and PI3K/Akt signaling pathway.

4. Materials and Methods

4.1. Pinocembrin Preparation

Pinocembrin was purchased from Sigma-Aldrich, St. Louis, MO, USA (Product Number: P5239-50 mg, Batch Number: MKCM4285). After purchase, Pinocembrin stock solution was prepared to be 195 mM in 100% DMSO, aliquoted, and stored at $-20\,°C$.

For each experiment, pinocembrin stock was directly diluted in cell culture media before each treatment.

4.2. Cell Lines and Cell Cultures

HaCaT keratinocytes were procured from CLS Cell Lines Service GmbH (Eppelheim, Baden-Wurttemberg, Germany). The cells were maintained in complete media, which was Dulbecco's modified Eagle's media (DMEM) (Gibco, New York, NY, USA), with the addition of 10% fetal bovine serum (Merck KGaA, Darmstadt, Germany), 100 U/mL penicillin, and 100 µg/mL streptomycin (both drugs from Thermo Fisher Scientific, Waltham, MA, USA). HaCaT cells were cultured in an incubator under a humidified atmosphere at 37 °C, 5% CO_2. Media were changed every 2–3 days, and sub-culture was performed when the cells reached approximately 90% confluence.

4.3. Cell Viability Assay

Following, 3-(4,5-dimethylthiazol-2-yl)-2,5-diphenyltetrazolium bromide (MTT) was used to evaluate the cell viability of pinocembrin-treated human keratinocytes. In 96-well plates (Thermo Fisher Scientific, USA), we seeded HaCaT cells at 2×10^5 cells per well (200 µL per well) in complete media overnight. Next day, pinocembrin was diluted in FBS-free media to a working concentration of 500 µM, then the concentration was further diluted by 2-fold dilution to create a concentration range of 0.5–500 µM. The adhered cells were treated with these varied concentrations of pinocembrin for 48 h in FBS-free media. DMSO (a vehicle control) was diluted in a similar way to make a concentration range of 0.001–0.05% control. After 48 h of pinocembrin exposure, MTT reagent (stock 5 mg/mL) was added to each well (25 µL per well), and cells were incubated in a CO_2 incubator for 1 h for formazan formation. After media were aspirated, formazan was dissolved with DMSO (µL per well). The difference in color intensity was determined by a microplate reader set at 570 nm.

4.4. Phase-Contrast Microscopy

Phase-contrast observation was performed to monitor keratinocyte colony expansion over time upon pinocembrin treatment. Human keratinocytes were seeded at 0.1×10^6 cells in 24-well plates in complete media overnight. Then, media were replaced to be FBS-free DMEM, and cells were treated with pinocembrin at 62.5 µM or DMSO. The micrograph of pinocembrin-treated human keratinocytes at various time points (0, 24, and 48 h) were captured with 10× magnification by using Axio Vert.A1 microscope (Carl Zeiss Suzhou Co., Ltd., Suzhou, China)

4.5. Direct Measurement of Cell Number

HaCaT cells were directly counted for measuring the changes in cell amount in different treating conditions. Human keratinocytes were seeded at 0.1×10^6 cells in 24-well plates in DMEM with FBS and incubated overnight. Adherent cells were then treated with 62.5 µM pinocembrin in media without FBS. The total number of cells were obtained at 0, 24, and 48 h by using CellDrop™ Automated Cell Counters (DeNovix Inc., Wilmington, DE, USA).

4.6. Cellular Wound-Healing Activity Assay

Human keratinocyte monolayer wound-healing assay was performed to investigate wound closure-accelerating effects of pinocembrin. The seeded HaCaT cells (0.02×10^6 cells) were allowed to attain confluence in complete media in 24-well plates. A scratch wound in a vertical and horizontal crossline fashion were created by using SPLScar™ Scratcher (SPL Life Sciences, Gyeonggi-do, Korea). Each well was washed one time with sterile phosphate buffer saline (PBS), and the cells were then treated with pinocembrin at 62.5 µM or DMSO in DMEM with no FBS. The changes in the wounded areas were observed and photographed at 0 h, 3 h, 6 h, 24 h, and 48 h using a phase-contrast Axio Vert.A1 microscope, with 10× magnification. In some experiments, a MEK-1 inhibitor (U0126) and a PI3K inhibitor (LY294002) were included to confirm the molecular mechanism of pinocembrin at the signaling level.

4.7. Western Blot Analysis

To investigate the possible mode of action of pinocembrin on cell proliferation signaling pathways and cell survival signaling pathways, we detected the phosphorylated forms of ERK1/2 kinases and protein kinase B (AKT) Western blotting as described in previous studies [18]. Human keratinocytes were seeded at 0.2×10^6 cells in 24-well plates overnight. The cells were then incubated with pinocembrin at various doses (15.6, 31.3, and 62.5 µM) for 15 min or treated with 62.5 µM at different time points (0 min, 2 min, 5 min, 15 min, 30 min, 1 h, 3 h, 6 h, 12 h, and 24 h). In some experiments, cells were exposed to U0126 or LY294002 for 2 h prior to treatment with pinocembrin or DMSO. Cell lysates were prepared with 1X reducing Laemmli buffer (150 µL), heated at 95 °C for 5 min in a heat box, and subjected to electrophoresis (SDS-PAGE) and electroblotting. Target proteins on the membranes were detected with specific antibodies (Cell Signaling Technology, Boston, MA, USA) which included antibodies against ERK1/2 (catalog no.9107), phosphorylated ERK1/2 (catalog no.4370), Akt (catalog no.2920), phosphorylated Akt (catalog no.4060), and actin (catalog no.3700) at 4 °C overnight, with gentle agitation. All antibodies were diluted as instructed by the company. After three washes with TBS-T, membranes were incubated with 1:10,000 of anti-mouse IgG-IRDye®800CW (catalog no.926–32210) or 1:10,000 of anti-rabbit IgG-IRDye®680RT (catalog no.926–68071) (LI−COR Biosciences, USA) for 2 h at room temperature. The signal of targeted protein on membranes were detected with an Odyssey® CLx Imaging System (LI−COR Biosciences, Lincoln, NE, USA). Densitometric analysis of each protein band was performed by using ImageJ software.

4.8. Immunofluorescence Study

To stain ERK and Akt phosphorylation signal in keratinocyte treated with pinocembrin, we performed immunostaining using the same primary antibodies as above. Human keratinocytes were seeded at 0.1×10^6 cells onto the sterile glass cover slips placed in 3 cm cell culture dishes overnight in complete media (DMEM). Cells were serum-starved for 24 h prior to treatment with 62.5 µM of pinocembrin for 15 min. Cells were then fixed with 4% paraformaldehyde or −20 °C absolute methanol (depending on the instruction of the company) for 15 min at room temperature. After three washes with PBS (each time for 5 min), paraformaldehyde-fixed cells were permeabilized with Triton X-100 (0.3% in sterile PBS) for 5 min at room temperature. Sample coverslips were incubated with 1% bovine serum albumin (diluted in PBS-T) for 1 h at room temperature to block non-specific binding. By following the instruction from the company, sample coverslips were incubated with certain primary antibodies at 4 °C overnight. All primary antibodies were the same ones used in Western blot analysis. After washing for three times with PBS, sample coverslips were incubated with anti-rabbit IgG-Alexa488 and 5 µg/mL of DAPI (nuclear staining) for 2 h at room temperature, in a light-protecting container. Sample coverslips were washed three times with PBS and one time with distilled water, and mounted with Fluoromount-G (SouthernBiotech, Birmingham, AL, USA). The fluorescent signal of the targeted proteins was visualized at 100× magnification and captured with Axio Vert.A1 microscope (Carl Zeiss Suzhou Co., Ltd., Suzhou, China), equipped with the Zen 2.6 (blue edition) Software for the Zeiss Axiocam 506 color microscope camera.

4.9. Statistical Analysis

Data from each experiment were obtained from at least three independent replicates, and presented as mean ± SD. One-way analysis of variance (ANOVA) with Tukey's post hoc multiple comparisons on raw data reads by using GraphPad Prism 8.0.1 (GraphPad Software Inc., San Diego, CA, USA) was applied. A p-value less than 0.05 indicates statistical significance.

5. Conclusions

We revealed that pinocembrin is an active compound with strong stimulating effects on human keratinocytes. Pinocembrin positively regulates growth and survival of the cells through activating ERK1/2 and Akt. The ability of pinocembrin in modulating the function of crucial signaling kinases at their post-translational modification level highlights its distinct regenerative properties. This evidence supports the use of pinocembrin-containing plants and natural products as an alternative means for skin regeneration and wound healing when some patients fail the currently available treatments, or when the cost of certain wound-healing agents, such as growth factors, is unaffordable.

Author Contributions: Conceptualization, W.N.; supervision, W.N.; project administration, W.N.; funding acquisition, W.N., N.W. and S.P.; writing—original draft preparation, W.N. and J.R.; investigation, J.R.; formal analysis, J.R.; resources, S.P. and N.W.; writing—review and editing, W.N., N.W. and S.P. All authors have read and agreed to the published version of the manuscript.

Funding: This research project is supported by the National Research Council of Thailand (NRCT): (N41A640202). This research project was also supported by Fundamental Fund 2022, Chiang Mai University (funding number FF65/042).

Institutional Review Board Statement: Not applicable.

Informed Consent Statement: Not applicable.

Data Availability Statement: Data is contained within the article.

Acknowledgments: J.R. was partly supported from the Teaching Assistant and Research Assistant (TA/RA) scholarships, Graduate School, Chiang Mai University, Chiang Mai, Thailand.

Conflicts of Interest: The authors declare no conflict of interest.

References

1. Kasuya, A.; Tokura, Y. Attempts to accelerate wound healing. *J. Dermatol. Sci.* **2014**, *76*, 169–172. [CrossRef] [PubMed]
2. Pastar, I.; Stojadinovic, O.; Yin, N.C.; Ramirez, H.; Nusbaum, A.G.; Sawaya, A.; Patel, S.B.; Khalid, L.; Isseroff, R.R.; Tomic-Canic, M. Epithelialization in Wound Healing: A Comprehensive Review. *Adv. Wound Care* **2014**, *3*, 445–464. [CrossRef] [PubMed]
3. Kirsner, R.S.; Eaglstein, W.H. The wound healing process. *Dermatol. Clin.* **1993**, *11*, 629–640. [CrossRef]
4. Shi, C.; Wang, C.; Liu, H.; Li, Q.; Li, R.; Zhang, Y.; Liu, Y.; Shao, Y.; Wang, J. Selection of Appropriate Wound Dressing for Various Wounds. *Front. Bioeng. Biotechnol.* **2020**, *8*, 182. [CrossRef]
5. Han, G.; Ceilley, R. Chronic Wound Healing: A Review of Current Management and Treatments. *Adv. Ther.* **2017**, *34*, 599–610. [CrossRef] [PubMed]
6. Hackam, D.J.; Ford, H.R. Cellular, biochemical, and clinical aspects of wound healing. *Surg. Infect.* **2002**, *3* (Suppl. S1), S23–S35. [CrossRef] [PubMed]
7. Kawasumi, A.; Sagawa, N.; Hayashi, S.; Yokoyama, H.; Tamura, K. Wound healing in mammals and amphibians: Toward limb regeneration in mammals. *Curr. Top. Microbiol. Immunol.* **2013**, *367*, 33–49. [CrossRef]
8. Goodson, W.H., 3rd; Hunt, T.K. Wound healing and aging. *J. Investig. Dermatol.* **1979**, *73*, 88–91. [CrossRef]
9. Gerstein, A.D.; Phillips, T.J.; Rogers, G.S.; Gilchrest, B.A. Wound healing and aging. *Dermatol. Clin.* **1993**, *11*, 749–757. [CrossRef]
10. Morikawa, T.; Funakoshi, K.; Ninomiya, K.; Yasuda, D.; Miyagawa, K.; Matsuda, H.; Yoshikawa, M. Medicinal foodstuffs. XXXIV. Structures of new prenylchalcones and prenylflavanones with TNF-alpha and aminopeptidase N inhibitory activities from Boesenbergia rotunda. *Chem. Pharm. Bull.* **2008**, *56*, 956–962. [CrossRef]
11. Eng-Chong, T.; Yean-Kee, L.; Chin-Fei, C.; Choon-Han, H.; Sher-Ming, W.; Li-Ping, C.T.; Gen-Teck, F.; Khalid, N.; Abd Rahman, N.; Karsani, S.A.; et al. Boesenbergia rotunda: From Ethnomedicine to Drug Discovery. *Evid. Based Complement. Alternat. Med.* **2012**, *2012*, 473637. [CrossRef] [PubMed]
12. Mazzotta, S.; Governa, P.; Borgonetti, V.; Marcolongo, P.; Nanni, C.; Gamberucci, A.; Manetti, F.; Pessina, F.; Carullo, G.; Brizzi, A.; et al. Pinocembrin and its linolenoyl ester derivative induce wound healing activity in HaCaT cell line potentially involving a GPR120/FFA4 mediated pathway. *Bioorg. Chem.* **2021**, *108*, 104657. [CrossRef] [PubMed]
13. Rasul, A.; Millimouno, F.M.; Ali Eltayb, W.; Ali, M.; Li, J.; Li, X. Pinocembrin: A Novel Natural Compound with Versatile Pharmacological and Biological Activities. *BioMed Res. Int.* **2013**, *2013*, 379850. [CrossRef]
14. Aguero, M.B.; Gonzalez, M.; Lima, B.; Svetaz, L.; Sanchez, M.; Zacchino, S.; Feresin, G.E.; Schmeda-Hirschmann, G.; Palermo, J.; Wunderlin, D.; et al. Argentinean propolis from Zuccagnia punctata Cav. (*Caesalpinieae*) exudates: Phytochemical characterization and antifungal activity. *J. Agric. Food Chem.* **2010**, *58*, 194–201. [CrossRef]

15. Kanchanapiboon, J.; Kongsa, U.; Pattamadilok, D.; Kamponchaidet, S.; Wachisunthon, D.; Poonsatha, S.; Tuntoaw, S. Boesenbergia rotunda extract inhibits Candida albicans biofilm formation by pinostrobin and pinocembrin. *J. Ethnopharmacol.* **2020**, *261*, 113193. [CrossRef] [PubMed]
16. María Belén Agüero, L.S.; Baroni, V.; Lima, B.; Luna, L.; Zacchino, S.; Saavedra, P.; Wunderlin, D.; Feresin, G.E.; Tapia, A. Urban propolis from San Juan province (Argentina): Ethnopharmacological uses and antifungal activity against Candida and dermatophytes. *Ind. Crops Prod.* **2014**, *57*, 166–173. [CrossRef]
17. Hooker, J.D. *The Flora of British India*; L. Reeve & Co.: London, UK, 1890; Volume 5. [CrossRef]
18. Ruttanapattanakul, J.; Wikan, N.; Okonogi, S.; Na Takuathung, M.; Buacheen, P.; Pitchakarn, P.; Potikanond, S.; Nimlamool, W. Boesenbergia rotunda extract accelerates human keratinocyte proliferation through activating ERK1/2 and PI3K/Akt kinases. *Biomed. Pharmacother.* **2021**, *133*, 111002. [CrossRef] [PubMed]
19. Punvittayagul, C.; Wongpoomchai, R.; Taya, S.; Pompimon, W. Effect of pinocembrin isolated from Boesenbergia pandurata on xenobiotic-metabolizing enzymes in rat liver. *Drug Metab. Lett.* **2011**, *5*, 1–5. [CrossRef]
20. Gosain, A.; DiPietro, L.A. Aging and wound healing. *World J. Surg.* **2004**, *28*, 321–326. [CrossRef]
21. Sorg, H.; Tilkorn, D.J.; Hager, S.; Hauser, J.; Mirastschijski, U. Skin Wound Healing: An Update on the Current Knowledge and Concepts. *Eur. Surg. Res.* **2017**, *58*, 81–94. [CrossRef]
22. Fisher, G.J.; Wang, Z.Q.; Datta, S.C.; Varani, J.; Kang, S.; Voorhees, J.J. Pathophysiology of premature skin aging induced by ultraviolet light. *N. Engl. J. Med.* **1997**, *337*, 1419–1428. [CrossRef] [PubMed]
23. Swift, M.E.; Burns, A.L.; Gray, K.L.; DiPietro, L.A. Age-related alterations in the inflammatory response to dermal injury. *J. Investig. Dermatol.* **2001**, *117*, 1027–1035. [CrossRef] [PubMed]
24. Swift, M.E.; Kleinman, H.K.; DiPietro, L.A. Impaired wound repair and delayed angiogenesis in aged mice. *Lab. Investig.* **1999**, *79*, 1479–1487. [PubMed]
25. Guo, S.; Dipietro, L.A. Factors affecting wound healing. *J. Dent. Res.* **2010**, *89*, 219–229. [CrossRef]
26. Fife, C.E.; Cartel, M.J.; Walker, D.; Thomson, B. Wound Care Outcomes and Associated Cost Among Patients Treated in US Outpatient Wound Centers: Data from the US Wound Registry. *Wounds* **2012**, *24*, 10–17.
27. Zhao, P.; Sui, B.D.; Liu, N.; Lv, Y.J.; Zheng, C.X.; Lu, Y.B.; Huang, W.T.; Zhou, C.H.; Chen, J.; Pang, D.L.; et al. Anti-aging pharmacology in cutaneous wound healing: Effects of metformin, resveratrol, and rapamycin by local application. *Aging Cell* **2017**, *16*, 1083–1093. [CrossRef]
28. Nimlamool, W.; Potikanond, S.; Ruttanapattanakul, J.; Wikan, N.; Okonogi, S.; Jantrapirom, S.; Pitchakarn, P.; Karinchai, J. Curcuma amarissima Extract Activates Growth and Survival Signal Transduction Networks to Stimulate Proliferation of Human Keratinocyte. *Biology* **2021**, *10*, 289. [CrossRef]
29. Nimlamool, W.; Chansakaow, S.; Potikanond, S.; Wikan, N.; Hankittichai, P.; Ruttanapattanakul, J.; Thaklaewphan, P. The Leaf Extract of *Mitrephora chulabhorniana* Suppresses Migration and Invasion and Induces Human Cervical Cancer Cell Apoptosis through Caspase-Dependent Pathway. *BioMed Res. Int.* **2022**, *2022*, 2028082. [CrossRef]
30. Ruttanapattanakul, J.; Wikan, N.; Chinda, K.; Jearanaikulvanich, T.; Krisanuruks, N.; Muangcha, M.; Okonogi, S.; Potikanond, S.; Nimlamool, W. Essential Oil from Zingiber ottensii Induces Human Cervical Cancer Cell Apoptosis and Inhibits MAPK and PI3K/AKT Signaling Cascades. *Plants* **2021**, *10*, 1419. [CrossRef] [PubMed]
31. Thaklaewphan, P.; Ruttanapattanakul, J.; Monkaew, S.; Buatoom, M.; Sookkhee, S.; Nimlamool, W.; Potikanond, S. Kaempferia parviflora extract inhibits TNF-alpha-induced release of MCP-1 in ovarian cancer cells through the suppression of NF-kappaB signaling. *Biomed. Pharmacother.* **2021**, *141*, 111911. [CrossRef] [PubMed]
32. Governa, P.; Carullo, G.; Biagi, M.; Rago, V.; Aiello, F. Evaluation of the In Vitro Wound-Healing Activity of Calabrian Honeys. *Antioxidants* **2019**, *8*, 36. [CrossRef]
33. Cui, Y.M.; Ao, M.Z.; Li, W.; Yu, L.J. Effect of glabridin from Glycyrrhiza glabra on learning and memory in mice. *Planta Med.* **2008**, *74*, 377–380. [CrossRef]
34. Drewes, S.E.; van Vuuren, S.F. Antimicrobial acylphloroglucinols and dibenzyloxy flavonoids from flowers of Helichrysum gymnocomum. *Phytochemistry* **2008**, *69*, 1745–1749. [CrossRef] [PubMed]
35. Park, Y.K.; Koo, M.H.; Abreu, J.A.; Ikegaki, M.; Cury, J.A.; Rosalen, P.L. Antimicrobial activity of propolis on oral microorganisms. *Curr. Microbiol.* **1998**, *36*, 24–28. [CrossRef] [PubMed]
36. Youn, K.; Jun, M. Biological Evaluation and Docking Analysis of Potent BACE1 Inhibitors from Boesenbergia rotunda. *Nutrients* **2019**, *11*, 662. [CrossRef] [PubMed]
37. Jost, M.; Huggett, T.M.; Kari, C.; Rodeck, U. Matrix-independent survival of human keratinocytes through an EGF receptor/MAPK-kinase-dependent pathway. *Mol. Biol. Cell* **2001**, *12*, 1519–1527. [CrossRef] [PubMed]
38. Deng, M.; Chen, W.L.; Takatori, A.; Peng, Z.; Zhang, L.; Mongan, M.; Parthasarathy, R.; Sartor, M.; Miller, M.; Yang, J.; et al. A role for the mitogen-activated protein kinase kinase kinase 1 in epithelial wound healing. *Mol. Biol. Cell* **2006**, *17*, 3446–3455. [CrossRef] [PubMed]
39. Czech, M.P. PIP2 and PIP3: Complex roles at the cell surface. *Cell* **2000**, *100*, 603–606. [CrossRef]
40. Insall, R.H.; Weiner, O.D. PIP3, PIP2, and cell movement—Similar messages, different meanings? *Dev. Cell* **2001**, *1*, 743–747. [CrossRef]

41. Wu, Q.; Wang, H.; Zhao, X.; Shi, Y.; Jin, M.; Wan, B.; Xu, H.; Cheng, Y.; Ge, H.; Zhang, Y. Identification of G-protein-coupled receptor 120 as a tumor-promoting receptor that induces angiogenesis and migration in human colorectal carcinoma. *Oncogene* **2013**, *32*, 5541–5550. [CrossRef]
42. Gao, B.; Huang, Q.; Jie, Q.; Lu, W.G.; Wang, L.; Li, X.J.; Sun, Z.; Hu, Y.Q.; Chen, L.; Liu, B.H.; et al. GPR120: A bi-potential mediator to modulate the osteogenic and adipogenic differentiation of BMMSCs. *Sci. Rep.* **2015**, *5*, 14080. [CrossRef] [PubMed]
43. Katsuma, S.; Hatae, N.; Yano, T.; Ruike, Y.; Kimura, M.; Hirasawa, A.; Tsujimoto, G. Free fatty acids inhibit serum deprivation-induced apoptosis through GPR120 in a murine enteroendocrine cell line STC-1. *J. Biol. Chem.* **2005**, *280*, 19507–19515. [CrossRef] [PubMed]
44. Chen, C.; Nimlamool, W.; Miller, C.J.; Lou, H.J.; Turk, B.E. Rational Redesign of a Functional Protein Kinase-Substrate Interaction. *ACS Chem. Biol.* **2017**, *12*, 1194–1198. [CrossRef] [PubMed]

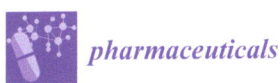

Article

Phenolic Secondary Metabolites and Antiradical and Antibacterial Activities of Different Extracts of *Usnea barbata* (L.) Weber ex F.H.Wigg from Călimani Mountains, Romania

Violeta Popovici [1,†], Laura Bucur [2,*], Cerasela Elena Gîrd [3,*], Antoanela Popescu [2,†], Elena Matei [4,†], Georgeta Camelia Cozaru [4,5,†], Verginica Schröder [6,*], Emma Adriana Ozon [7,*], Ancuța Cătălina Fița [7,*], Dumitru Lupuliasa [7,‡], Mariana Aschie [4,5,‡], Aureliana Caraiane [8,‡], Mihaela Botnarciuc [9,‡] and Victoria Badea [1,‡]

1. Department of Microbiology and Immunology, Faculty of Dental Medicine, Ovidius University of Constanta, 7 Ilarie Voronca Street, 900684 Constanta, Romania; violeta.popovici@365.univ-ovidius.ro (V.P.); victoria.badea@365.univ-ovidius.ro (V.B.)
2. Department of Pharmacognosy, Faculty of Pharmacy, Ovidius University of Constanta, 6 Capitan Al. Serbanescu Street, 900001 Constanta, Romania; antoanela.popescu@365.univ-ovidius.ro
3. Department of Pharmacognosy, Phytochemistry, and Phytotherapy, Faculty of Pharmacy, Carol Davila University of Medicine and Pharmacy, 6 Traian Vuia Street, 020956 Bucharest, Romania
4. Center for Research and Development of the Morphological and Genetic Studies of Malignant Pathology, Ovidius University of Constanta, CEDMOG, 145 Tomis Blvd., 900591 Constanta, Romania; sogorescuelena@gmail.com (E.M.); drcozaru@yahoo.com (G.C.C.); aschiemariana@yahoo.com (M.A.)
5. Clinical Service of Pathology, Sf. Apostol Andrei Emergency County Hospital, 145 Tomis Blvd., 900591 Constanta, Romania
6. Department of Cellular and Molecular Biology, Faculty of Pharmacy, Ovidius University of Constanta, 6 Capitan Al. Serbanescu Street, 900001 Constanta, Romania
7. Department of Pharmaceutical Technology and Biopharmacy, Faculty of Pharmacy, Carol Davila University of Medicine and Pharmacy, 6 Traian Vuia Street, 020956 Bucharest, Romania; dumitru.lupuliasa@umfcd.ro
8. Department of Oral Rehabilitation, Faculty of Dental Medicine, Ovidius University of Constanta, 7 Ilarie Voronca Street, 900684 Constanta, Romania; aureliana.caraiane@365.univ-ovidius.ro
9. Department of Microbiology, Faculty of Medicine, Ovidius University of Constanta, 1 University Street, 900470 Constanta, Romania; mihaela.botnarciuc@365.univ-ovidius.ro
* Correspondence: laurabucur@univ-ovidius.ro (L.B.); cerasela.gird@umfcd.ro (C.E.G.); verginica.schroder@univ-ovidius.ro (V.S.); emma.budura@umfcd.ro (E.A.O.); catalina.fita@umfcd.ro (A.C.F.)
† These authors contributed equally to this work.
‡ These authors contributed equally to this work.

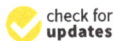

Citation: Popovici, V.; Bucur, L.; Gîrd, C.E.; Popescu, A.; Matei, E.; Cozaru, G.C.; Schröder, V.; Ozon, E.A.; Fița, A.C.; Lupuliasa, D.; et al. Phenolic Secondary Metabolites and Antiradical and Antibacterial Activities of Different Extracts of *Usnea barbata* (L.) Weber ex F.H.Wigg from Călimani Mountains, Romania. *Pharmaceuticals* **2022**, *15*, 829. https://doi.org/10.3390/ph15070829

Academic Editors: Fernando Calzada and Miguel Valdes

Received: 6 June 2022
Accepted: 1 July 2022
Published: 4 July 2022

Publisher's Note: MDPI stays neutral with regard to jurisdictional claims in published maps and institutional affiliations.

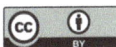

Copyright: © 2022 by the authors. Licensee MDPI, Basel, Switzerland. This article is an open access article distributed under the terms and conditions of the Creative Commons Attribution (CC BY) license (https://creativecommons.org/licenses/by/4.0/).

Abstract: Phenolic compounds represent an essential bioactive metabolites group with numerous pharmaceutical applications. Our study aims to identify and quantify phenolic constituents of various liquid and dry extracts of *Usnea barbata* (L.) Weber ex F.H. Wigg (*U. barbata*) from Calimani Mountains, Romania, and investigate their bioactivities. The extracts in acetone, 96% ethanol, and water with the same dried lichen/solvent ratio (w/v) were obtained through two conventional techniques: maceration (*m*UBA, *m*UBE, and *m*UBW) and Soxhlet extraction (*d*UBA, *d*UBE, and *d*UBW). High-performance liquid chromatography with diode-array detection (HPLC-DAD) was performed for usnic acid (UA) and different polyphenols quantification. Then, the total phenolic content (TPC) and 2,2-diphenyl-1-picrylhydrazyl (DPPH) free-radical scavenging activity (AA) were determined through spectrophotometric methods. Using the disc diffusion method (DDM), the antibacterial activity was evaluated against Gram-positive and Gram-negative bacteria known for their pathogenicity: *Staphylococcus aureus* (ATCC 25923), *Streptococcus pneumoniae* (ATCC 49619), *Pseudomonas aeruginosa* (ATCC 27853), and *Klebsiella pneumoniae* (ATCC 13883). All extracts contain phenolic compounds expressed as TPC values. Five lichen extracts display various UA contents; this significant metabolite was not detected in *d*UBW. Six polyphenols from the standards mixture were quantified only in ethanol and water extracts; *m*UBE has all individual polyphenols, while *d*UBE shows only two. Three polyphenols were detected in *m*UBW, but none was found in *d*UBW. All *U. barbata* extracts had antiradical activity; however, only ethanol and acetone extracts proved inhibitory activity against *P. aeruginosa*, *S. pneumoniae*, and *S. aureus*. In contrast, *K. pneumoniae* was strongly resistant (IZD = 0). Data analysis evidenced a high positive correlation between the phenolic constituents and bioactivities of each *U. barbata* extract. Associating these extracts' properties with both conventional techniques used for their preparation revealed the extraction conditions' significant influence on lichen extracts metabolites profiling, with a powerful impact on their pharmacological potential.

Keywords: *Usnea barbata* (L.) Weber ex F.H. Wigg extracts; phenolic secondary metabolites; usnic acid; polyphenols; DPPH free-radical scavenging activity; antibacterial activity

1. Introduction

Phenolic compounds are essential plant secondary metabolites with numerous pharmaceutical applications [1]. As unique symbionts between fungi and algae, lichens are distinguished in the plants' world by their specific secondary metabolites with phenolic structures (depsides, depsidones, dibenzofurans, anthraquinones, and xanthones) [2]. These constituents are deposited as crystals on fungal hyphae in the cortex or medulla; the different distribution in the thallus layers is correlated with their biological actions [3]. The lichen's most significant pharmacological activities are antioxidant [4], antimicrobial [5], anticancer [6], photoprotective [7], and anti-inflammatory [8]. Therefore, they are considered important representatives with biopharmaceutical potential [9]. Due to remarkable antioxidant [10] and antibacterial [11] properties, lichens represent a promising source of protective [12–14] and antibiotic drugs [15–17].

With numerous pharmacological activities, the lichens of the genus *Usnea* (Parmeliaceae) are appreciated as powerful phytomedicines, used for therapeutical purposes for thousands of years [18]. The most known secondary metabolite in *Usnea* sp. is usnic acid—a phenolic compound with a dibenzofuran structure. As yellow crystals, it is found on cortex fungal hyphae, exhibiting a photoprotective action [19]. Usnic acid is found as a (+) enantiomer in *Usnea* lichens [20]. A valuable representative of this genus, known for its antioxidant [21], antibacterial [22], and photoprotective [7] effects, is *U. barbata*. Usnic acid is the main secondary metabolite responsible for its pharmacological potential [23]. The pharmaceutical applications of UA as an antibacterial agent are limited by its poor water solubility [24] and significant hepatotoxicity [25]. Therefore, the nanosystems with usnic acid must be able to increase its bio-disponibility, tolerance, and antibacterial effects [26]. Interesting nano-formulations were performed: liposomal UA-cyclodextrin inclusion complexes, which increase usnic acid solubility in water [27], glycosylated cationic liposomes, promoting usnic acid penetration in the bacterial biofilm matrix [28], and magnetic nanoparticles [29] with antimicrobial activity and antibiofilm activity against Gram-positive bacteria (*S. aureus* and *E. faecalis*) and Gram-negative ones (*P. aeruginosa*). Balaz et al. [30] recently proposed a bio-mechanochemical synthesis of silver nanoparticles using *U. antarctica* and other lichen species. Using $AgNO_3$ (as a silver precursor) and lichens (as reduction agents), they performed techniques of mechanochemistry (ball milling) and obtained nanoparticles with an intense antibacterial effect against *S. aureus*. This described procedure overcomes the lichen secondary metabolites' low solubility in water. Siddiqi et al. [31] demonstrated the antimicrobial properties of *U. longissima*-driven silver nanoparticles through the denaturation of ribosomes, leading to enzyme inactivation and protein denaturation, resulting in bacterial apoptosis.

U. barbata also contains bioactive polyphenols with pharmaceutical applications; different nanotechnologies were described to enhance their bioavailability and biocompatibility [32]. They can be used as nanoparticles to increase their antioxidant and antibacterial potential or other activities [33–38].

Numerous studies investigated the antibacterial effects of *Usnea* sp. Extracts—obtained through conventional and green extraction techniques—for pharmaceutical applications [39]. Thus, Tosun et al. [40] explored the antimycobacterial action of *U. barbata* fractions in petroleum ether, chloroform, methanol, and water. Bate et al. [41] studied the antibacterial activity of *U. articulata* and *U. florida* methanol macerates against MDR bacteria (*Staphylococcus* sp., *P aeruginosa*, *Salmonella* sp., and *E. coli*). Zizovic et al. [42] proved the strong antibacterial action of *U. barbata* supercritical fluid extracts (SFE). One year later, Ivanovic et al. [43] analyzed the influence of various extraction conditions (temperature, pressure) and pre-treatment methods on bactericidal effects against *S. aureus* strains. Basiouni et al. [44] evaluated the *U. barbata* sunflower oil extract inhibitory activity on bacterial strains isolates from poultry. In a previous study, Matvieva et al. [15] analyzed the antimicrobial properties of the ethanol, isopropanol, acetone, DMSO, and water extracts of *Usnea* sp against *S. aureus*, *B. subtilis*, and *E coli*.

We propose to investigate the antibacterial and antiradical properties of *U barbata* extracts in the same solvents, obtained by two low-cost and easy-to-use conventional techniques. Our study novelty consists of a comparative analysis of fluid and dry *U. barbata* extracts in ethanol, acetone, and water, obtained by maceration and Soxhlet extraction [34], determining their phenolic constituents and evaluating the free radical scavenging activity and antibacterial effects. Our results revealed that, despite the same ratio between the dried lichen and the solvent (w/v), all *U. barbata* extracts display significant differences in the phenolic metabolites' diversity and amount due to extraction conditions, with a substantial impact on their bioactivities.

2. Results

2.1. Lichen Extracts

All data regarding the obtained *U. barbata* extracts are displayed in Table 1 and Figure S1 from Supplementary Materials.

Table 1. Extraction conditions and *U. barbata* extracts color.

Extraction Solvent	*U. barbata* Extract	Temperature of Extraction (°C)	Yield (%)	*U. barbata* Extract's Color
Acetone	*d*UBA	55–60	5.55 [b]	Yellow-brown
	*m*UBA	20–22	n/a	Yellow
Ethanol	*d*UBE	75–80	11.15 [a]	Light brown
	*m*UBE	20–22	n/a	Light brown
Water	*d*UBW	95–100	1.76 [c]	Dark brown-reddish
	*m*UBW	20–22	n/a	Brown reddish

UBA—*U. barbata* acetone extract, UBE—*U. barbata* ethanol extract, UBW—*U. barbata* water extract; *m*—macerate, *d*—dry extract, n/a—not applicable. The yield values followed by superscript letters are statistically significant ($p < 0.05$).

Data from Table 1 show that the extraction temperature for liquid extracts was 20–22 °C, and their color varies from yellow (*m*UBA) to light brown (*m*UBE) and brown-reddish (*m*UBW).

At Soxhlet extraction, the temperature value increased from *d*UBA (55–60 °C) to *d*UBE (75–80 °C) and *d*UBW (95–100 °C). The highest yield (11.15%) was obtained for *d*UBE; its value decreased to 5.55% for *d*UBA and 1.76% for *d*UBW. Moreover, the dry extracts color changed from yellow-brown (*d*UBA) to light brown (*d*UBE) and dark brown-reddish (*d*UBW).

2.2. HPLC-DAD Determination of Usnic Acid Content

The usnic acid contents in all *U. barbata* extracts are displayed in Table 2.

All liquid extracts contain UA. Thus, *m*UBA had the highest UA content (211.9 mg/g extract equivalent to 21.19 mg/g dried lichen), following in decreasing order *m*UBE (0.257 mg/g, corresponding to 0.025 mg/g dried lichen) and *m*UBW (0.045 mg/g corresponding to 0.004 mg/g dried lichen). According to https://pubchem.ncbi.nlm.nih.gov/compound/Usnic-acid (accessed on 20 May 2022), usnic acid solubility significantly decreases in order: acetone > ethanol > water; these data can explain our results.

Table 2. Usnic acid content in fluid and dry *U. barbata* extracts.

U. barbata Extract		UAC	
		mg/g Lichen Extract	mg/g Dried Lichen
Acetone	mUBA	211.900 ± 0.002 [b]	21.190 [f]
	dUBA	241.830 ± 0.172 [a]	13.418 [g]
Ethanol	mUBE	0.257 ± 0.002 [d]	0.025 [i]
	dUBE	108.742 ± 0.703 [c]	12.125 [h]
Water	mUBW	0.045 ± 0.002 [e]	0.004 [j]
	dUBW	ND	n/a

UAC—usnic acid content, UBA—*U. barbata* acetone extract, UBE—*U. barbata* ethanol extract, UBW—*U. barbata* water extract; m—macerate, d—dry extract, ND—non-detected, n/a—not applicable; the mean values followed by superscript letters are statistically significant ($p < 0.05$).

The chromatograms of usnic acid standard and *U. barbata* extracts in all three solvents are displayed in Figure 1.

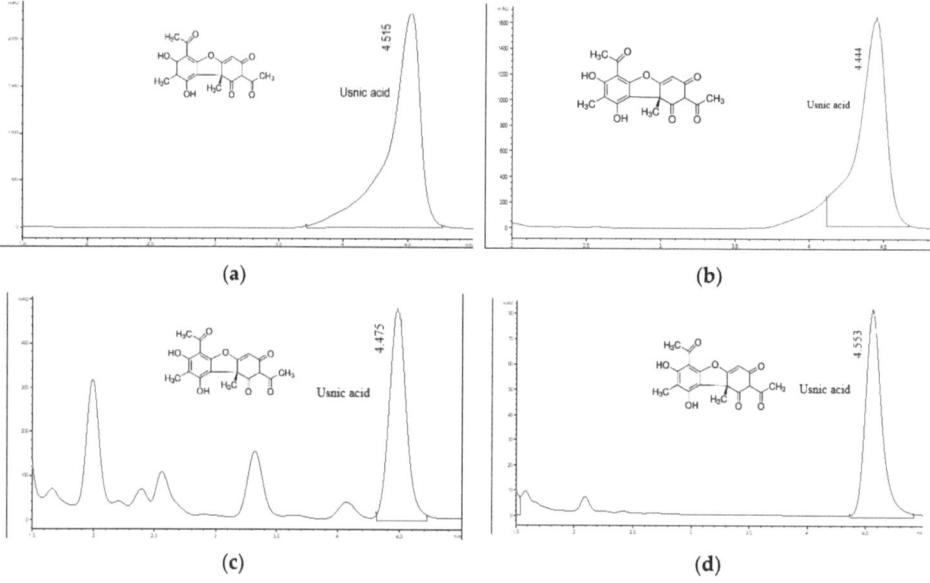

Figure 1. Chromatograms of usnic acid standard (**a**), mUBA (**b**), mUBE (**c**), mUBW (**d**). The red lines mark the significant peak areas.

Data from Table 2 show that only two dry extracts contain UA because in dUBW it was non-detected. Dry acetone extract contains UA of 241.773 mg/g, corresponding to 13.418 mg/g dried lichen. The usnic acid content in dUBE is 108.752 mg/g (12.125 mg/g dried lichen).

2.3. HPLC-DAD Determination of Polyphenols

The polyphenols contents are displayed in Table 3.
The chromatograms of *U. barbata* extracts are displayed in Figures 2–5.

Table 3. Polyphenols contents in *U. barbata* fluid and dry extracts in ethanol and water.

U. barbata Extracts	*m*UBE	*m*UBW	*d*UBE	*d*UBW
Polyphenols	Polyphenols Content mg/g Lichen Extract			
Caffeic acid (CA)	0.414 ± 0.005	ND	ND	ND
p-coumaric acid (pCA)	0.312 ± 0.001 [b]	0.749 ± 0.049 [a]	ND	ND
Ellagic acid (EA)	230.819 ± 0.264 [c]	ND	0.605 ± 0.007 [d]	ND
Chlorogenic acid (ChA)	0.512 ± 0.006 [f]	0.627 ± 0.006 [e]	ND	ND
Gallic acid (GA)	27.487 ± 0.459 [h]	60.358 ± 0.363 [g]	0.870 ± 0.008 [k]	ND
Cinnamic acid (CiA)	17.948 ± 0.114	ND	ND	ND

UBA—*U. barbata* acetone extract, UBE—*U. barbata* ethanol extract, UBW—*U. barbata* water extract; *m*—macerate, *d*—dry; pCA—*p*-coumaric acid, ChA—chlorogenic acid, CA—caffeic acid, CiA—cinnamic acid, EA—ellagic acid, GA—gallic acid, ND—non-detected; the mean values followed by superscript letters are statistically significant ($p < 0.05$).

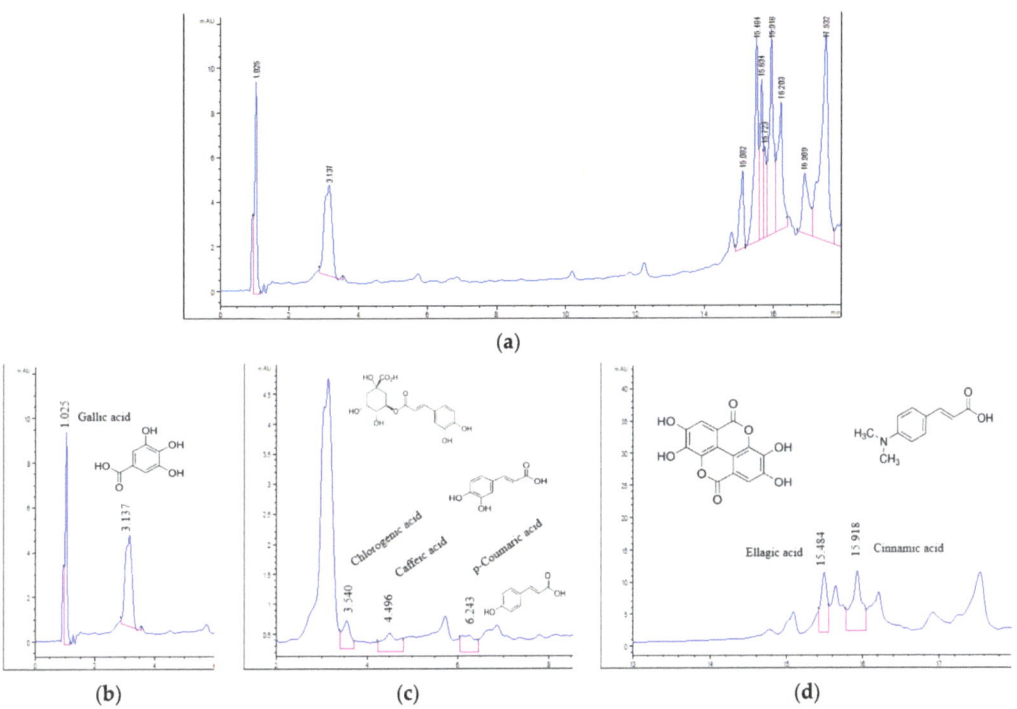

Figure 2. Chromatograms of *m*UBE (**a**); polyphenols in *m*UBE: gallic acid (**b**); chlorogenic, caffeic, and *p*-coumaric acids (**c**); ellagic and cinnamic acids (**d**). The red lines mark the significant peak areas, UBE—*U. barbata* ethanol extract, *m*—macerate.

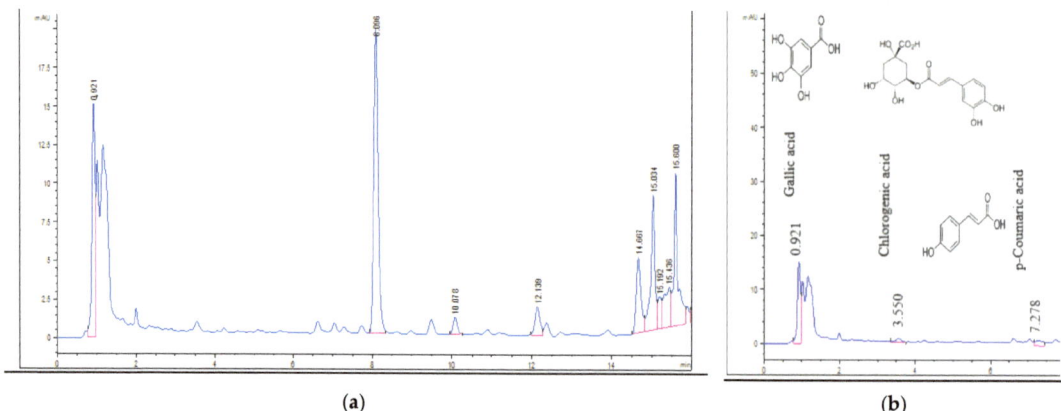

Figure 3. Chromatograms of *m*UBW (**a**); polyphenols in *m*UBW (**b**). The red lines mark the significant peak areas; UBW—*U. barbata* water extract, *m*—macerate.

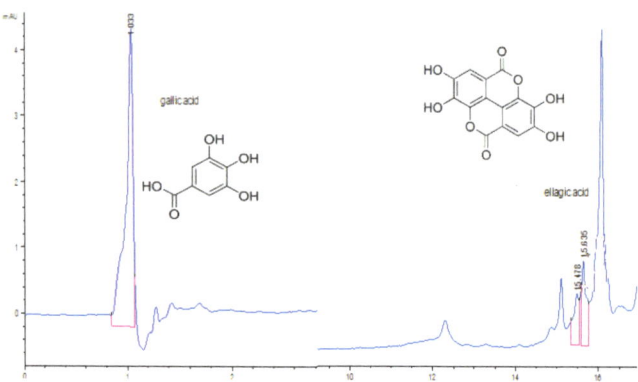

Figure 4. Gallic acid and ellagic acid in *d*UBE. The red lines mark the significant peak areas.

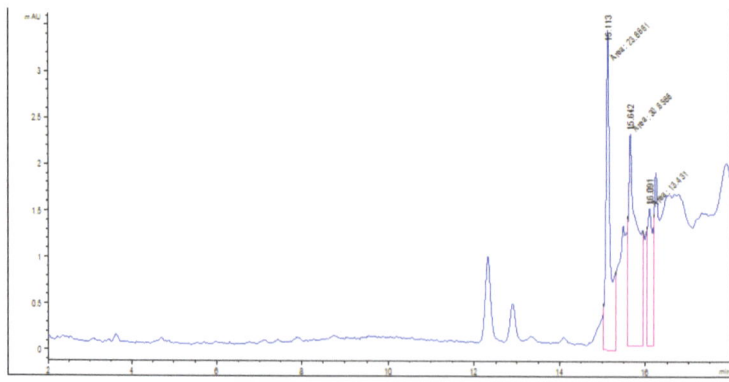

Figure 5. Chromatogram of *d*UBW. The red lines mark the significant peak areas.

As can be seen, six polyphenols of the standard mixture were identified only in ethanol and water fluid extracts; their high solubility in polar solvents could justify their absence in acetone extracts (Table 3 and Figures 2 and 3).

Of all six polyphenols identified in mUBE: caffeic acid (CA), p-coumaric acid (pCA), ellagic acid (EA), chlorogenic acid (ChA), gallic acid (GA), and cinnamic acid (CiA), only two (EA and GA) were found in dUBE, and three (pCA, ChA, and GA) in mUBW (Figures 2–4). The common polyphenol for all three extracts is GA, with the highest content in mUBW (60.358 mg/g), followed by mUBE (27.487 mg/g) and dUBE (0.870 mg/g). Ellagic acid content is 230.819 mg/g in mUBE and 0.605 mg/g in dUBE (Table 3, Figure 4).

The common polyphenols for mUBW and mUBE were pCA and ChA; their amounts were higher in mUBW (0.749 and 0.627 mg/g) than mUBE (0.312 and 0.512 mg/g). The other two polyphenols—CA (0.414 mg/g) and CiA (17.948 mg/g)—were identified exclusively in mUBE (Table 3, Figure 2).

The dUBW chromatogram (Figure 5) shows three peaks at the following retention times (RT): 15.113 min, 15.642 min, and 16.091 min; these RT values differed from standard polyphenols' ones. Their absence in dUBW could be due to their thermolability; the Soxhlet extraction involves prolonged heating for 8 h at 95–100 °C [45].

The polyphenols from the standard mixture were also non-detected in both U. barbata acetone extracts (Table 3) because their solubility is lower in this solvent than in ethanol or water.

2.4. Total Phenolic Content

It can be observed that the highest total phenolic content (TPC) values belong to dry U. barbata extracts (Table 4). The dUBA had the highest TPC (862.843 mg PyE/g); it is followed in decreasing order by dUBE (573.234 mg PyE/g) and dUBW (111.626 mg PyE/g). The TPC values in fluid extracts decreased in the following order: mUBE (276.603 mg PyE/mL), mUBA (220.597 mg PyE/mL), and mUBW (176.129 mg PyE/mL). TPC includes usnic acid, identified polyphenols, and unidentified phenolic constituents of each U. barbata extract.

Table 4. Total phenolic content (TPC) and free-radical scavenging activity of U. barbata extracts.

	U. barbata Extract	TPC (mg PyE/g Extract)	DPPH-Free Radical Scavenging%
Acetone	mUBA	220.597 ± 24.527 [d]	11.146 ± 0.577 [k]
	dUBA	862.843 ± 33.727 [a]	15.471 ± 0.629 [h]
Ethanol	mUBE	276.603 ± 15.025 [c]	12.162 ± 0.396 [j]
	dUBE	573.234 ± 42.308 [b]	16.728 ± 0.284 [g]
Water	mUBW	176.129 ± 24.169 [e]	6.429 ± 0.286 [l]
	dUBW	111.626 ± 11.132 [f]	3.951 ± 0.297 [m]

TPC—total phenolic content, UBA—U. barbata acetone extract, UBE—U. barbata ethanol extract, UBW—U. barbata water extract; m—macerate, d—dry extract, mg PyE—mg equivalents pyrogallol. The mean values followed by superscript letters are statistically significant ($p < 0.05$).

2.5. Free-Radical Scavenging Activity Assay

The results are displayed in Table 4.

Data from Table 4 show that all U. barbata extracts have antiradical activity. This effect was higher for dry ethanol and acetone extracts (16.728% for dUBE, 15.471% for dUBA) than fluid ones (12.162% for mUBE, 11.146% for mUBA). Only for water extracts, the antiradical activity of dUBW (3.951%) is lower than the mUBW one (6.429%).

2.6. Antibacterial Activity

The obtained results proved that the negative control (DMSO 0.1%) has no inhibitory effect on the bacteria tested (IZD = 0 mm). Only U. barbata extracts in acetone and ethanol inhibited bacterial strains' growth. (Figure S2, Supplementary Materials). Neither UBWs have any inhibitory effect on the tested bacteria (IZD = 0 mm).

Given that usnic acid is the major secondary metabolite of the genus Usnea, we considered this phenolic compound as a positive control. For the optimal interpretation of the obtained IZD values, we used two bactericidal antibiotics with different mechanisms of action and breakpoints: ofloxacin (OFL) and ceftriaxone (CTR).

The data displayed in Table 5 show the IZD values (mm) for all *U. barbata* extracts, UA, and standard antibiotics drugs (OFL and CTR).

Table 5. Antibacterial activity of *U. barbata* extracts.

Bacteria			S. aureus	S. pneumoniae	P. aeruginosa	K. pneumoniae
				Inhibition Zone Diameter—IZD (mm)		
UA			16.33 ± 0.82	17.33 ± 0.47	16.67 ± 0.47	0
				Liquid extracts		
mUBA			12.00 ± 0.82 [b]	17.67 ± 0.47	17.33 ± 1.25	0
mUBE			11.00 ± 0.82 [d]	18.67 ± 0.47	20.33 ± 1.70	0
mUBW			0	0	0	0
				Dry extracts		
dUBA			13.66 ± 0.47 [a]	18.00 ± 1.63	17.00 ± 1.63	0
dUBE			12.33 ± 1.25 [c]	18.33 ± 0.47	20.00 ± 1.63	0
dUBW			0	0	0	0
				Standard antibacterial drugs inhibitory activity		
OFL 5			26.33 ± 1.70	19.00 ± 1.63	19.33 ± 1.70	30.00 ± 0.82
CTR 30			25.00 ± 2.45	32.33 ± 2.05	21.00 ± 2.16	32.33 ± 2.49
				Standard antibacterial drugs breakpoints *		
				Ofloxacin		
		S *	≥18 *	≥16 *	≥16 *	≥16 *
OFL 5		I *	17–15 *	15–13 *	15–13 *	15–13 *
		R *	≤14 *	≤12 *	≤12 *	≤12 *
				Ceftriaxone		
		S *	≥21 *	≥26 *		≥23 *
CTR 30		I *			17–15 *	22–20 *
		R *	≤20 *	≤25 *	≤14 *	≤19 *

UBA—*U. barbata* acetone extract, UBE—*U. barbata* ethanol extract, UBW—*U. barbata* water extract; m—macerate, d—dry extract, UA—usnic acid (positive control), * Data adapted from CLSI breakpoints analyzed by Humphries et al. [46]; OFL—ofloxacin, CTR—ceftriaxone; 5, 30 μg—the antibiotic amount from the standard antibiotic disc; S—sensitivity, I—intermediate (dose-dependent action), R—resistance. The superscripts letters noted the statistically significant IZD mean values ($p < 0.05$).

Therefore, comparing the IZD values of the *U. barbata* extracts to those of both standard antibiotics on *S. aureus*, none had antibacterial action (IZD = 11.00–13.66 mm). Only usnic acid has an IZD (16.33 mm) in the "I" range of ofloxacin (17–15 mm); this means that antibacterial activity on *S. aureus* is dose dependent. Compared to ceftriaxone, the IZD value for UA belongs to the resistance range (<20 mm).

S. pneumoniae is sensitive to all *U. barbata* extracts as well as to usnic acid (IZD = 17.33–18.67 mm) when IZD values are compared to ofloxacin (S ≥ 16 mm *). However, it could be considered resistant when IZD values were compared to CTR (S ≥ 26 mm *).

Among Gram-negative bacteria, *P. aeruginosa* proves the highest sensitivity; all lichen extracts showed antibacterial action on *P. aeruginosa* (IZD = 16.77–20.33 mm), compared to ofloxacin (S ≥ 16 mm *). Only ethanol extracts (IZD = 20.00–20.33 mm) had an antibacterial effect related to ceftriaxone (S ≥ 18 mm *); the others are active in a dose-dependent manner (I = 17–15 mm). Contrariwise, no *U. barbata* extract inhibited the growth of *K. pneumoniae* colonies (IZD = 0 mm).

Considering the data registered in Table 5, we calculated the antibacterial activity index (AI), reporting the IZD values (mm) of lichen extracts to the ones of the standard antibiotic drugs [47]. It can be noted that dry and fluid *U. barbata* acetone and ethanol extracts had similar inhibitory effects (Table 6).

Table 6. Antibacterial activity index of *U. barbata* extracts and UA compared to both standard antibiotic drugs.

Bacteria	AI Values (Adim)					AB
	*m*UBA	*d*UBA	*m*UBE	*d*UBE	UA	
S. aureus	0.455	0.519	0.417	0.468	0.620	OFL5
	0.480	0.546	0.440	0.490	0.693	CTR30
S. pneumoniae	0.930 [a]	0.947 [a]	0.982 [a]	0.964 [a]	0.912 [a]	OFL5
	0.546 [b]	0.556 [b]	0.577 [b]	0.566 [b]	0.536 [b]	CTR30
P. aeruginosa	0.896	0.879	1.051	1.034	0.862	OFL5
	0.825	0.809	0.968	0.952	0.793	CTR30

AI—antibacterial activity index, adim—without measure unit, UBA—*U. barbata* acetone extract, UBE—*U. barbata* ethanol extract, *m*—macerate, *d*—dry extract, UA—usnic acid, AB—standard antibiotic drug, OFL—ofloxacin, CTR—ceftriaxone. 5, 30 μg—the antibiotic amount from the standard antibiotic disc. The AI values noted with superscripts letters are statistically significant ($p < 0.05$).

The presence of similar bioactive secondary metabolites, the fluid extracts used after solvent evaporation, and the additional presence of the polyphenols known for their strong antibacterial action could explain the results registered in Tables 5 and 6. Thus, UA had the highest inhibitory activity on *S. aureus*, showing a dose-dependent antibacterial effect and the highest AI values; the following are the extracts with a high usnic acid content, respectively UBA. *U. barbata* ethanol extracts show the lowest inhibitory effect because usnic acid is known for its highest inhibition levels on *S. aureus*; both UBEs have lower UAC values than the corresponding UBAs ones (Table 5).

On *S. pneumoniae* and *P. aeruginosa*, the lichen extracts in ethanol indicated the most significant inhibitory levels. Antibacterial activities of individual polyphenols could justify these results. They showed an antibacterial action against *S. pneumoniae* similar to ofloxacin. On *S. pneumoniae*, the AI values compared to OFL are statistically different from those linked to CTR (Table 6). In this case, for all *U. barbata* extracts, AI ≥ 0.912, proving that their antibacterial activity is similar to OFL. Against *P. aeruginosa*, *m*UBA and *d*UBA reported AI values higher than OFL (AI > 1) and similar to CTR (AI ≥ 0.952) (Table 6).

2.7. Data Analysis

We obtained *U. barbata* extracts performing two easy-to-use and low-cost conventional techniques mentioned in Romanian Pharmacopoeia X [48]: maceration for fluid extracts and Soxhlet extraction for dry ones. They have been one of the most used extraction procedures for herbal bioactive compounds [49]. According to the green chemistry concept, the solvents used for lichen extraction are "preferable," having low toxicity and significant safety [50]. Our entire study's data were synthesized in Table 7.

From the beginning, the same ratio—1:10 (w/v) between dried lichen and solvent—was maintained for all extracts. The fluid extracts were obtained at room temperature (20–22 °C). The Soxhlet extraction was performed by prolonged heating, and the requested temperature values registered in Table 7 were maintained for 8 h.

The phenolic metabolites contents were strongly influenced by extraction conditions, as shown in Table 7. Usnic acid content and TPC significantly increase in acetone and ethanol dry extracts than in fluid ones; UBAs have higher UAC and TPC than UBEs. The *m*UBW had the lowest TPC and UAC. However, after 8 h of Soxhlet extraction at 100 °C, *d*UBW shows diminished TPC values and no UAC.

The individual polyphenols were quantified only in ethanol and water *U. barbata* extracts. The *m*UBE contains all six polyphenols (CA, CiA, pCA, EA, GA, and ChA) and *m*UBW—only three (pCA, GA, and ChA). Regarding the corresponding dry extracts, in *d*UBE only two polyphenols (EA and GA) were found in lower content than *m*UBE; *d*UBW has no polyphenols.

Table 7. Characteristics of U. barbata extracts in ethanol, acetone, and water obtained by two different conventional techniques, regarding the extraction conditions, phenolic metabolites, and bioactivities.

U. barbata Extract		mUBE	dUBE	mUBA	dUBA	mUBW	dUBW
		\multicolumn{6}{c}{Extraction conditions}					
	Solvent	\multicolumn{2}{c}{96% ethanol}	\multicolumn{2}{c}{Acetone}	\multicolumn{2}{c}{Water}			
	Ratio (w/v)			\multicolumn{2}{c}{1:10}					
	Temperature (°C)	20–22	75–80	20–22	55–60	20–22	95–100
	Yield (%)		11.150		5.550		1.760
		\multicolumn{6}{c}{Phenolic metabolites (mg/g extract)}					
UA	TPC	276.603	573.234	220.597	862.843	176.129	111.626
	mg/g extract	0.257	108.74	211.190	241.830	0.045	
	% in dried lichen	0.002	1.212	2.119	1.341	0.0004	
	CA	0.414					
	pCA	0.312				0.749	
	EA	230.820	0.605				
	GA	27.487	0.870			60.358	
	CiA	17.948					
	ChA	0.513				0.627	
		\multicolumn{6}{c}{Antibacterial activity—IZD (mm)}					
	S.a.	11.000	12.330	12.000	13.670		
	S.p.	18.670	18.330	17.670	18.000		
	P.a.	20.330	20.000	17.330	17.000		
		\multicolumn{6}{c}{DPPH free radical scavenging activity (%)}					
AA		12.162	16.728	11.146	15.471	6.429	3.951

pCA—p-coumaric acid, ChA—chlorogenic acid, CA—caffeic acid, CiA—cinnamic acid, EA—ellagic acid, GA—gallic acid, UA—usnic acid, TPC—total phenolic content, AA—antiradical activity, P.a.—inhibitory activity against *P. aeruginosa*, S.a.—inhibitory activity against *S. aureus*, S.p.—inhibitory activity against *S. pneumoniae*; UBA—*U. barbata* acetone extract, UBE—*U. barbata* ethanol extract, UBW—*U. barbata* water extract; mUBE, mUBA, mUBW—obtained by maceration; dUBE, dUBA, dUBW—obtained by Soxhlet extraction.

These detailed aspects could be explained in the first step by the solubility differences of phenolic compounds in each extraction solvent. Polyphenols are soluble in polar solvents (ethanol, water); however, they are affected by prolonged heating [45]; thus, it can justify their decreasing or absence in the dry extracts after Soxhlet extraction for 8 h at 75–80 °C (dUBE) and 95–100 °C (dUBA). The lowest solubility of usnic acid in water underlies the minimal UAC value in mUBW. The high temperature of extraction (100 °C for 8 h) affects usnic acid stability; thus, the absence of UA in dUBW could be justified. According to https://www.biocrick.com/Usnic-acid-BCN4306.html (accessed on 2 May 2022), usnic acid storage requests desiccation and freezing (−20 °C); this information supports our results.

On the other hand, it can be seen that the dry extracts are obtained with a considerably low yield. When all UAC values are reported to the dried lichen amount used for each extract preparation, 2.119% corresponds to mUBA and only 1.341% for dUBA.

Principal Component Analysis

Principal component analysis (PCA) was performed for all *U. barbata* liquid and dry extracts and variable parameters—according to the correlation matrix from Supplementary Materials—and illustrated in Figure 6.

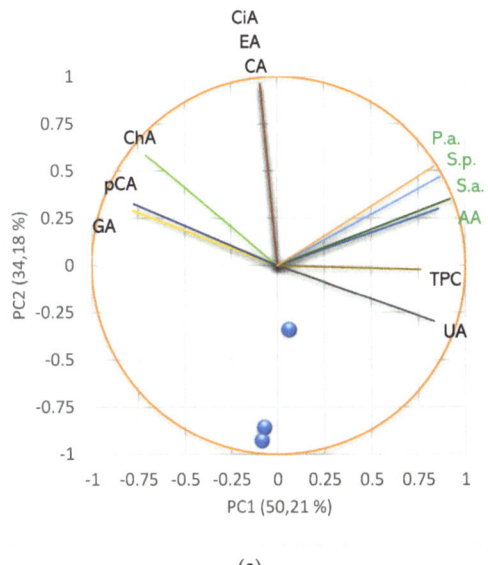 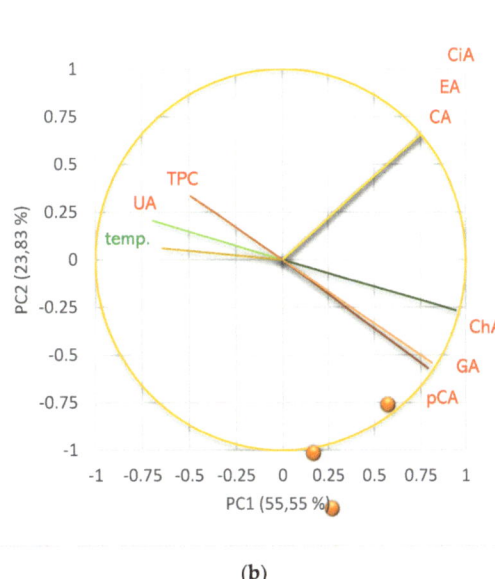

Figure 6. Principal component analysis (PCA): PCA-Correlation circle between phenolic metabolites and bioactivities of *U. barbata* extracts (**a**); PCA-Correlation circle between phenolic metabolites and extraction temperature (**b**). pCA—*p*-coumaric acid, ChA—chlorogenic acid, CA—caffeic acid, CiA—cinnamic acid, EA—ellagic acid, GA—gallic acid, UA—usnic acid, TPC—total phenolic content, AA—antiradical activity, P.a.—inhibitory activity against *P. aeruginosa*, S.a.—inhibitory activity against *S. aureus*, S.p.—inhibitory activity against *S. pneumoniae*, temp—extraction temperature.

The PCA-Correlation circle from Figure 6a explains 84.40% of the data variances [51] and correlates the lichen extracts metabolites with their bioactivities. It can be observed that the horizontal axis (PC1) is linked to pCA, GA, and ChA, usnic acid content, TPC, AA, and antibacterial activities. PC2 is associated with CA, EA, and CiA. Figure 6a shows that UA moderately correlates with the lichen extracts bioactivities: AA ($r = 0.626$, $p > 0.05$), S.a. ($r = 0.728$, $p > 0.05$), S.p. ($r = 0.625$, $p > 0.05$), and P.a. ($r = 0.545$, $p > 0.05$). TPC displays a good positive correlation with AA ($r = 0.822$, $p < 0.05$) and the moderate ones with antibacterial activities—r values decrease from 0.693 (S.a.) to 0.603 (S.p.) and 0.563 (P.a.), $p > 0.05$. We can also observe that AA is highly correlated with antibacterial activities—r values are 0.923 (S.a.), 0.900 (S.p.), and 0.897 (P.a.), $p < 0.05$—because in both effects involve the phenolic metabolites, with their phenolic -OH groups (Figure 6a). The individual polyphenols are insignificantly (positively or negatively) correlated with both bioactivities for all lichen extracts because these compounds were quantified only in three *U. barbata* extracts (Figure 6a).

The PCA-Correlation circle from Figure 6b explains 79.38% of the data variances and correlates the lichen extracts metabolites with extraction temperature. All parameters (except TPC, $r = 0.209$) are negatively correlated with the temperature ($p > 0.05$). The temperature values moderately correlate with pCA ($r = -0.587$), ChA ($r = 0.652$) and GA ($r = 0.594$). Other variable parameters reported a low negative correlation with extraction temperature (detailed data in Supplementary Materials). Usnic acid with temperature registered the lowest negative correlation ($r = -0.042$).

The lichen extracts' phytoconstituents significantly influence their pharmacological potential. Hence, we explored the metabolites content to explain the differences in the obtained results regarding antiradical and antibacterial effects. Then, we determined the correlations between these bioactivities and phenolic metabolites quantified in each lichen extract. All data are displayed in Figures 7–10 and detailed in Supplementary Materials.

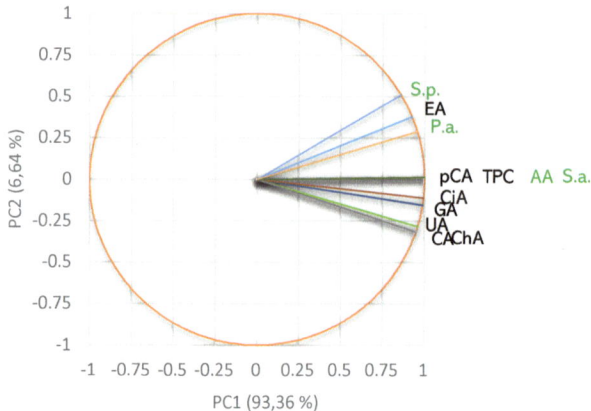

Figure 7. PCA-Correlation circle between TPC, UA, and individual polyphenols in *m*UBE and antibacterial and antiradical activities. *m*UBE—*U. barbata* liquid ethanol extract, pCA—*p*-coumaric acid, ChA—chlorogenic acid, CA—caffeic acid, CiA—cinnamic acid, EA—ellagic acid, GA—gallic acid, UA—usnic acid, TPC—total phenolic content, AA—antiradical activity, P.a.—inhibitory activity against *P. aeruginosa*, S.a.—inhibitory activity against *S. aureus*, S.p.—inhibitory activity against *S. pneumoniae*.

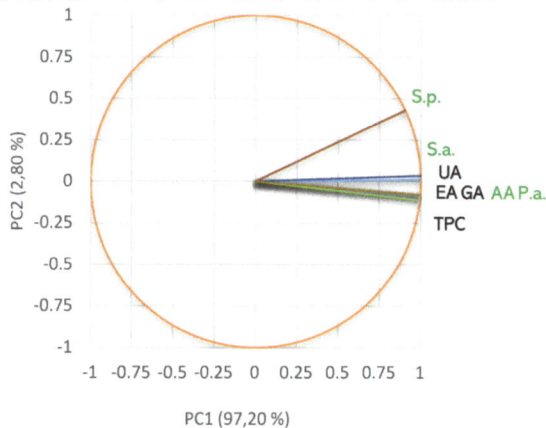

Figure 8. PCA-Correlation circle between TPC, UA, and individual polyphenols in *d*UBE and antibacterial and antiradical activities. *d*UBE—*U. barbata* dry ethanol extract, EA—ellagic acid, GA—gallic acid, UA—usnic acid, TPC—total phenolic content, AA—antiradical activity, P.a.—inhibitory activity against *P. aeruginosa*, S.a.—inhibitory activity against *S. aureus*, S.p.—inhibitory activity against *S. pneumoniae*.

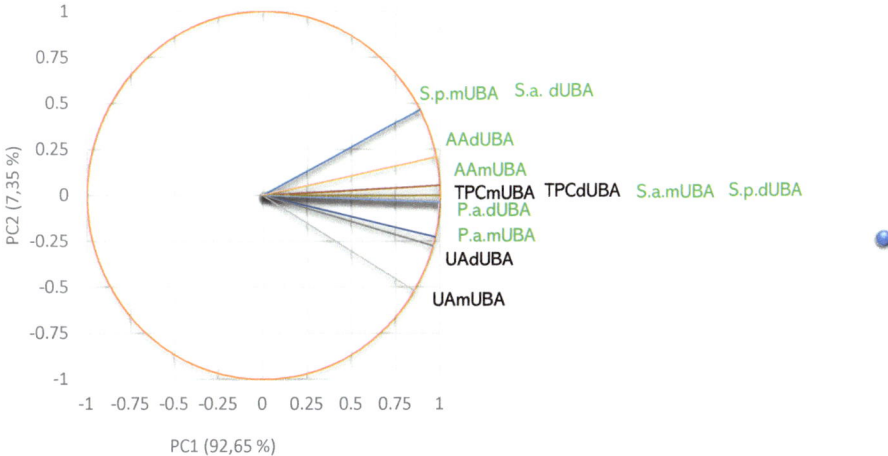

Figure 9. PCA-Correlation circle between TPC, UA, and individual polyphenols in *m*UBA and *d*UBA and antibacterial and antiradical activities; UBA—*U. barbata* acetone extract, *m*—macerate, *d*—dry; UA—usnic acid, TPC—total phenolic content, AA—antiradical activity, P.a.—inhibitory activity against *P. aeruginosa*, S.a.—inhibitory activity against *S. aureus*, S.p.—inhibitory activity against *S. pneumoniae*.

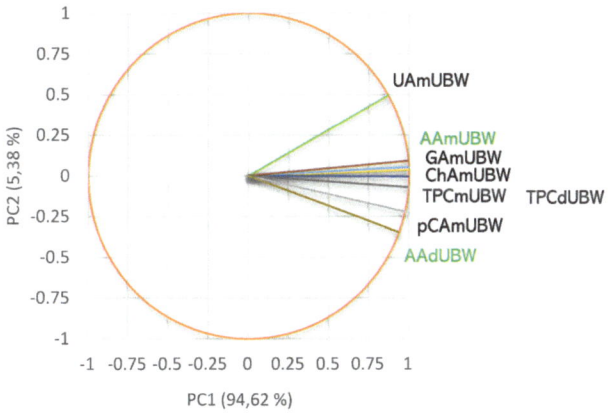

Figure 10. PCA-Correlation circle between TPC, UA, and individual polyphenols in *m*UBW and only between TPC in *d*UBW and antiradical activities; UBW—*U. barbata* water extract, *m*—macerate, *d*—dry; pCA—*p*-coumaric acid, ChA—chlorogenic acid, GA—gallic acid, UA—usnic acid, TPC—total phenolic content, AA—antiradical activity.

In *m*UBE, all quantified phenolic secondary metabolites significantly correlate with DPPH free radical scavenging ability (AA, $r \geq 0.930$) and antibacterial activities (Figure 7).

As expected, Figure 7 shows a high correlation ($r = 0.999$, $p < 0.05$) between pCA and TPC and AA and S.a. Ellagic acid remarkably correlates with AA ($r = 0.930$, $p > 0.05$) and all antibacterial effects—r value decreases from 0.996 (P.a.) to 0.989 (S.p.) and 0.930 (S.a.), $p > 0.05$. The phenolic compounds correlate with the inhibitory effect against *S. aureus* registering the highest correlation index values ($r \geq 0.930$, $p > 0.05$), followed by the one against P. aeruginosa ($r = 0.817$–0.996, $p > 0.05$) and S. pneumoniae (in the most cases, a moderate correlation, $r = 0.655$–0.867, $p > 0.05$). UA shows the highest correlation with S.a. ($r = 0.945$, $p > 0.05$), followed by P.a. ($r = 0.817$, $p > 0.05$) and S.p. ($r = 0.655$, $p > 0.05$). Moreover, AA is considerably correlated with all antibacterial activities, S.a. ($r = 0.999$, $p < 0.05$), P.a. ($r = 0.961$, $p > 0.05$) and S.p. ($r = 0.866$, $p > 0.05$).

In dUBE, we identified two polyphenols (gallic acid and ellagic acid) and UA. The phenolic metabolites remarkably correlate with both bioactivities ($r \geq 0.848$, $p </> 0.05$, Figure 8).

Data illustrated in Figure 8 highlight the strongest correlation ($r = 0.999$, $p < 0.05$) between phenolic compounds (EA, GA, and TPC) and AA and P.a. On P. aeruginosa, the powerful action of ellagic acid and gallic acid is due to phenolic compound general mechanisms and biofilm inhibition [52]. The same correlation ($r = 0.999$, $p < 0.05$) can be noticed between UA and S.a.; UA is a valuable antibacterial compound against S. aureus and, as a positive control, had a dose-dependent antibacterial effect. Both activities—AA and P.a.—are also highly correlated ($r = 0.999$, $p < 0.05$).

TPC of mUBA and dUBA are positively correlated with antibacterial effects (Figure 9). In mUBA, TPC correlates with S.a. ($r = 0.999$, $p < 0.05$); it also corellates with S.p. and P.a. in dUBA. UA moderately corellates with S.p. ($r = 0.515$, $p < 0.05$) in mUBA and S.a. in dUBA ($r = 0.723$, $p > 0.05$). In both UBAs, UA ($r = 0.827$ and 0.884, $p > 0.05$) and TPC ($r = 0.996$ and 0.978, $p > 0.05$) display a high correlation with AA. These correlations are evidenced in Figure 9. Furthermore, in both UBAs, DPPH free-radical scavenging activity and antibacterial effects are strongly correlated ($r = 0.906$, 0.962 and 0.970, $p > 0.05$, Figure 9).

These correlations associated with the bio-activities of all quantified metabolites could explain the similar inhibitory activity on bacterial strains growing of both U barbata extracts in ethanol and acetone. Moreover, in these extracts, all phenolic metabolites could synergistically act.

The PCA-correlation circle for UBWs is displayed in Figure 10.

Data from Figure 10 show that usnic acid ($r = 0.910$, $p > 0.05$) and individual polyphenols—pCA ($r = 0.951$, $p > 0.05$), GA and ChA ($r = 0.999$, $p < 0.05$) highly correlate with AA in liquid water extract. Furthermore, in both UBWs, TPC show a powerful correlation with AA ($r = 0.995$, and 0.961, $p < 0.05$). However, because the phenolic compounds with known antibacterial action were extracted in water in minimal quantities, both UBWs did not exhibit any inhibitory effect on bacteria tested (IZD = 0).

Our study deeply analyzed six U. barbata extracts in three solvents, from the description of extraction conditions to phenolic constituents' determination and the evaluation of their biological activities. A detailed data analysis was performed on the correlations between phenolic metabolites and biological activities for each U. barbata extract, aiming to explain the obtained results. We correlated phenolic metabolites with antiradical and antibacterial activities and with extraction temperature for all six U. barbata extracts. The extraction temperature's significant role was highlighted by comparing the liquid and dry extracts in the same solvent. Thus, we evidenced the strong influence of the extraction temperature on phenolic metabolites diversity and content and, consequently, the strong impact on antiradical and antibacterial activities.

Correlating and interpreting all data, we made each lichen extract characterization, highlighting the similar and different properties compared to the others (Figure 11).

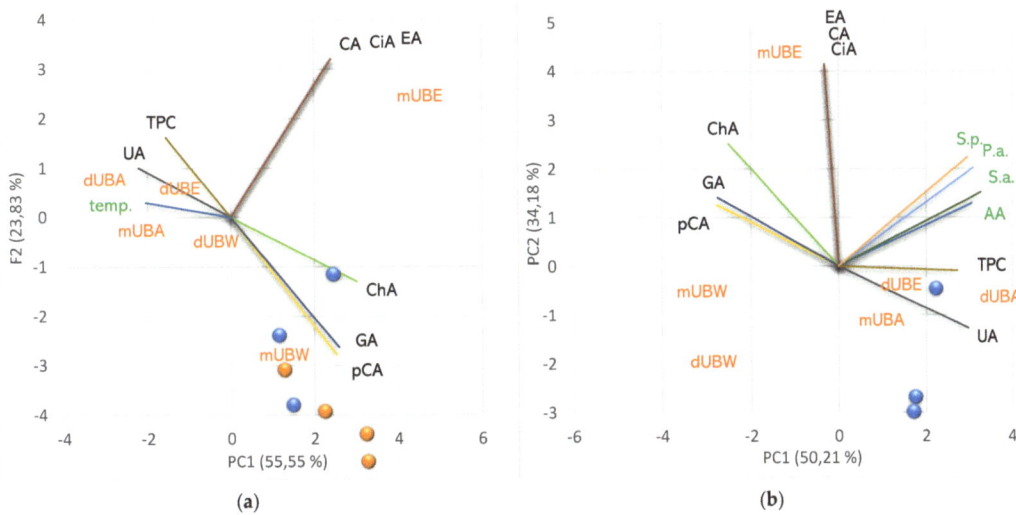

Figure 11. Characterization of *U. barbata* extracts by positioning each lichen extract according to its phenolic metabolites correlated with temperature (**a**) and bioactivities (**b**). pCA—*p*-coumaric acid, ChA—chlorogenic acid, CA—caffeic acid, CiA—cinnamic acid, EA—ellagic acid, GA—gallic acid, UA—usnic acid, TPC—total phenolic content, AA—antiradical activity; P.a.—inhibitory activity against *P. aeruginosa*, S.a.—inhibitory activity against *S. aureus*, S.p.—inhibitory activity against *S. pneumoniae*; temp—extraction temperature. UBA—*U. barbata* acetone extract, UBE—*U. barbata* ethanol extract, UBW—*U. barbata* water extract; *m*—macerate, *d*—dry extract.

Figure 11a shows that the fluid UBE (obtained at room temperature) contains UA in a low content and all six polyphenols in an appreciable amount. It can be noticed that CA, EA, and CiA are associated exclusively with *m*UBE; moreover, it shares ChA, GA, and pCA with *m*UBW. Individual polyphenols contribute considerably to the *m*UBE's TPC value (Figure 11a). These constituents could synergistically act, leading to their significant antiradical and antibacterial potential (Figure 11b). The Soxhlet extraction at 75–80 °C significantly diminished the polyphenols content; thus, *d*UBE reported low concentrations of only two polyphenols (EA and GA, Figure 11a). Moreover, UA and other phenolic secondary metabolites were resistant to prolonged heating and detected in dry acetone extract (Figure 11a). Therefore, *d*UBE shows a higher AA than *m*UBE and similar antibacterial effects. The fluid water extract (*m*UBW) shows the lowest content of phenolic metabolites compared to other macerates. It contains three individual polyphenols (pCA, GA, ChA) and usnic acid (Figure 11a). Despite the antibacterial properties of all phenolic constituents, their content is too low, and *m*UBW does not inhibit bacterial strains' growth; it has only moderate antiradical activity (Figure 11b). The prolonged heating at 100 °C during Soxhlet extraction diminished phenolics content; UA and individual polyphenols from *m*UBW were not detected in *d*UBW (Figure 11a), and AA decreased.

Both acetone extracts (*m*UBA and *d*UBA) have the same metabolites (UA and TPC) and bioactivities (Figure 11b); the temperature and yield have a quantitative influence, increasing UAC and TPC in *d*UBA. Therefore, AA augments and antibacterial properties are similar. In Figure 11a,b, both UBAs and *d*UBE are positioned at low distances; both UBWs are located in the same quarter of the PCA–biplot, thus evidencing their similar properties.

3. Discussion

The low yields associated with diminished UAC in dried lichen can also be observed in other studies on *U. barbata* extracts obtained in various conditions [42,43,53,54]. The most relevant data are displayed in Table 8.

Table 8. Various *U. barbata* extracts with different extraction conditions correlated with the yield and usnic acid content expressed as mg/g extract, and % UA in dried lichen.

U. barbata Extract	Extraction Solvent	Conditions of Extraction				Yield %	UAC (mg/g in Extract)	% UA in Dried Lichen *
		Pressure (Mpa)	Temperature (°C)	CO_2 Pressure (m^3/kg)	Pretreatment			
UBDEA [a]	Ethyl acetate		75–80			6.27	376.73	2.362
UB-SFE [b]	99% CO_2	30	60			0.38	594.80	2.226
UB-SFE [b]	99% CO_2	30	40			0.60	364.90	2.190
UBO [c]	Canola oil		22				0.915	2.162
UBDA [a]	Acetone		55–60			6.36	282.78	1.798
UBDE [a]	96% ethanol		75–80			12.52	127.21	1.592
UBDM [a]	Methanol		65			11.29	137.60	1.553
UB-SFE [d]	99% CO_2	50	40	992	CM	2.28	545	1.243
					RM	1.67	585	0.977
					UM + RGD	1.50	645	0.968
		30	40	911	UM	1.27	617	0.806
					UM + RGD	1.46	423	0.618
					UM	0.85	648	0.551
					RM	0.78	634.5	0.481
					CM	0.86	558.1	0.479

UB SFE—*U. barbata* extract obtained by supercritical fluid extraction with CO_2, UBDEA—*U. barbata* dry extract in ethyl acetate, UBDA—*U. barbata* dry extract in acetone, UBDE—*U. barbata* dry extract in ethanol, UBDM—*U. barbata* dry extract in methanol, UBO—*U. barbata* extract in canola oil, RM—roller mill; UM—ultra-centrifugal mill; CM—cutting mill; RGD—rapid gas decompression. * Data registered in decreasing order; superscript letters evidenced the data adapted from: [a] [53], [b] [42], [c] [54], [d] [43].

The data from Table 8 indicate that the UAC (%) in dried lichen generally decreases directly proportional to the extraction yield when the same solvent is used.

The usnic acid chemical structure strongly relates to *U. barbata* antiradical and antibacterial activities [22]. Due to protonophore and uncoupling action, all three phenolic OH groups of UA are essential [55], leading to bacterial membrane potential dissipation, associated with bacterial colonies growing inhibition. Maciag-Dorszynska et al. [56] proved that usnic acid produces a rapid and strong inhibition of nucleic acids synthesis in Gram-positive bacteria (*S. aureus* and *B. subtilis*). It could also inhibit Group A Streptococcus (*Streptococcus pyogenes*) biofilm formation [57], reducing biofilm biomass and depleting the biofilm-forming cells' proteins and fatty acids. Sinha et al. [58] proved that UA could act synergistically with norfloxacin and modify *S. aureus* methicillin-resistant (MRSA) drug resistance. This effect involves efflux pump inhibition, oxidative stress induction, and down-regulation of peptidoglycans and fatty acids biosynthesis. These mechanisms alter membrane potential and perturb cell respiration and metabolic activity.

The polyphenols could synergistically act with usnic acid and other secondary metabolites in *U. barbata* extracts' antiradical and antibacterial activities. The antibacterial effects of polyphenols implicate various mechanisms. Thus, Lou et al. [59] proved that the *p*-coumaric acid bactericidal effect against *S. aureus* and *S. pneumoniae* involves irreversible permeability changes in bacterial cell walls and binding to bacterial genomic DNA; as a result, it occurs cell function inhibition followed by bacteria cell death. Caffeic acid (CA) acts as an antibacterial drug through various mechanisms; it produces cell membrane depolarization and disruption, reduces the respiratory activity of bacteria, decreases efflux activity, affects intracellular redox processes, donates protons, and increases intracellular acidity [34]. Moreover, CA proved to have an appreciable inhibitory effect against *S. aureus* (IZD = 12 mm) [34]. Cinnamic acid (CiA) preferentially acts against Gram-negative bacteria (*P. aeruginosa*), determining cell membrane damage, affecting its lipidic profile, and leading to protein loss and denaturation [60]. Chlorogenic acid (ChA) antibacterial mechanisms involve outer cell membrane bounding and disrupting, intracellular potential exhausting, and loss of cytoplasm macromolecules, leading to cell death [61]. On *S. pneumoniae*, ChA inhibits a key virulence factor (neuraminidase) [62]. Gallic acid (GA) has a significant antibacterial effect against Gram-positive bacteria (*S. aureus, Streptococcus* sp.), increasing their ability to accept electrons. On Gram-negative bacteria, this property could decrease, indicating that GA is an electrophilic compound interacting with bacterial surface components [63–65]. Ellagic acid (EA) acts on *S. aureus* damaging the bacteria cell membrane, leading to significant leakage of proteins and nucleic acids. Its antibacterial activity could inhibit protein synthesis, inducing great morphological changes in bacterial cell structure [66]. Both phenolic acids (GA and EA) also proved bactericidal effects against *P. aeruginosa* [52]. In encapsulated form, their antibacterial potential could increase [38].

Numerous researchers analyzed the antibacterial activity of *U. barbata* and *Usnea* sp.; generally, their results were similar to those obtained in our study [39]. The sensibility of Gram-positive bacteria to usnic acid and various *Usnea* sp. extracts is most known. Idamokoro et al. [67] analyzed the effect of *U. barbata* extracts in methanol and ethyl-acetate against 13 isolated *Staphylococcus* sp. involved in cow mastitis. They evidenced ethyl-acetate extract's lower inhibitory activity than methanol ones. On *S. aureus*, they reported an IZD value = 14 mm for methanol extract, similar to our *d*UBA (IZD = 13.66 mm). Mesta et al. [68] indicated the IZD values of 12 mm—for *U. ghatensis* ethanol extract 15 mg/mL against *S. aureus*—and 18 mm—for *U. undullata* ethanol extract 15 mg/mL on *S. pneumoniae*; both values are similar to those for *m/d*UBE obtained in the present study. In a previous study [69], we evaluated the antibacterial activity of *U. barbata* liquid extracts against two other *Streptococcus* sp. (*S. oralis* and *S. intermedius*) isolated from the oral cavity. Those obtained IZD values proved that *m*UBE had a stronger action for both *Streptococcus* sp. than *m*UBA; *m*UBW did not show any inhibitory effect. No inhibitory effects (IZD = 0) displayed the extracts of *U. pectinata, U. coraline*, and *U. baileyi* in methanol and dichloromethane against *K. pneumoniae* [5]. The methanol extracts of *U. articulata* (IZD = 28 mm) and *U. florida* (IZD = 18 mm) highlighted a remarkable antibacterial action against *P. aeruginosa* [41]. *U. florida* extract in methanol also proved significant activity on *S. aureus* (IZD = 30). Boisova et al. [70] optimized the conditions of UA SFE extraction from *U. subfloridana* (for 80 min, at a temperature of 85 °C and pressure of 150 atm). Their obtained extract proved an intense antibacterial activity against *S. aureus*.

4. Materials and Methods

4.1. Materials

Our study's chemicals, reagents, and standards were of analytical grade. Usnic acid standard 98.1% purity, phenolic standards (Z-resveratrol, caffeic acid, E-resveratrol, chlorogenic acid, ferulic acid, gallic acid, ellagic acid, p-coumaric acid, vanillin, 3-methyl gallic acid, cinnamic acid) were purchased from Sigma (Sigma-Aldrich Chemie GmbH., Taufkirchen, Germany). Folin–Ciocâlteu reagent, Pyrogallol, DPPH, acetone, and ethanol were supplied by Merck (Merck KGaA, Darmstadt, Germany).

The bacterial lines were obtained from Microbiology Department, S.C. Synevo Romania SRL, Constanta Laboratory, in partnership agreement No 1060/25.01.2018 with the Faculty of Pharmacy, Ovidius University of Constanta. Culture media Mueller–Hinton agar simple and one with 5% defibrinated sheep blood were supplied by Thermo Fisher Scientific, GmbH, Dreieich, Germany.

4.2. Lichen Extracts

U. barbata was harvested from Călimani Mountains, Romania (47°28′ N, 25°10′ E, 900 m altitude) in March 2021. The lichen was dried at a constant temperature below 25 °C in an airy room, protected from the sunlight. After drying, the obtained herbal product was preserved for a long time in the same conditions for use in subsequent studies. The lichen was identified using standard methods by the Department of Pharmaceutical Botany of the Faculty of Pharmacy, Ovidius University of Constanta. A voucher specimen (*Popovici 3/2021 Ph/UOC*) [71] can be found at the Department of Pharmacognosy, Faculty of Pharmacy, Ovidius University of Constanta.

The dried lichen was ground in an LM 120 laboratory mill (PerkinElmer, Waltham, MA, USA) and passed through the no. 5 sieve [19]. The obtained moderately fine lichen powder (particle size $\leq$ 315 μm) was subjected to extraction in acetone, 96% ethanol, and water (dried lichen: solvent ratio (w/v) = 1:10) using two conventional techniques.

The first procedure was maceration—three samples of 10 g ground dried lichen were extracted with 100 mL solvent (water, acetone, and 96% ethanol) in a dark place at room temperature (20–22 °C) for 10 days, with manual shaking 3–4 times/day. The resulting extractive solutions were filtered and made up of a 100 mL volumetric flask with each solvent. These fluid extracts (*m*UBA, *m*UBE, and *m*UBW) were preserved in dark-glass recipients with sealed plugs in the same conditions until processing.

The second one was Soxhlet extraction for 8 h, with the temperature values around each solvent's boiling point. Thus, three samples of 20 g ground dried lichen were refluxed at Soxhlet for eight hours with 200 mL of each solvent. Acetone and 96% ethanol were evaporated at the rotary evaporator TURBOVAP 500 (Caliper Life Sciences Inc., Hopkinton, MA, USA). Then, these extracts were kept for 16 h in a chemical exhaust hood for optimal solvent evaporation. After filtration with filter paper, UBW was concentrated on a Rotavapor R-215 with a vacuum controller V-850 (BÜCHI Labortechnik AG, Flawil, Switzerland), and lyophilized with a freeze-dryer Christ Alpha 1-2L (Martin Christ Gefriertrocknungsanlagen GmbH, Osterode am Harz, Germany) connected to a vacuum pump RZ 2.5 (VACUUBRAND GmbH, Wertheim, Germany) [72]. All these dry extracts (*d*UBA, *d*UBE, *d*UBW) were transferred in sealed-glass containers and preserved in freezer (Sirge® Elettrodomestici—S.A.C. Rappresentanze, Torino, Avigliana, Italy) at -18 °C [73] until processing.

4.3. HPLC-DAD Determination of Usnic Acid Content

A previously validated HPLC-DAD method was adapted for quantifying usnic acid [53].

4.3.1. Equipment and Chromatographic Conditions

This analytic method used an Agilent 1200 HPLC (Agilent Technologies, Santa Clara, CA, USA) with a G1311 quaternary pump, Agilent 1200 G1315B diode array detector (DAD), G1316 thermostatted column compartment, G1322 vacuum degassing system, G1329 autosampler.

The system has a Zorbax C18 analytical column 150 mm/4.6 mm; 5 µm (Agilent Technologies, Santa Clara, CA, USA). As a mobile phase, isocratic methanol: water: acetic acid = 80:15:5 was selected for 6 min per run, at an injection volume of 20 µL at a flow rate = 1.5 mL/min. The oven temperature was established at 25 °C, and the detection was performed at 282 nm.

4.3.2. Sample, Blank, Standard Solutions

All requested solutions were prepared using acetone as a solvent. The standard was usnic acid dissolved in acetone at concentrations of 2.5, 5, 10, 20, 50 µg/mL, with which the calibration curve (Figure S3, Supplementary Materials) was drawn (y = 39.672x − 3.8228; R^2 = 0.999). Each dilution was injected 6 times (20 µL) in the chromatographic system, and the obtained retention time value was 4.463 ± 0.008 min.

4.3.3. Data Processing

Data processing was achieved using the Waters Empower 2 chromatography data software with ICS 1.05 (Waters Corporation, Milford, MA, USA).

4.4. HPLC-DAD Determination of Polyphenols

The polyphenols quantification was achieved using a standardized HPLC method. It was described by the USP 30-NF25 monograph and previously validated [74].

4.4.1. Equipment and Chromatographic Conditions

The Agilent HPLC-DAD system was the analytical platform, with the same Zorbax C18 column, 150 mm 4.6 mm; 5 µm. As a mobile phase, two solutions were used: solution A: 0.1% phosphoric acid and solution B: acetonitrile, with gradient elution, at 22 min per run, with the same injection volume and flow The temperature was set at 35 °C and the detection was performed at UV 310 nm.

4.4.2. Sample, Blank, Standard Solutions

The standard solutions were 70% methanol solutions with various concentrations of: Z-resveratrol (0.22 mg/mL), caffeic acid (0.36 mg/mL), E-resveratrol (0.37 mg/mL), chlorogenic acid (0.37 mg/mL), ferulic acid (0.38 mg/mL), gallic acid (0.39 mg/mL), ellagic acid (0.40 mg/mL), p-coumaric acid (0.41 mg/mL), vanillin (0.42 mg/mL), 3-methyl gallic acid (0.51 mg/mL), cinnamic acid (0.58 mg/mL). The retention time values (minutes), established after 6 injections with each standard were displayed in Figure S4 and Table S1, Supplementary Materials; all phenolic standards have R^2 values > 0.99, as admissibility condition. The samples were the *U. barbata* extracts in different solvents (their preparation was mentioned in the Section 4.2).

4.5. Total Phenolic Content

The total phenolic content was determined using Folin–Ciocâlteu reagent through a spectrophotometric method detailed in a previous study [53]. Pyrogallol was selected as the standard, the TPC values being calculated as mg of pyrogallol equivalents (PyE) per gram extract.

4.6. DPPH Free-Radical Scavenging Activity Assay

The *U. barbata* extracts free radical scavenging activity (AA) was determined spectrophotometrically through the DPPH free-radical scavenging assay previously described [19].

4.7. Antibacterial Activity

The antibacterial effects were evaluated by an adapted disc diffusion method (DDM) from the Clinical and Laboratory Standard Institute (CLSI) [75], previously described [76].

4.7.1. Microorganisms and Media

We obtained all bacteria strains from the American Type Culture Collection (ATCC). Their identification was performed at the Department of Microbiology and Immunology, Faculty of Dental Medicine, Ovidius University of Constanta. The Gram-positive bacteria were *S. aureus* (ATCC 25923) and *S. pneumoniae* (ATCC 49619); the Gram-negative ones were *Pseudomonas aeruginosa* (ATCC 27853) and *K. pneumoniae* (ATCC 13883). As a culture medium for all bacterial strains, Mueller–Hinton agar was used.

4.7.2. Inoculum Preparation

We prepared the bacterial inoculum using the direct colony suspension method (CLSI). Thus, we obtained a 0.9% saline suspension of bacterial colonies selected from a 24 h agar plate, according to the 0.5 McFarland standard, with around 10^8 CFU/mL (CFU—colony-forming unit).

4.7.3. Lichen Samples Preparations

The fluid extracts were subjected to solvent evaporation in the rotary evaporator TURBOVAP 500. These concentrated extracts were kept for 2 h in a chemical exhaust hood for each optimal solvent evaporation. Then, all *U. barbata* extracts were redissolved in 0.1% DMSO [77], obtaining a final solution of 15 mg/mL concentration.

The dry lichen extracts were dissolved in 0.1% DMSO, resulting in 15 mg/mL concentration solutions.

4.7.4. Disc Diffusion Method

The 15 mg/mL lichen extracts in 0.1% DMSO were applied on Whatman® filter paper discs (6 mm, Merk KGaA, Darmstadt, Germany). The negative control was the solvent (0.1% DMSO); UA of 15 mg/mL in 0.1% DMSO was the positive control for all extracts. We impregnated each filter paper disc with 10 µL control and sample solutions. The standard antibiotic discs (6 mm) with ofloxacin 5 µg and ceftriaxone 30 µg (Oxoid, Thermo Fisher Scientific GmbH, Dreieich, Germany) were selected for antimicrobial activity evaluation. These blank discs were stored in a freezer at $-14\ °C$ and incubated for 2 h before analysis at room temperature.

Each inoculum was applied over the entire surface of the plate with the suitable culture media using a sterile cotton swab. After 15 min of drying, the filter paper discs were applied to the inoculated plates; they were incubated at 37 °C for 24 h.

4.7.5. Reading Plates

Circular zones of a microorganism growing inhibition around several discs could be observed, examining the plates after 24 h incubation. The results of the disc diffusion assay are expressed in the inhibition zone diameter (IZD) measured in mm. These IZD values quantify bacterial strains' susceptibility levels after 24 h incubation [78].

4.7.6. Interpretation of Disc Diffusion Method results

Usnic acid and *U. barbata* extracts' IZD were compared to the IZD values of the positive controls represented by the blank antibiotic discs, ofloxacin 5 ug and ceftriaxone 30 ug [78]. In DDM, IZD values inversely correlate with minimum inhibitory concentrations (MIC) from standard dilution tests. According to CLSI [78], the interpretive categories are as follows: susceptible ("S"), intermediate—dose-dependent susceptibility ("I"), and resistant ("R") [46].

4.7.7. Activity Index

The activity index (AI) [47] is calculated using the following formula:

$$AI = \frac{IZD\ sample}{IZD\ standard} \quad (1)$$

where IZD sample—inhibition zone diameter for each *U. barbata* extract, and IZD standard—inhibition zone diameter for each antibacterial drug, used as standard.

4.8. Data Analysis, Software

All analyses were accomplished in triplicate, and the results are expressed as the mean (n = 3) ± SD, calculated by Microsoft 365 Office Excel (Redmond, Washington, DC, USA). The p-values were calculated with the one-way ANOVA test; when the p-value was <0.05, the differences between the obtained mean values were considered significant. The principal component analysis (PCA) [51] was performed using XLSTAT 2022.2.1. by Addinsoft (New York, NY, USA) [79].

5. Conclusions

Our study analyzed the phenolic constituents and bioactivities of six *U. barbata* lichen extracts obtained through two low-cost conventional techniques widely used in pharmaceutical laboratories. Despite the same ratio between the dried lichen and the solvent (w/v), all lichen extracts displayed significant differences regarding the phenolic metabolites' diversity and amount due to extraction conditions, with a substantial impact on their bioactivities. All *U. barbata* extracts show antiradical activity; the antibacterial study proves that the *U. barbata* extracts in acetone and ethanol obtained through both methods considerably inhibit bacterial colony growth. Both Gram-positive bacteria and *P. aeruginosa* of Gram-negative ones reveal the highest sensibility.

Our results suggest that further research could extend the antibacterial studies, exploring their effects on other bacteria species. Future studies could optimize both extraction processes to obtain *U. barbata* extracts with valuable bioactivities for potential pharmaceutical applications.

Supplementary Materials: The following supporting information can be downloaded at: https://www.mdpi.com/article/10.3390/ph15070829/s1, Figure S1. (a). *U. barbata* fluid extracts: A. *m*UBW, B. *m*UBA, C. *m*UBE; (b–d) *U. barbata* dry extracts: (b) *d*UBW, (c) *d*UBA, (d) *d*UBE; Figure S2. Antibacterial activity of usnic acid (1) and *U. barbata* extracts: *m*UBA (2), *d*UBA (3), *m*UBE (4), *d*UBE (5), *m*UBW (6), on *S. aureus* (a), *S. pneumoniae* (b), *P. aeruginosa* (c), *K. pneumoniae* (d); Figure S3. Calibration curve for usnic acid; Figure S4. Polyphenols standards: mixture (a), ellagic acid (b), *p*-coumaric acid (c), cis-resveratrol, and trans-resveratrol (d); Table S1. Concentration, retention time, and correlation coefficient (R^2) values for all phenolic standards used in the HPLC-DAD method.

Author Contributions: Conceptualization, V.P., L.B. and A.P.; methodology, L.B., C.E.G., A.P., E.M., G.C.C., M.A., V.S., E.A.O., A.C.F., D.L. and V.B.; software, V.P., L.B. and A.P.; validation, L.B., C.E.G., A.P., M.B. and V.B.; formal analysis, C.E.G., E.M., G.C.C., M.A., V.S. and D.L.; investigation, E.M., G.C.C., M.A., E.A.O., A.C.F., D.L., A.C. and M.B.; resources, V.P., L.B., C.E.G., A.P., E.M., G.C.C., M.A., E.A.O., A.C.F., D.L., M.B. and V.B.; data curation, E.M., G.C.C., M.A., E.A.O., V.S. and A.C.; writing—original draft preparation, V.P., L.B., C.E.G., A.P. and V.B.; writing—review and editing, V.P., L.B., C.E.G., E.A.O., A.C.F. and V.B.; visualization, L.B., C.E.G., A.P., E.M., G.C.C., M.A., V.S., E.A.O., A.C.F., D.L., A.C., M.B. and V.B.; supervision, L.B., C.E.G., A.P., E.A.O., A.C.F., D.L., A.C. and V.B.; project administration, V.B.; funding acquisition, V.P. All authors have read and agreed to the published version of the manuscript.

Funding: This work is supported by the project ANTREPRENORDOC, in the framework of Human Resources Development Operational Programme 2014–2020, financed from the European Social Fund under the contract number 36355/23.05.2019 HRD OP/380/6/13—SMIS Code: 123847.

Institutional Review Board Statement: Not applicable.

Informed Consent Statement: Not applicable.

Data Availability Statement: Data are contained within the article.

Acknowledgments: This project is performed in collaboration with the Department of Pharmacognosy, Phytochemistry, and Phytotherapy, and Department of Pharmaceutical Technology and Biopharmacy, Faculty of Pharmacy, Carol Davila University of Medicine and Pharmacy, 6 Traian Vuia Street, 020956 Bucharest, Romania, and Center for Research and Development of the Morphological and Genetic Studies of Malignant Pathology, Ovidius University of Constanta, CEDMOG, 145 Tomis Blvd., 900591 Constanta, Romania.

Conflicts of Interest: The authors declare no conflict of interest.

References

1. Ge, L.; Li, S.P.; Lisak, G. Advanced sensing technologies of phenolic compounds for pharmaceutical and biomedical analysis. *J. Pharm. Biomed. Anal.* **2020**, *179*, 112913. [CrossRef] [PubMed]
2. Albornoz, L.; Torres-Benítez, A.; Moreno-Palacios, M.; Simirgiotis, M.J.; Montoya-Serrano, S.A.; Sepulveda, B.; Stashenko, E.; García-Beltrán, O.; Areche, C. Phylogenetic Studies and Metabolite Analysis of *Sticta* Species from Colombia and Chile by Ultra-High Performance Liquid Chromatography-High Resolution-Q-Orbitrap-Mass Spectrometry. *Metabolites* **2022**, *12*, 560. [CrossRef] [PubMed]
3. Stocker-Wörgötter, E.; Cordeiro, L.M.C.; Iacomini, M. Accumulation of potential pharmaceutically relevant lichen metabolites in lichens and cultured lichen symbionts. In *Studies in Natural Products Chemistry*; Atta-ur-Rahman, Ed.; Elsevier: Amsterdam, The Netherlands, 2013; Volume 39, pp. 337–380.
4. Fernández-Moriano, C.; Gómez-Serranillos, M.P.; Crespo, A. Antioxidant potential of lichen species and their secondary metabolites. A systematic review. *Pharm. Biol.* **2016**, *54*, 1–17. [CrossRef] [PubMed]
5. Jha, B.N.; Shrestha, M.; Pandey, D.P.; Bhattarai, T.; Bhattarai, H.D.; Paudel, B. Investigation of antioxidant, antimicrobial and toxicity activities of lichens from high altitude regions of Nepal. *BMC Complement. Altern. Med.* **2017**, *17*, 282. [CrossRef]
6. Kello, M.; Kuruc, T.; Petrova, K.; Goga, M.; Michalova, Z.; Coma, M.; Rucova, D.; Mojzis, J. Pro-apoptotic potential of *Pseudevernia furfuracea* (L.) Zopf extract and isolated physodic acid in acute lymphoblastic leukemia model in vitro. *Pharmaceutics* **2021**, *13*, 2173. [CrossRef]
7. Varol, M.; Tay, T.; Candan, M.; Türk, A.; Koparal, A.T. Evaluation of the sunscreen lichen substances usnic acid and atranorin. *Biocell* **2015**, *39*, 25–31.
8. Varol, M. Lichens as a Promising Source of Unique and Functional Small Molecules for Human Health and Well-Being. In *Studies in Natural Products Chemistry*; Atta-ur-Rahman, Ed.; Elsevier: Amsterdam, The Netherlands, 2018; Volume 60, pp. 425–458.

9. Tas, I.; Yildirim, A.B.; Ozkan, E.; Ozyigitoglu, G.C.; Yavuz, M.Z.; Turker, A.U. Evaluation of pharmaceutical potential and phytochemical analysis of selected traditional lichen species. *Farmacia* **2021**, *69*, 1101–1106. [CrossRef]
10. Elečko, J.; Vilková, M.; Frenák, R.; Routray, D.; Ručová, D.; Bačkor, M.; Goga, M. A Comparative Study of Isolated Secondary Metabolites from Lichens and Their Antioxidative Properties. *Plants* **2022**, *11*, 1077. [CrossRef]
11. Gunasekaran, S.; Pillai Rajan, V.; Ramanathan, S.; Murugaiyah, V.; Samsudin, M.W.; Din, L. Antibacterial and Antioxidant Activity of Lichens *Usnea rubrotincta, Ramalina dumeticola, Cladonia verticillata* and Their Chemical Constituents. *Malays. J. Anal. Sci.* **2016**, *20*, 1–13. [CrossRef]
12. Areche, C.; Parra, J.R.; Sepulveda, B.; Garc, O.; Simirgiotis, M.J. UHPLC-MS Metabolomic Fingerprinting, Antioxidant, and Enzyme Inhibition Activities of *Himantormia lugubris* from Antarctica. *Metabolites* **2022**, *12*, 560. [CrossRef]
13. Odabasoglu, F.; Cakir, A.; Suleyman, H.; Aslan, A.; Bayir, Y.; Halici, M.; Kazaz, C. Gastroprotective and antioxidant effects of usnic acid on indomethacin-induced gastric ulcer in rats. *J. Ethnopharmacol.* **2006**, *103*, 59–65. [CrossRef] [PubMed]
14. Fitriani, L.; Fista, B.; Ismed, F.; Zaini, E. Membrane of Usnic Acid in Solid Dispersion and Effectiveness in Burn Healing. *Adv. Health Sci. Res.* **2021**, *40*, 323–329.
15. Matvieieva, N.A.; Pasichnyk, L.A.; Zhytkevych, N.V.; Pabón, G.G.; Pidgorskyi, V.S. Antimicrobial Activity of Extracts from Ecuadorian Lichens. *Mikrobiol. Z.* **2015**, *77*, 23–27. [CrossRef] [PubMed]
16. Oh, J.M.; Kim, Y.J.; Gang, H.S.; Han, J.; Ha, H.H.; Kim, H. Antimicrobial Activity of Divaricatic Acid Isolated from the Lichen *Evernia mesomorpha* against Methicillin-Resistant *Staphylococcus aureus*. *Molecules* **2018**, *23*, 3068. [CrossRef]
17. Fitriani, L.; Afifah; Ismed, F.; Bakhtiar, A. Hydrogel formulation of usnic acid and antibacterial activity test against *Propionibacterium acne*. *Sci. Pharm.* **2019**, *87*, 1. [CrossRef]
18. Prateeksha Paliya, B.S.; Bajpai, R.; Jadaun, V.; Kumar, J.; Kumar, S.; Upreti, D.K.; Singh, B.N.R.; Nayaka, S.; Joshi, Y.; Brahma Singh, N.; et al. The genus *Usnea*: A potent phytomedicine with multifarious ethnobotany, phytochemistry and pharmacology. *RSC Adv.* **2016**, *6*, 21672–21696. [CrossRef]
19. Popovici, V.; Bucur, L.; Gîrd, C.E.; Calcan, S.I.; Cucolea, E.I.; Costache, T.; Rambu, D.; Oroian, M.; Mironeasa, S.; Schröder, V.; et al. Advances in the Characterization of *Usnea barbata* (L.) Weber ex F.H. Wigg from Călimani Mountains, Romania. *Appl. Sci.* **2022**, *12*, 4234. [CrossRef]
20. Galanty, A.; Paśko, P.; Podolak, I. Enantioselective activity of usnic acid: A comprehensive review and future perspectives. *Phytochem. Rev.* **2019**, *18*, 527–548. [CrossRef]
21. Maulidiyah, M.; Darmawan, A.; Ahmad, E.; Musdalifah, A.; Wibowo, D.; Salim, L.O.A.; Arham, Z.; Mustapa, F.; Nurdin, I.F.A.; Nurdin, M. Antioxidant activity-guided isolation of usnic acid and diffractaic acid compounds from lichen genus *Usnea* sp. *J. Appl. Pharm. Sci.* **2021**, *11*, 075–083. [CrossRef]
22. Bachtiar, E.; Hermawati, E.; Juliawaty, L.D.; Syah, Y.M. Antibacterial properties of usnic acid against vibriosis. *Res. J. Chem. Environ.* **2020**, *24*, 100–101.
23. White, P.A.S.; Oliveira, R.C.M.; Oliveira, A.P.; Serafini, M.R.; Araújo, A.A.S.; Gelain, D.P.; Moreira, J.C.F.; Almeida, J.R.G.S.; Quintans, J.S.S.; Quintans-Junior, L.J.; et al. Antioxidant activity and mechanisms of action of natural compounds isolated from lichens: A systematic review. *Molecules* **2014**, *19*, 14496–14527. [CrossRef] [PubMed]
24. Kristmundsdóttir, T.; Jónsdóttir, E.; Ögmundsdóttir, H.M.; Ingólfsdóttir, K. Solubilization of poorly soluble lichen metabolites for biological testing on cell lines. *Eur. J. Pharm. Sci.* **2005**, *24*, 539–543. [CrossRef] [PubMed]
25. Kwong, S.P.; Wang, C. Review: Usnic acid-induced hepatotoxicity and cell death. *Environ. Toxicol. Pharmacol.* **2020**, *80*, 103493. [CrossRef] [PubMed]
26. Macedo, D.C.S.; Almeida, F.J.F.; Wanderley, M.S.O.; Ferraz, M.S.; Santos, N.P.S.; López, A.M.Q.; Santos-Magalhães, N.S.; Lira-Nogueira, M.C.B. Usnic acid: From an ancient lichen derivative to promising biological and nanotechnology applications. *Phytochem. Rev.* **2021**, *20*, 609–630. [CrossRef]
27. Lira, M.C.B.; Ferraz, M.S.; da Silva, D.G.V.C.; Cortes, M.E.; Teixeira, K.I.; Caetano, N.P.; Sinisterra, R.D.; Ponchel, G.; Santos-Magalhães, N.S. Inclusion complex of usnic acid with β-cyclodextrin: Characterization and nanoencapsulation into liposomes. *J. Incl. Phenom. Macrocycl. Chem.* **2009**, *64*, 215–224. [CrossRef]
28. Francolini, I.; Giansanti, L.; Piozzi, A.; Altieri, B.; Mauceri, A.; Mancini, G. Glucosylated liposomes as drug delivery systems of usnic acid to address bacterial infections. *Colloids Surf. B Biointerfaces* **2019**, *181*, 632–638. [CrossRef]
29. Grumezescu, A.M.; Cotar, A.I.; Andronescu, E.; Ficai, A.; Ghitulica, C.D.; Grumezescu, V.; Vasile, B.S.; Chifiriuc, M.C. In vitro activity of the new water-dispersible Fe_3O_4@usnic acid nanostructure against planktonic and sessile bacterial cells. *J. Nanoparticle Res.* **2013**, *15*, 1766. [CrossRef]
30. Baláž, M.; Goga, M.; Hegedüs, M.; Daneu, N.; Kováčová, M.; Tkáčiková, L.; Balážová, L.; Bačkor, M. Biomechanochemical Solid-State Synthesis of Silver Nanoparticles with Antibacterial Activity Using Lichens. *ACS Sustain. Chem. Eng.* **2020**, *8*, 13945–13955. [CrossRef]
31. Siddiqi, K.S.; Rashid, M.; Rahman, A.; Husen, A.; Rehman, S. Biogenic fabrication and characterization of silver nanoparticles using aqueous-ethanolic extract of lichen (*Usnea longissima*) and their antimicrobial activity. *Biomater. Res.* **2018**, *22*, 23. [CrossRef]
32. Mariadoss, A.V.A.; Saravanakumar, K.; Sathiyaseelan, A.; Karthikkumar, V.; Wang, M.H. Smart drug delivery of p-Coumaric acid loaded aptamer conjugated starch nanoparticles for effective triple-negative breast cancer therapy. *Int. J. Biol. Macromol.* **2022**, *195*, 22–29. [CrossRef]

33. Mitrea, D.R.; Malkey, R.; Florian, T.L.; Filip, A.; Clichici, S.; Bidian, C.; Moldovan, R.; Hoteiuc, O.A.; Toader, A.M.; Baldea, I. Daily oral administration of chlorogenic acid prevents the experimental carrageenan-induced oxidative stress. *J. Physiol. Pharmacol.* **2020**, *71*, 74–81.
34. Khan, F.; Bamunuarachchi, N.I.; Tabassum, N.; Kim, Y.M. Caffeic Acid and Its Derivatives: Antimicrobial Drugs toward Microbial Pathogens. *J. Agric. Food Chem.* **2021**, *69*, 2979–3004. [CrossRef] [PubMed]
35. Boo, Y.C. p-coumaric acid as an active ingredient in cosmetics: A review focusing on its antimelanogenic effects. *Antioxidants* **2019**, *8*, 275. [CrossRef] [PubMed]
36. Abozaid, O.A.R.; Moawed, F.S.M.; Ahmed, E.S.A.; Ibrahim, Z.A. Cinnamic acid nanoparticles modulate redox signal and inflammatory response in gamma irradiated rats suffering from acute pancreatitis. *Biochim. Biophys. Acta—Mol. Basis Dis.* **2020**, *1866*, 165904. [CrossRef] [PubMed]
37. Yu, Z.; Song, F.; Jin, Y.C.; Zhang, W.M.; Zhang, Y.; Liu, E.J.; Zhou, D.; Bi, L.L.; Yang, Q.; Li, H.; et al. Comparative pharmacokinetics of gallic acid after oral administration of Gallic acid monohydrate in normal and isoproterenol-induced myocardial infarcted rats. *Front. Pharmacol.* **2018**, *9*, 328. [CrossRef]
38. De Souza Tavares, W.; Pena, G.R.; Martin-Pastor, M.; de Sousa, F.F.O. Design and characterization of ellagic acid-loaded zein nanoparticles and their effect on the antioxidant and antibacterial activities. *J. Mol. Liq.* **2021**, *341*, 116915. [CrossRef]
39. Cansaran, D.; Kahya, D.; Yurdakulol, E.; Atakol, O. Identification and quantitation of usnic acid from the lichen *Usnea* species of Anatolia and antimicrobial activity. *Z. Fur Naturforsch.—Sect. C. J. Biosci.* **2006**, *61*, 773–776. [CrossRef]
40. Tosun, F.; Kizilay, Ç.A.; Şener, B.; Vural, M. The evaluation of plants from Turkey for in Vitro antimycobacterial activity. *Pharm. Biol.* **2005**, *43*, 58–63. [CrossRef]
41. Bate, P.N.N.; Orock, A.E.; Nyongbela, K.D.; Babiaka, S.B.; Kukwah, A.; Ngemenya, M.N. In vitro activity against multi-drug resistant bacteria and cytotoxicity of lichens collected from Mount Cameroon. *J. King Saud Univ.—Sci.* **2020**, *32*, 614–619. [CrossRef]
42. Zizovic, I.; Ivanovic, J.; Misic, D.; Stamenic, M.; Djordjevic, S.; Kukic-Markovic, J.; Petrovic, S.D. SFE as a superior technique for isolation of extracts with strong antibacterial activities from lichen *Usnea barbata* L. *J. Supercrit. Fluids* **2012**, *72*, 7–14. [CrossRef]
43. Ivanovic, J.; Meyer, F.; Misic, D.; Asanin, J.; Jaeger, P.; Zizovic, I.; Eggers, R. Influence of different pre-treatment methods on isolation of extracts with strong antibacterial activity from lichen Usnea barbata using carbon dioxide as a solvent. *J. Supercrit. Fluids* **2013**, *76*, 1–9. [CrossRef]
44. Basiouni, S.; Fayed, M.A.A.; Tarabees, R.; El-Sayed, M.; Elkhatam, A.; Töllner, K.R.; Hessel, M.; Geisberger, T.; Huber, C.; Eisenreich, W.; et al. Characterization of sunflower oil extracts from the lichen *Usnea barbata*. *Metabolites* **2020**, *10*, 353. [CrossRef] [PubMed]
45. Ghafoor, K.; Ahmed, I.A.M.; Doğu, S.; Uslu, N.; Gbemisola Jamiu, F.; Al Juhaimi, F.; Babiker, E.E.; Özcan, M.M. The Effect of Heating Temperature on Total Phenolic Content, Antioxidant Activity, and Phenolic Compounds of Plum and Mahaleb Fruits. *Int. J. Food Eng.* **2019**, *15*, 11–12. [CrossRef]
46. Humphries, R.M.; Abbott, A.N.; Hindler, J.A. Understanding and addressing CLSI breakpoint revisions: A primer for clinical laboratories. *J. Clin. Microbiol.* **2019**, *57*, e00203–e00219. [CrossRef] [PubMed]
47. Shiromi, P.S.A.I.; Hewawasam, R.P.; Jayalal, R.G.U.; Rathnayake, H.; Wijayaratne, W.M.D.G.B.; Wanniarachchi, D. Chemical Composition and Antimicrobial Activity of Two Sri Lankan Lichens, *Parmotrema rampoddense*, and *Parmotrema tinctorum* against Methicillin-Sensitive and Methicillin-Resistant Staphylococcus aureus. *Evid.—Based Complement. Altern. Med.* **2021**, 9985325. [CrossRef]
48. Farmacopeea Rom. 10th ed. 1993; pp. 419–421. Available online: https://ro.scribd.com/doc/215542717/Farmacopeea-Romana-X (accessed on 26 May 2022).
49. Malik, J.; Mandal, S.C. Extraction of herbal biomolecules. In *Herbal Biomolecules in Healthcare Applications*; Mandal, S.C., Nayak, A.K., Dhara, A.K., Eds.; Academic Press: Cambridge, MA, USA, 2022; pp. 21–46.
50. Joshi, D.R.; Adhikari, N. An Overview on Common Organic Solvents and Their Toxicity. *J. Pharm. Res. Int.* **2019**, *28*, 1–18. [CrossRef]
51. Sawicki, T.; Starowicz, M.; Kłębukowska, L.; Hanus, P. The Profile of Polyphenolic Compounds, Contents of Total Phenolics and Flavonoids, and Antioxidant and Antimicrobial Properties of Bee Products. *Molecules* **2022**, *27*, 1301. [CrossRef]
52. Kosuru, R.Y.; Aashique, M.; Fathima, A.; Roy, A.; Bera, S. Revealing the dual role of gallic acid in modulating ampicillin sensitivity of Pseudomonas aeruginosa biofilms. *Future Microbiol.* **2018**, *13*, 297–312. [CrossRef]
53. Popovici, V.; Bucur, L.; Popescu, A.; Schröder, V.; Costache, T.; Rambu, D.; Cucolea, I.E.; Gîrd, C.E.; Caraiane, A.; Gherghel, D.; et al. Antioxidant and cytotoxic activities of *Usnea barbata* (L.) F.H. Wigg. dry extracts in different solvents. *Plants* **2021**, *10*, 909. [CrossRef]
54. Popovici, V.; Bucur, L.; Gîrd, C.E.; Rambu, D.; Calcan, S.I.; Cucolea, E.I.; Costache, T.; Ungureanu-Iuga, M.; Oroian, M.; Mironeasa, S.; et al. Antioxidant, Cytotoxic, and Rheological Properties of Canola Oil Extract of *Usnea barbata* (L.) Weber ex F. H. Wigg from Călimani Mountains, Romania. *Plants* **2022**, *11*, 854. [CrossRef]
55. Antonenko, Y.N.; Khailova, L.S.; Rokitskaya, T.I.; Nosikova, E.S.; Nazarov, P.A.; Luzina, O.A.; Salakhutdinov, N.F.; Kotova, E.A. Mechanism of action of an old antibiotic revisited: Role of calcium ions in protonophoric activity of usnic acid. *Biochim. Biophys. Acta—Bioenerg.* **2019**, *1860*, 310–316. [CrossRef] [PubMed]

56. Maciag-Dorszyńska, M.; Wegrzyn, G.; Guzow-Krzemińska, B. Antibacterial activity of lichen secondary metabolite usnic acid is primarily caused by inhibition of RNA and DNA synthesis. *FEMS Microbiol. Lett.* **2014**, *353*, 57–62. [CrossRef] [PubMed]
57. Nithyanand, P.; Beema Shafreen, R.M.; Muthamil, S.; Karutha Pandian, S. Usnic acid, a lichen secondary metabolite inhibits Group A *Streptococcus* biofilms. *Antonie Van Leeuwenhoek Int. J. Gen. Mol. Microbiol.* **2015**, *107*, 263–272. [CrossRef] [PubMed]
58. Sinha, S.; Gupta, V.K.; Kumar, P.; Kumar, R.; Joshi, R.; Pal, A.; Darokar, M.P. Usnic acid modifies MRSA drug resistance through down-regulation of proteins involved in peptidoglycan and fatty acid biosynthesis. *FEBS Open Bio.* **2019**, *9*, 2025–2040. [CrossRef] [PubMed]
59. Lou, Z.; Wang, H.; Rao, S.; Sun, J.; Ma, C.; Li, J. P-Coumaric acid kills bacteria through dual damage mechanisms. *Food Control* **2012**, *25*, 550–554. [CrossRef]
60. Vasconcelos, N.G.; Croda, J.; Simionatto, S. Antibacterial mechanisms of cinnamon and its constituents: A review. *Microb. Pathog.* **2018**, *120*, 198–203. [CrossRef]
61. Lou, Z.; Wang, H.; Zhu, S.; Ma, C.; Wang, Z. Antibacterial activity and mechanism of action of chlorogenic acid. *J. Food Sci.* **2011**, *76*, 398–403. [CrossRef]
62. Guan, S.; Zhu, K.; Dong, Y.; Li, H.; Yang, S.; Wang, S.; Shan, Y. Exploration of binding mechanism of a potential *Streptococcus pneumoniae* neuraminidase inhibitor from herbaceous plants by molecular simulation. *Int. J. Mol. Sci.* **2020**, *21*, 1003. [CrossRef]
63. Selim, S.; Abdel-Mawgoud, M.; Al-Sharary, T.; Almuhayawi, M.S.; Alruhaili, M.H.; Al Jaouni, S.K.; Warrad, M.; Mohamed, H.S.; Akhtar, N.; Abdelgawad, H. Pits of date palm: Bioactive composition, antibacterial activity and antimutagenicity potentials. *Agronomy* **2022**, *12*, 54. [CrossRef]
64. Štumpf, S.; Hostnik, G.; Primožič, M.; Leitgeb, M.; Bren, U. Generation Times of *E. coli* Prolong with Increasing Tannin Concentration while the Lag Phase Extends Exponentially. *Plants* **2020**, *9*, 1680. [CrossRef]
65. Štumpf, S.; Hostnik, G.; Primožič, M.; Leitgeb, M.; Salminen, J.P.; Bren, U. The effect of growth medium strength on minimum inhibitory concentrations of tannins and tannin extracts against *E coli*. *Molecules* **2020**, *25*, 2947. [CrossRef] [PubMed]
66. Zhou, D.; Liu, Z.H.; Wang, D.M.; Li, D.W.; Yang, L.N.; Wang, W. Chemical composition, antibacterial activity and related mechanism of valonia and shell from *Quercus variabilis* Blume (Fagaceae) against Salmonella paratyphi a and Staphylococcus aureus. *BMC Complement. Altern. Med.* **2019**, *19*, 271. [CrossRef] [PubMed]
67. Idamokoro, E.M.; Masika, P.J.; Muchenje, V.; Falta, D.; Green, E. In-vitro antibacterial sensitivity of *Usnea barbata* lichen extracted with methanol and ethyl-acetate against selected Staphylococcus species from milk of cows with mastitis. *Arch. Anim. Breed.* **2014**, *57*, 25. [CrossRef]
68. Mesta, A.R.; Rajeswari, N.; Kanivebagilu, V.S. Assessment of Antimicrobial Activity of Ethanolic Extraction of *Usnea ghattensis* and *Usn Undulata*. *Int. J. Res. Ayurveda Pharm.* **2020**, *11*, 75–77. [CrossRef]
69. Popovici, V.; Bucur, L.; Popescu, A.; Caraiane, A.; Badea, V. Evaluation of the Antibacterial Action of the *Usnea barbata* L. Extracts, on Streptococcus Species from the Oro-Dental Cavity. In Proceedings of the Romanian National Congress of Pharmacy, Bucharest, Romania, 26–29 September 2018. 17th ed..
70. Boitsova, T.A.; Brovko, O.S.; Ivakhnov, A.D.; Zhil'tsov, D.V. Optimizing Supercritical Fluid Extraction of Usnic Acid from the Lichen Species *Usn Subfloridana*. *Russ. J. Phys. Chem. B* **2020**, *14*, 1135–1141. [CrossRef]
71. Stern, W.L.; Chambers, K.L. The Citation of Wood Specimens and Herbarium Vouchers in Anatomical. *Int. Assoc. Plant Taxon.* **2018**, *9*, 7–13. Available online: https://www.jstor.org/stable/1217349 (accessed on 20 May 2022). [CrossRef]
72. Popovici, V.; Bucur, L.; Costache, T.; Gherghel, D.; Vochita, G.; Mihai, C.T.C.T.; Rotinberg, P.; Schroder, V.; Badea, F.C.F.C.; Badea, V.; et al. Studies on Preparation and UHPLC Analysis of the *Usnea barbata* (L.) F.H.Wigg Dry acetone extract. *Rev. Chim.* **2019**, *70*, 3775–3777. [CrossRef]
73. Ranković, B.; Kosanić, M.; Stanojković, T.; Vasiljević, P.; Manojlović, N. Biological activities of *Toninia candida* and *Usnea barbata* together with their norstictic acid and usnic acid constituents. *Int. J. Mol. Sci.* **2012**, *13*, 14707–14722. [CrossRef]
74. Popovici, V.; Bucur, L.; Popescu, A.; Caraiane, A.; Badea, V. Determination of the content in usnic acid and polyphenols from the extracts of *Usnea barbata* L. and the evaluation of their antioxidant activity. *Farmacia* **2018**, *66*, 337–341.
75. Hudzicki, J. Kirby-Bauer Disk Diffusion Susceptibility Test Protocol Author Information. *Am. Soc. Microbiol.* **2009**, *15*, 55–63.
76. Popovici, V.; Bucur, L.; Calcan, S.I.; Cucolea, E.I.; Costache, T.; Rambu, D.; Schröder, V.; Gîrd, C.E.; Gherghel, D.; Vochita, G.; et al. Elemental Analysis and In Vitro Evaluation of Antibacterial and Antifungal Activities of *Usnea barbata* (L.) Weber ex F.H. Wigg from C ă limani Mountains, Romania. *Plants* **2022**, *11*, 32. [CrossRef] [PubMed]
77. Timm, M.; Saaby, L.; Moesby, L.; Hansen, E.W. Considerations regarding use of solvents in in vitro cell based assays. *Cytotechnology* **2013**, *65*, 887–894. [CrossRef] [PubMed]
78. Kassim, A.; Omuse, G.; Premji, Z.; Revathi, G. Comparison of Clinical Laboratory Standards Institute and European Committee on Antimicrobial Susceptibility Testing guidelines for the interpretation of antibiotic susceptibility at a University teaching hospital in Nairobi, Kenya: A cross-sectional study. *Ann. Clin. Microbiol. Antimicrob.* **2016**, *15*, 21. [CrossRef] [PubMed]
79. Vidal, N.P.; Manful, C.F.; Pham, T.H.; Stewart, P.; Keough, D.; Thomas, R.H. The use of XLSTAT in conducting principal component analysis (PCA) when evaluating the relationships between sensory and quality attributes in grilled foods. *MethodsX* **2020**, *302*, 125326. [CrossRef] [PubMed]

MDPI AG
Grosspeteranlage 5
4052 Basel
Switzerland
Tel.: +41 61 683 77 34

Pharmaceuticals Editorial Office
E-mail: pharmaceuticals@mdpi.com
www.mdpi.com/journal/pharmaceuticals

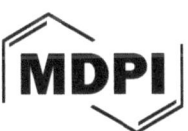

Disclaimer/Publisher's Note: The title and front matter of this reprint are at the discretion of the Guest Editors. The publisher is not responsible for their content or any associated concerns. The statements, opinions and data contained in all individual articles are solely those of the individual Editors and contributors and not of MDPI. MDPI disclaims responsibility for any injury to people or property resulting from any ideas, methods, instructions or products referred to in the content.